Medical Management of Type 2 Diabetes

Medical Management of Type 2 Diabetes

Editor: Vanessa Artiga

AMERICAN
MEDICAL PUBLISHERS
www.americanmedicalpublishers.com

AMERICAN
MEDICAL PUBLISHERS
www.americanmedicalpublishers.com

Cataloging-in-Publication Data

Medical management of type 2 diabetes / edited by Vanessa Artiga.
p. cm.
Includes bibliographical references and index.
ISBN 978-1-63927-719-3
1. Type 2 diabetes. 2. Type 2 diabetes--Treatment. 3. Type 2 diabetes--Treatment--Methodology.
4. Type 2 diabetes--Complications. 5. Type 2 diabetes--Diagnosis. 6. Disease management.
I. Artiga, Vanessa.
RC662.18 .M43 2023
616.462--dc23

American Medical Publishers,
41 Flatbush Avenue,
1st Floor, New York,
NY 11217, USA

ISBN 978-1-63927-719-3 (Hardback)

Contents

Preface

This book was inspired by the evolution of our times; to answer the curiosity of inquisitive minds. Many developments have occurred across the globe in the recent past which has transformed the progress in the field.

A disease that occurs due to high blood sugar levels is called diabetes. There are three major types of diabetes, namely, type 1 diabetes, type 2 diabetes, and gestational diabetes. Of these, the most prominent type of diabetes is the type 2 diabetes. In type 2 diabetes, the pancreas produces insulin but the body is not able to use the insulin, the way it should be used. This long-term condition causes high level of sugar circulating in the bloodstream that results in circulatory, nervous, and immune system disorders. The symptoms of type 2 diabetes are increased thirst, frequent urination, increased hunger, fatigue, blurred vision, frequent infections, etc. It is caused due to two interrelated problems. The first problem is insulin resistance developed by cells in muscle, fat and the liver which leads to lower amount of sugar. The second issue is the inability of the pancreas to produce enough insulin to manage blood sugar levels. Certain lifestyle changes such as eating healthy foods, losing weight, and avoiding inactivity for long periods are some measures to prevent or manage the disease. This book explores all the important aspects of type 2 diabetes and its medical management in the present day scenario. It will serve as a reference to a broad spectrum of readers.

This book was developed from a mere concept to drafts to chapters and finally compiled together as a complete text to benefit the readers across all nations. To ensure the quality of the content we instilled two significant steps in our procedure. The first was to appoint an editorial team that would verify the data and statistics provided in the book and also select the most appropriate and valuable contributions from the plentiful contributions we received from authors worldwide. The next step was to appoint an expert of the topic as the Editor-in-Chief, who would head the project and finally make the necessary amendments and modifications to make the text reader-friendly. I was then commissioned to examine all the material to present the topics in the most comprehensible and productive format.

I would like to take this opportunity to thank all the contributing authors who were supportive enough to contribute their time and knowledge to this project. I also wish to convey my regards to my family who have been extremely supportive during the entire project.

Editor

An Almond-Based Low Carbohydrate Diet Improves Depression and Glycometabolism in Patients with Type 2 Diabetes through Modulating Gut Microbiota and GLP-1

Mengxiao Ren [1], Huaiyu Zhang [2], Jindan Qi [1], Anni Hu [1], Qing Jiang [1], Yunying Hou [1], Qianqian Feng [1], Omorogieva Ojo [3] and Xiaohua Wang [1,*]

1 School of Nursing, Medical College, Soochow University, Suzhou 215006, China; 20185231008@stu.suda.edu.cn (M.R.); 20184231002@stu.suda.edu.cn (J.Q.); 20174231001@stu.suda.edu.cn (A.H.); jiangqing2015@suda.edu.cn (Q.J.); houyunying@suda.edu.cn (Y.H.); 20195231027@stu.suda.edu.cn (Q.F.)

2 School of Medicine, University of California, San Francisco, CA 94110, USA; huaiyu.zhang@ucsf.edu

3 School of Health Sciences, Faculty of Education, Health and Human Sciences, University of Greenwich, London SE9 2UG, UK; o.ojo@greenwich.ac.uk

* Correspondence: wangxiaohua@suda.edu.cn

Abstract: Background: Alow carbohydrate diet (LCD) is more beneficial for the glycometabolism in type 2 diabetes (T2DM) and may be effective in reducing depression. Almond, which is a common nut, has been shown to effectively improve hyperglycemia and depression symptoms. This study aimed to determine the effect of an almond-based LCD (a-LCD) on depression and glycometabolism, as well as gut microbiota and fasting glucagon-like peptide 1 (GLP-1) in patients with T2DM. Methods: This was a randomized controlled trial which compared an a-LCD with a low-fat diet (LFD). Forty-five participants with T2DM at a diabetes club and the Endocrine Division of the First and Second Affiliated Hospital of Soochow University between December 2018 to December 2019 completed each dietary intervention for 3 months, including 22 in the a-LCD group and 23 in the LFD group. The indicators for depression and biochemical indicators including glycosylated hemoglobin (HbA1c), gut microbiota, and GLP-1 concentration were assessed at the baseline and third month and compared between the two groups. Results: A-LCD significantly improved depression and HbA1c ($p < 0.01$). Meanwhile, a-LCD significantly increased the short chain fatty acid (SCFAs)-producing bacteria *Roseburia*, *Ruminococcus* and *Eubacterium*. The GLP-1 concentration in the a-LCD group was higher than that in the LFD group ($p < 0.05$). Conclusions: A-LCD could exert a beneficial effect on depression and glycometabolism in patients with T2DM. We speculate that the role of a-LCD in improving depression in patients with T2DM may be associated with it stimulating the growth of SCFAs-producing bacteria, increasing SCFAs production and GPR43 activation, and further maintaining GLP-1 secretion. In future studies, the SCFAs and GPR43 activation should be further examined.

Keywords: type 2 diabetes; diet; carbohydrate; almond; depression; HbA1c; microbiota; short-chain fatty acids; GLP-1

1. Introduction

Type 2 diabetes mellitus (T2DM) is a heterogenous set of disorders characterized by glycometabolism abnormalities. According to a report of the International Diabetes Federation (IDF), there are currently around 415 million people with diabetes worldwide, a figure likely to increase to 629 million by 2045 [1]. Diabetes is associated with several complications such as mental health-related disorders, particularly depressive disorders [2]. A meta-analysis revealed that the prevalence of depression in patients with diabetes was considerably higher than in non-diabetic subjects (17.6% vs. 9.8%) [3].Furthermore, epidemiological evidence indicated that patients with T2DM are almost three times as likely to be affected by depression compared with the general population [4]. A bidirectional relationship exists between T2DM and depression; depression increases the risk of the development of T2DM and the subsequent risks of hyperglycemia, insulin resistance, and micro and macro vascular complications. Conversely, a diagnosis of T2DM increases the risk of incident depression and can contribute to a more severe course of depression [2]. The American Diabetes Association (ADA) [5] and IDF [6] emphasize that: management of mental health is an important aspect of diabetes treatment. However, the tricyclic antidepressant commonly used in clinical practice has an adverse effect on glucose homeostasis control by reducing the insulin secretory rate [7].

Medical nutrition therapy is an essential measure to prevent and control diabetes at any stage of its natural course, and it improves blood glucose by regulating the nutrient and energy intake. Nevertheless, most available nutritional therapy mainly focuses on improving glycometabolism, and little attention is paid to improving the depression in T2DM patients. In China, low-fat diet (LFD) is recommended by ***Guideline for prevention and control of type 2 diabetes in China (2017 Edition)*** to help improve blood glucose levels in patients with T2DM [8]. However, a meta-analysis which included a total of nine studies and pooled results suggested a reasonable low-carbohydrate diet (LCD) is more beneficial for T2DM [9]. LCD refers to a dietary strategy that reduces the energy supply ratio of carbohydrates and increases the energy supply ratio of fats and proteins [10]. According to the energy supply ratio of carbohydrates, it can be divided into two modes: very low LCD (<26%), LCD (26~45%) [11].

In terms of the relationship between the proportion of carbohydrate intake and depression, the results remain controversial. Most studies support a protective effect of a low fat-high carbohydrate diet on depression. Pellegrin et al. [12] showed that daily carbohydrate intake was negatively correlated with depression score ($R = -0.33$, $p < 0.01$) in obese women. Deijen et al. [13] found that long-term consumption of LCD would aggravate negative psychology such as depression. A randomized controlled trial (RCT) by Rosenthal et al. [14] showed that a carbohydrate-rich meal could reduce depression level in patients with seasonal affective disorder. However, for T2DM patients, carbohydrate is by far the greatest dietary contributor to blood glucose rise, as expected, dietary carbohydrate restriction reliably reduces glucose profile [9]. So, it is crucial to explore a diet regimen that is beneficial to both depression and glycometabolism.

Nuts as part of LCD have been shown to effectively improve glycosylated hemoglobin (HbA1c) levels and fasting blood glucoses (FBG) in T2DM patients [15]. In addition, the synergy and interaction of all the nutrients and other bioactive components in nuts have a beneficial effect on brain, cognition, and neuropsychiatric disorders [16,17]. Various interventions [18,19], along with two recently published cohort studies [20,21], have found higher nut consumption was associated with lower depression scores. A cohort study in Tianjin, China indicated that nut consumption may be beneficial in the prevention of depressive symptoms [21]. In a large, parallel-group, multicenter, RCT using a Mediterranean diet supplemented with 30 g mixed nuts (15 g walnuts, 7.5 g hazelnuts, and 7.5 g almonds) including 7447 participants for 3 years, the result indicated that the inverse association with depression was not significant (RR = 0.78, 95% CI 0.55–1.10) in the whole cohort. However, when the analysis was restricted to participants with T2DM, a 40% lower risk of depression in participants with T2DM (RR = 0.59, 95% CI 0.36–0.98) was reported [18].

Almond is the most consumed and studied nut. It possesses potential prebiotic properties; its ingestion leads to an improvement in the gut microbiota profile and a modification of the gut microbiota activities [22].The study of Liu et al. [23] indicated that almond supplementation could significantly increase the populations of *Bifidobacterium* and *Lactobacillus*, which may potentially contribute to increased production of short-chain fatty acids(SCFAs) [24]. SCFAs are the ligand of G protein-coupled receptor43 (GPR43), and its combination with GPR43 can promote the secretion of glucagon-like peptide 1 (GLP-1) [25]. GLP-1 is an important regulator of microbiota–gut–brain signaling in health and stress-related psychiatric illnesses, which has been proven to have antidepressant effect [26].

In our previous preliminary study, we replaced 150 g/d staple food with 56 g/d almond to form an almond-based LCD (a-LCD) [15]. There are very few studies that have explored the role of a-LCD on both the depression and glycometabolism in T2DM patients. Based on the above, we hypothesized that a-LCD could improve depression and glycometabolism in patients with T2DM through modulating gut microbiota and GLP-1. In this study, we further explored the effect of a-LCD on the depression, HbA1c, gut microbiota and GLP-1.

2. Materials and Methods

2.1. Study Design

This was a 3-month, prospective RCT performed at a diabetes club and the Endocrine Division of the First and Second Affiliated Hospital of Soochow University from December 2018 to December 2019. The recruited participants were randomly allocated to either an intervention or control group using a table of computer-producing random numbers. The random numbers were concealed by someone who was not responsible for this study, so both the researcher and the participants were blinded prior to assignment. Before intervention, all participants underwent a one-week washout period to diminish the effect of background diets [27]. In this regard, participants who met the inclusion criteria were asked to stop eating nuts for >4 d/w before the intervention. This study followed the Declaration of Helsinki and the Guidelines for Good Clinical Practice and was approved by the ethics committee of the Soochow University (No. 2019000147). All enrolled patients signed consent form.

2.2. Study Participants

Inclusion criteria of this study were as follows: patients (1) had been diagnosed with T2DM; (2) were older than 18 years; (3) had no change in oral anti-diabetic drugs or insulin in half a month before the intervention; (4) were able to communicate with others; (5) had volunteered to participate in this study, and (6) were able to provide informed consent. Patients were excluded from this study if they (1) ate nuts regularly (>4 days/week) [28]; (2) were allergic to nuts or received other dietary interventions; (3) had difficulty in chewing nuts; (4) had severe conditions including digestive dysfunction, heart failure, renal failure, malignant tumors, severe cerebrovascular diseases, ketosis, hyperthyroidism, liver dysfunction, or severe gallbladder and pancreatic diseases; (5) their FBG were more than 16.7 mmol/L [15];(7) suffered from mental illness; (8) used anti-depressant, anxiety, neurological or psychiatric medication [29]; (9) pregnant or lactating [29]; (10) used GLP-1 receptor agonists or Dipeptidyl Peptidase-4 (DPP-4) inhibitors;(11) regularly took glucocorticoids;(12) regularly took antibiotics, supplementations (e.g., prebiotics) and yogurt within 3 weeks which were known to alter gut microbiota [30]. Patients were withdrawn from the study if the following occurred: patients (1) ate almond <4 d/w (56 g/d) in the a-LCD group and ate almond in the LFD group >2d/w (56 g/d); (2) were unable to follow the diet plan; (3) suffered from major life events; (4) had adverse effect occurred during the intervention (e.g., intolerance to almonds).

2.3. Sample Size Calculation

Evidence from the literature showed that the mean difference of the changes in the depression score was 2 between the LCD and the LFD group [31]. Therefore, we calculated 23 participants for each group, with $\alpha = 0.05$ and power = 0.80. Considering the 10% sample loss rate, the increase of sample size according to the actual situation is expected to be 25 cases in each group.

2.4. Intervention

The control group adopted an LFD education program which is a named six-point formula [15] developed by our research team based on the diabetes dietary guideline. The detailed contents of the six-point formula included: 1 jin vegetables/days; 2 liang staple food/meal (300 g/day); 3 tablespoons of oil/day; eating fruits under 4 conditions (stable glycemia, low glycemic index fruit, between two meals, adding energy fruit provided to the total calories); 5 kinds of protein food/day (1 carton of milk (220 mL), 1 egg, 1 liang fish or shrimp, 1 liang soybean production, 1 liang meat); 6 g salt/day. The a-LCD group consumed 56 g/day almond which replaced 150 g/d staple food (1 liang staple foods/meal) that is rich in carbohydrate, and the remaining of the dietary regimen kept the same as those of LFD. Almonds were uniformly purchased, weighed, vacuum-packed, and distributed every two weeks. The participants were instructed to consume almonds between meals or with breakfast, or when hungry. For those whose FBG were higher than normal (>6.1 mmol/L), the almonds were required to be consumed before 10:00 a.m. [32]. The participants were instructed to consume 50% of the nuts before bedtime if there was a risk of a nocturnal hypoglycemic event. Participants were followed up once a week, including where we: collected the information about the implementation of dietary regimen and almond adherence to understand the dietary adherence; strengthened their compliance and excluded participants with poor compliance; collected information of anti-diabetics; asked if they had any adverse reactions, hypoglycemic events, and major life events.

2.5. Outcomes

2.5.1. Glycated Hemoglobin (HbA1c)

Blood samples were obtained to measure HbA1c at the nursing School of Soochow University and measured by high-performance liquid chromatography using Afinion AS100 Analyzer (Alere, Inc., Shanghai, China) in the molecular laboratory of the nursing school of Soochow University.

2.5.2. Depression

Depression score was assessed through PROMIS short form v1.0-Depression 8b [33], which are universal rather than disease-specific. The PROMIS Depression item banks assess self-reported negative mood (sadness, guilt), views of self (self-criticism, worthlessness), and social cognition (loneliness, interpersonal alienation), as well as decreased positive affect and engagement (loss of interest, meaning, and purpose). Our team investigated local patients with T2DM and found that its cronbach's α was 0.879. The total scores ranged from 37.1 to 81.1 points. The higher the score of the scale, the more serious the depressive symptoms.

2.5.3. Anthropometric Measurements

The weight and height were measured bya unified measuring device at the nursing school of Soochow University.Body mass index (BMI) was calculated as weight (in kilograms) divided by height (in meterssquared).

2.5.4. Dietary Record

Patients maintained a dietary record, including a detailed diet of one day of the weekend and two working days, and then *Feihua nutrition software V2.72 version* (Bowen Shixun Technology, Beijing, China) was used to calculate the proportion of three macro-nutrients per day to evaluate the implementation of the dietary plan of the subjects. An almond adherence record table was used to measure the compliance of almond intake, and consumption ≥4 days/week indicates good compliance.

2.5.5. Fasting GLP-1 Concentration

GLP-1 was measured byenzyme-linked immunosorbent assay (ELISA). The fasting peripheral venous blood of participants was collected by vacuum blood vessels containing EDTA anticoagulants, DPP-4 inhibitors were added immediately after blood collection at bedside to prevent GLP-1 degradation. The blood samples were centrifuged at 2~8 °C 1000× g for 15 min within 30 min after collection and thesupernatant was retained and stored at −20 °C or −80 °C, but repeated freeze-thaw was avoided.

2.5.6. Gut Microbiota

The fecal specimens of all participants were taken. Researchers instructed the participants to put the feces on the thick sterile pad. The sterile cotton swab was used to take about 20 g fresh fecesfrom participants into the sterile feces collection tubes. After the specimen was collected, it was immediately put into the portable liquid nitrogen tank and frozen for 15 min. The specimens were transferred to the −80 °C refrigerator within 24 h for preservation. For each fecal specimen, DNA was extracted and purified, and the V3-V4 region of the 16S rRNA genes was polymerase chain reaction (PCR)-amplified using modified universal bacterial primers [34]. Purified PCR products were sequenced with the Hiseq2500 PE250 platform [35]. Sequence data were compiled and processed using QIIME [36]. Sequence data were screened and filtered for quality and then aligned to the full-length 16S rRNA gene, using the SILVA reference alignment as a template [37]. Sequences were grouped into operational taxonomic units (OTUs) of 97% similarity. Phylogenetic classification was used to describe the intestinal composition of each participant [38]. The following alpha-diversity measures were assessed: (1) Chao1 index, a measure of species richness that is particularly applied to low abundance datasets; (2) Faith's Phylogenetic Diversity (Faith's PD), the most commonly used measure of phylogenetic diversity. The principal co-ordinates analysis (PCoA) of the weighted Unifrac (quantitative, i.e., weighs branches of phylogenetic tree based on abundance) distances was used to compare the overall microbiota structures in the two groups.

2.6. Statistical Analysis

A statistical analysis was performed using SPSS 25.0 software (SPSS, Inc., Chicago, IL, USA). For continuous variables, the results were described as the mean ± standard deviation (SD) and comparisons were performed using Independent Samples t-test, Paired Samples t-test or the Mann–Whitney U test, and Wilcoxon rank-sum test. For categorical variables, the results were presented as frequency (percentages); comparisons between groups were made using the Chi-squared test. To eliminate the problem of confounding factors, the comparisons of outcomes between the groups after the intervention were performed using a covariance analysis (covariate: age, protein, baseline level for depression and HbA1c, the rate of change of anti-diabetics).The intention-to-treat (ITT) of depression and HbA1c were performed so as to ensure the reliability of the research results. The proportion of three macro-nutrients in relation to energy supply, representing participants' dietary adherence, which were assessed once a week during the intervention have been presented as a pie chart. The comparisons of gut microbiota between two groups were evaluated with theMann–Whitney U test, within group differences were analyzed using Wilcoxonrank test. A p value of <0.05 was considered statistically significant. A corrected false discovery rate (FDR) <0.2 was considered as significant [39].

3. Results

3.1. Study Participants

On the basis of inclusion and exclusion criteria, 50 participants with T2DM were recruited and randomly allocated to the a-LCD group (n =25) and the LFD group (n =25). Three participants (1 who did not like almond, 2 with difficulty chewing) in the a-LCD group and two participants (1 who ate almond <4 day/week, another who was lost during follow-up) in the LFD group withdrew from the study. Finally, the data of 22 participants in the a-LCD group and 23 in the LFD group were analyzed (Figure 1). The mean age of participants was (71.98 ± 5.63 years) and 25 (55.6%) were female. The general characteristics of the enrolled participants in each group are shown in Table 1. There were no statistically significant differences in any of the parameters between the two groups ($p > 0.05$).

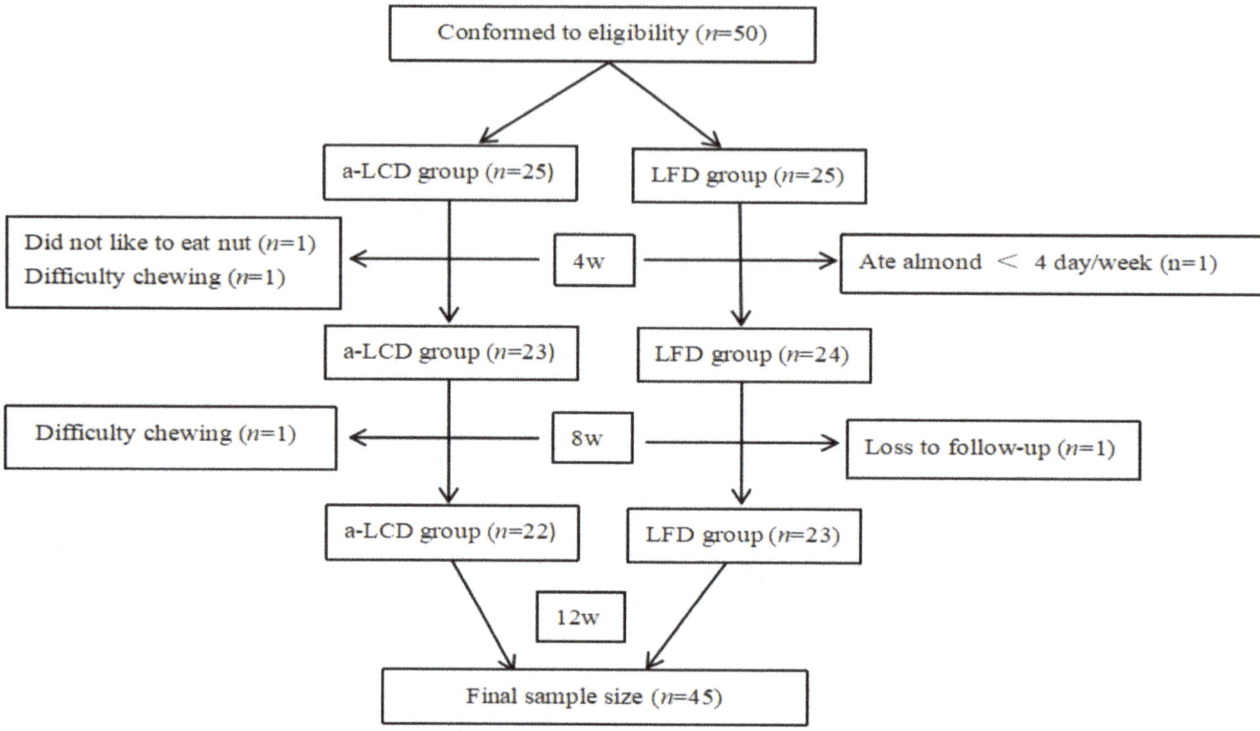

Figure 1. Flow diagram of the participants included in the study (a-LCD (almond-based low carbohydrate diet); LFD (low fat diet).

Table 1. Baseline characteristic.

Variables		a-LCD (n = 22)	LFD (n = 23)	t/x^2/Z	p
		x ± SD/n(%)/ M (P25,P50)	x ± SD/n(%)/ M (P25,P50)		
Demographic data					
Age (years)		73.55 ± 4.99	70.48 ± 5.91	−1.877 [a]	0.067
Gender-male		9 (40.9%)	11 (47.8%)	0.218 [b]	0.641
Marital status (married)		20 (90.9%)	21 (91.3%)	0.002 [c]	0.963
Education	Primary and below	2 (9.1%)	2 (8.7%)	4.037 [b]	0.258
	Journal high school	4 (18.2%)	10 (43.5%)		
	Technical and senior high school	11 (50.0%)	9 (39.1%)		
	Journal college school and above	5 (22.7%)	2 (8.7%)		
Payment	Medical insurance	22 (100%)	21 (91.3%)	2.002 [c]	0.157
Monthly income (thousand yuan)	<2	0 (0%)	3 (13.0%)	3.950 [b]	0.139
	2~5	19 (86.4%)	15 (65.2%)		
	≥5	3 (13.6%)	5 (21.7%)		
Occupation status	Retire	22 (100%)	22 (95.7%)	0.978 [c]	0.323
	On the job	0 (0%)	1 (4.3%)		
Residential status	Living by oneself	2 (9%)	2 (8%)	0.311 [b]	0.856
	Living with spouse	19 (86%)	19 (83%)		
	Living with children	1 (5%)	2 (9%)		
Exercise intensity (d)	Low intensity	19 (86.4%)	18 (78.3%)	0.505 [b]	0.477
	Moderate intensity	3 (13.6%)	5 (21.7%)		
Exercise time/(minute)		315.00 (210.00,420.00)	360.00 (210.00,420.00)	−0.537 [d]	0.591

Table 1. *Cont.*

Variables		a-LCD (n = 22)	LFD (n = 23)	t/χ^2/Z	p
Clinical data					
Smoking (Yes)		1 (4.5%)	2 (8.7%)	0.311 [c]	0.577
Drinking (Yes)		4 (18.2%)	3 (13.0%)	0.226 [c]	0.634
Diabetes duration (years)		14.18 ± 7.06	15.65 ± 7.02	0.700 [a]	0.487
Family history of diabetes (Yes)		12 (54.5%)	11 (47.8%)	0.203 [b]	0.652
Diabetic complication (Yes)		9 (40.9%)	11 (59.3%)	0.573 [b]	0.449
Accompanying disease (Yes)		16 (72.7%)	17 (73.9%)	0.008 [b]	0.928
Therapy method	None	1 (4.5%)	1 (4.3%)	1.825 [b]	0.610
	Only Hypoglycemic drugs	12 (54.5%)	14 (60.9%)		
	Only Insulin	1 (4.5%)	3 (13.0%)		
	Hypoglycemic drugs + insulin	8 (36.4%)	5 (21.7%)		
Number of combination medication	0	2 (8.7%)	4 (14.8%)	5.022 [b]	0.170
	1	8 (34.8%)	4 (14.8%)		
	2	13 (56.5%)	16 (59.3%)		
	3	0 (0%)	3 (11.1%)		

a-LCD (almond-based low carbohydrate diet); LFD (low fat diet); [a] Independent-samples T test; [b] Pearson chi-square; [c] Yates' correction chi-square; [d] Mann–Whitney U. M(P25,P50): median (25th and 75th percentile).

3.2. Dietary Adherence

3.2.1. Proportions of Calories from Three Macro-Nutrients the Patients Consumed

The results of the three macro-nutrients allocated between the a-LCD and the LFD group based on three days diet record showed that at the baseline, the total energy and the proportions of calories from the three macro-nutrients were not significantly different between the two groups. At the third month, the total energy was not significantly different between the two groups. However, compared to the LFD group, the calories from carbohydrates decreased, while those from fat significantly increased in the a-LCD group ($p < 0.01$) (Table 2). In addition, after the intervention, the percentage of the calories from carbohydrates (40%) met the standard of LCD in the a-LCD group, while the calories from fat (25%) met the standard of LFD in the LFD group (Figure 2).

Table 2. Comparison of the calories from three macro-nutrients consumed by the patients.

	Variables	a-LCD (n =22)	LFD (n =23)	t	p
Baseline	Total calorie intake/day	1686.34 ± 231.25	1781.91 ± 280.91	−1.232	0.184
	Carbohydrate-calorie (Kcal)	974.95 ± 148.22	1007.61 ± 136.32	−0.761	0.504
	Fat-calorie (Kcal)	406.76 ± 143.88	478.29 ± 149.97	−1.614	0.085
	Protein-calorie (Kcal)	318.45 ± 63.19	292.38 ± 65.12	1.348	0.524
Third month	Total calorie intake/day	1642.08 ± 227.74	1764.77 ± 297.40	−1.536	0.114
	Carbohydrate-calorie (Kcal)	673.14 ± 91.80	1042.10 ± 195.41	−8.016	<0.01 **
	Fat-calorie (Kcal)	648.19 ± 128.93	433.01 ± 137.39	5.357	<0.01 **
	Protein-calorie (Kcal)	372.03 ± 64.45	288.94 ± 64.34	1.962	0.067

p Value for comparison by independent sample t-test. **: $p < 0.01$.

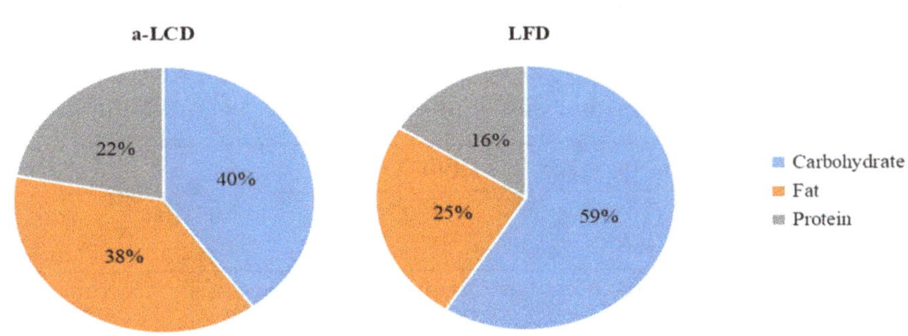

Figure 2. Three macro-nutrient energy supply ratios of two groups after intervention.

3.2.2. Almond Adherence

The almond adherence of the a-LCD group is shown in Figure 3. A fold line diagram was performed to describe the changing trend of almond adherence in the a-LCD group. The result indicated that the frequency of almond consumption was stable and good.

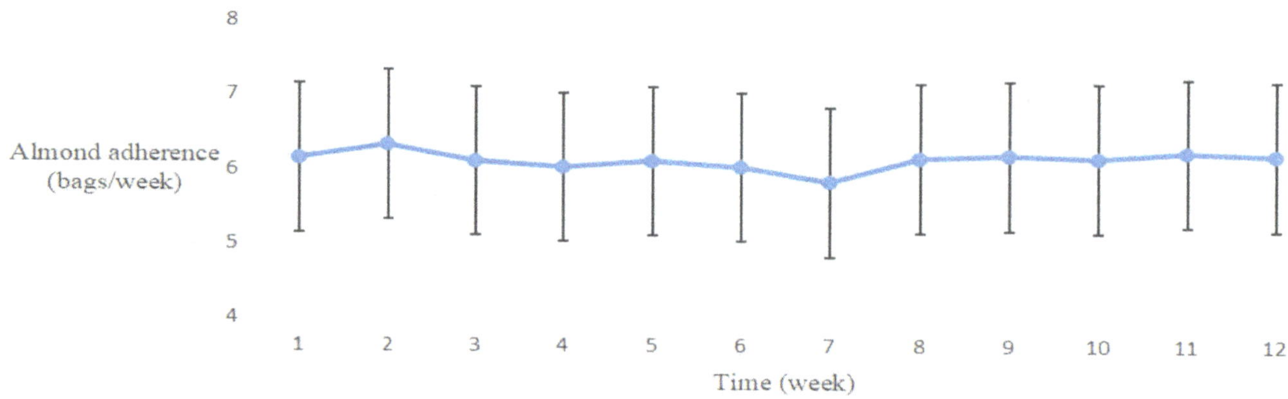

Figure 3. The changing trends of almond adherence in the a-LCD group.

3.3. *Effect of a-LCD on Glycated Hemoglobin (HbA1c)*

At the baseline, HbA1c levels were not significantly different between the two groups. Compared to the baseline, HbA1c levels in both groups decreased significantly ($p < 0.01$, $p < 0.05$) during the study period. At the third month, the HbA1c level in the a-LCD group decreased more than that in the LFD group ($p < 0.01$, Table 3). The ITT, in relation to HbA1c levels, was performed to ensure the stability of the above results. The result of ITT was found to be in agreement with the findings above (Supplementary Table S1).

Table 3. Comparison of glycated hemoglobin (%) between the two groups.

Study Period	a-LCD (n =22)	LFD (n =23)	t/F	p
Baseline	7.67 ± 1.60	7.54 ± 1.31	−0.287 [a]	0.776
Third month	6.85 ± 1.02 (adjusted:6.77 ± 0.13)	7.37 ± 1.29 (adjusted:7.44 ± 0.12)	14.111 [b]	<0.01 **
t	4.081 [c]	2.614 [c]		
p	<0.01 **	0.016 *		

[a] Independent-samples T test for between-groupdifferencesat the baseline; [b] covariance analysis for between-groupdifferences at the third month, with adjusted data presented as mean ± standard error (covariate: age, baseline HbA1c, protein, the rate of change of anti-diabetics); [c] paired sample T test for within-group difference. * $p < 0.05$; ** $p < 0.01$.

3.4. *Effect of a-LCD on the Changes of Anti-Diabetics*

During the intervention, three in the LCD group and five in the LFD group had anti-diabetic dosage reduced, while the other participants remained unchanged, but there was no significant difference between the two groups in the third month ($p > 0.05$, Table 4)

Table 4. Comparison of other anti-diabetic drugs between the two groups.

	a-LCD (n = 22)	LFD (n = 23)	χ^2	p
Reduction	3 (14%)	5 (22%)	0.019	0.889
No change	19 (86%)	18 (78%)		

p value for comparison between treatments diets by Chi-square test.

3.5. Effect of a-LCD on Weight and BMI

At the third month, weight and BMI showed no significant difference between the two groups ($p > 0.05$, Table 5). Compared to the baseline, weight and BMI of a-LCD group improved significantly at the third month ($p < 0.05$, Table 5).

Table 5. Comparison of weight and BMI between the two groups.

Variables		a-LCD ($n = 22$)	LFD ($n = 23$)	t	p
Weight (Kg)	Baseline	66.60 ± 8.81	63.07 ± 12.88	0.784 [a]	0.459
	Third month	59.34 ± 8.90	62.58 ± 13.12	0.967 [a]	0.339
	t	2.164 [b]	1.397[b]		
	p	0.042 *	0.176		
BMI (Kg/m^2)	Baseline	23.53 ± 2.33	23.69 ± 2.83	0.216	0.830
	Third month	23.02 ± 2.45	23.53 ± 3.04	0.641	0.524
	t	−2.261	−1.283		
	p	0.034 *	0.211		

p value for comparison between two groups by Independent Samples t-test and paired sample T test. [a] Independent-samples T test for between-group differencesat the baseline and third month; [b] paired sample T test for within-group difference. * $p < 0.05$.

3.6. Effect of a-LCD on Depression

At baseline, the depression scores were not significantly different between the two groups. Compared to the baseline, depression score in the a-LCD group decreased significantly ($p < 0.01$) in the third month, while there was no decrease in the LFD group ($p > 0.05$). At the third month, the depression score in the a-LCD group was significantly lower than that in the LFD group ($p < 0.01$, Table 6). The ITT, in relation to depression scores, was performed to ensure the stability of the above results. The ITT result was found to be in agreement with the earlier findings (Supplementary Table S2).

Table 6. Comparison of depression scores between the two groups.

Study Period	a-LCD ($n = 22$)	LFD ($n = 23$)	t/F	p
Baseline	48.41 ± 8.05	49.57 ± 8.46	0.471 [a]	0.640
Third month	42.07 ± 5.80(adjusted:42.58 ± 0.89)	48.65 ± 7.69(adjusted:48.16 ± 0.87)	19.308 [b]	<0.01 **
t	6.196 [c]	0.838 [c]		
p	<0.01 **	0.411		

[a] Independent-samples T test for between-group differencesat the baseline; [b] covariance analysis for between-group differences at the third month, with adjusted data presented as mean ± standard error (covariate: age, baseline depression scores, protein); [c] paired sample T test for within-group difference. * $p < 0.01$.

3.7. Fasting Plasma GLP-1 Concentration

Compared to the baseline, we found that GLP-1 did not significantly change in both groups at the third month. However, GLP-1 in the a-LCD group was significantly higher than that in the LFD group after intervention ($p < 0.05$). (Table 7)

Table 7. Comparison of GLP-1[M(P25,P75)], (pmol/L)] in the two groups.

Study Period	a-LCD (n =22)	LFD (n =23)	Z	p
Baseline	1.381 (0.697,3.157)	1.190 (0.804,1.896)	−0.409	0.683
Third month	1.092 (0.886,2.671)	0.630 (0.261,1.997)	−2.396	0.017 *
Z	−0.221	−1.339		
p	0.833	0.162		

Z-value and p-value for comparisons by Mann–Whitney U or Wilcoxon for between or within group differences at the baseline and third month, the result presented as M(P25, P75). * $p < 0.05$; M(P25,P50): median (25th and 75th percentile).

3.8. *Gut Microbiota*

A total of 2,981,481 quality reads of 90 samples were generated with an average of 33,128 ± 2868 reads per sample.

3.8.1. Alpha-Adversity

The alpha-diversity of the gut microbiota community indicated that compared with the baseline, the Chao 1 and PD index of both groups increased significantly ($p< 0.01$) (Supplementary Figures S1 and S2).

3.8.2. Beta-Diversity

The PCoA of the weighted Unifrac distances was used to compare the overall microbiota structures in the two groups and the results are shown in Supplementary Figures S3 and S4.The more similar the samples of community microbials are, the closer they are to each other.The result revealed there was no extremelyapparent separation in gut microbiota structure between and within the groups at the baseline and the third month.

3.8.3. The Comparison of the Composition of Gut Microbiota in the Two Groups

The overall microbial compositions between two groups at baseline and three months are shown in the Figures 4 and 5. To determine if the a-LCD affected the gut microbiota, we compared the composition of gut microbiota in the two groups at baseline and the third month (Table 8). At the phylum level, *Firmicutes* in the a-LCD group was significantly lower than that in the LFD group by the third month ($p < 0.05$, FDR = 0.026). Compared to the baseline, *Bacteroidetes* ($p < 0.05$, FDR = 0.016) decreased significantly in the a-LCD group. At the genus level, *Roseburia* ($p < 0.01$, FDR <0.01,) and *Ruminococcus* ($p < 0.05$, FDR = 0.073)in the a-LCD group were significantly higher than those in the LFD group by the third month; compared to the baseline: *Eubacterium*($p < 0.01$, FDR = 0.013), *Roseburia* increased significantly($p < 0.05$, FDR = 0.021) and *Bacteroides*($p < 0.05$, FDR = 0.013)decreased significantly in the a-LCD group.

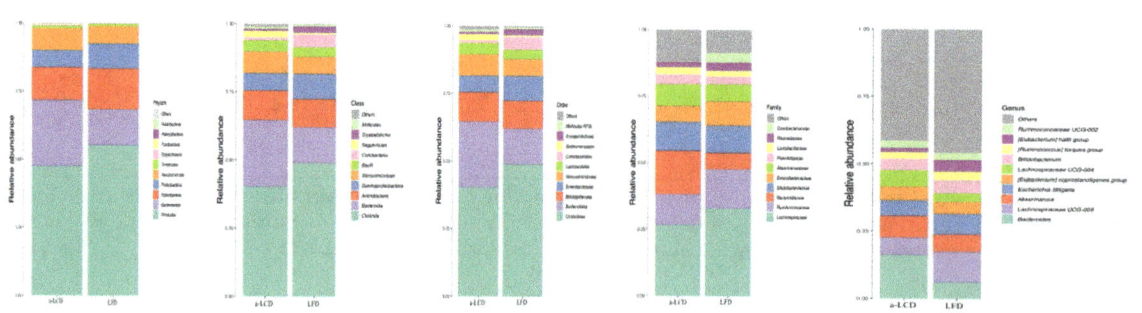

Figure 4. The comparison of the overall microbial composition between the two groups at the baseline. Only taxonomic groups 1% or greater are shown.

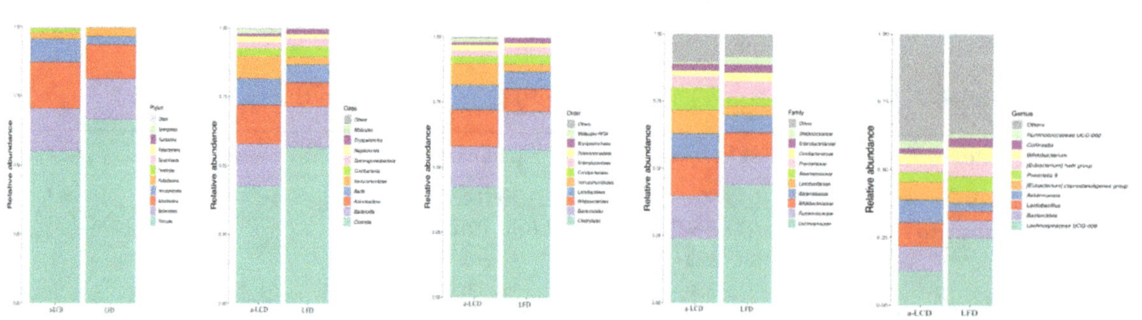

Figure 5. The comparison of the overall microbial composition between the two groups at the third month. Only taxonomic groups 1% or greater are shown.

Table 8. Comparison of the composition of gut microbiota [M(P25,P75)] in the two groups.

Phylum	Genus	Study Period	a-LCD (n =22)	LFD (n =23)	Z	p(adj. val.)
Firmicutes		Baseline	0.389 (0.283,0.729)	0.544 (0.455,0.671)	−1.317	0.188 (0.194)
		Third month	0.580 (0.371,0.672)	0.684 (0.561,0.778)	−2.317	0.021 * (0.026)
		Z	−1.282	−2.281		
		p(adj. val.)	0.200 (0.213)	0.023 * (0.038)		
	Roseburia	Baseline	0.002 (0.000,0.005)	0.009 (0.005,0.024)	−1.892	<0.01 ** (<0.01)
		Third month	0.005 (0.000,0.006)	0.000 (0.000,0.001)	−2.626	<0.01 ** (<0.01)
		Z	−2.193	−4.075		
		p(adj. val.)	0.028 * (0.021)	<0.01 ** (<0.01)		
	Eubacterium	Baseline	0.008 (0.004,0.0220)	0.037 (0.018,0.070)	−3.747	<0.01 ** (<0.01)
		Third month	0.026 (0.004,0.057)	0.042 (0.024,0.099)	−2.082	0.037 * (0.073)
		Z	−2.678	−1.734		
		p(adj. val.)	<0.01 ** (0.013)	0.083 (0.052)		
	Ruminococcus	Baseline	0.017 (0.011,0.033)	0.020 (0.005,0.037)	−0.829	0.470 (0.407)
		Third month	0.026 (0.005,0.044)	0.005 (0.000,0.019)	−2.015	0.044 * (0.073)
		Z	−0.341	−2.312		
		p	0.733 (0.308)	0.021 * (0.020)		
	Lactobacillus	Baseline	0.007 (0.003,0.049)	0.005 (0.002,0.012)	−1.420	0.156 (0.223)
		Third month	0.007 (0.000,0.068)	0.000 (0.000,0.047)	−1.666	0.096 (0.245)
		Z	−1.150	−0.973		
		p(adj. val.)	0.130 (0.073)	0.330 (0.167)		
Bacteroidetes		Baseline	0.249 (0.120,0.323)	0.110 (0.072,0.180)	−2.793	<0.01 ** (0.011)
		Third month	0.151 (0.061,0.256)	0.108 (0.042,0.236)	−0.591	0.555 (0.415)
		Z	−2.451	−1.004		
		p(adj. val.)	0.014 * (0.016)	0.361 (0.188)		
	Bacteroides	Baseline	0.144 (0.057,0.256)	0.047 (0.023,0.119)	−3.244	<0.01 ** (<0.01)
		Third month	0.064 (0.027,0.106)	0.057 (0.009,0.085)	−0.978	0.328 (0.364)
		Z	−2.354	−0.335		
		p(adj. val.)	0.019 * (0.013)	0.735 (0.308)		

Z-value and p-value for comparisons by Mann–Whitney U or Wilcoxon for between or within group differences at the baseline and third month, the result presented as M (P25,P75). * $p < 0.05$; ** $p < 0.01$; M(P25,P50): median (25th and 75th percentile). P value (adj. val.), FDR < 0.2 was considered as significant.

4. Discussion

Until now, only few studies have reported whether a diet regimen is beneficial to both depression and glycometabolism in T2DM patients. Almond is rich in some nutrients and it may be protective against the development of depression.Based on our previous study of a-LCD improving glucose [15], we further explored the effect of this diet regimen on both depression and glycometabolism in T2DM patients.

4.1. *Effect of a-LCD on Glycemic Control and Anti-Diabetics*

For diabetes patients with depression, the primary clinical concern is still on the control of glycometabolism. HbA1c level can reflect mean blood glucose level over the last 8–12 weeks and long-term glycemic control of T2DM patients [8]. It could be used as the main indicator to establish glycemic control. Over 3 months, our study found that both a-LCD ($p < 0.01$) and LFD ($p < 0.05$) improved HbA1c level, while better HbA1c level was seen in the a-LCD group($p < 0.01$), which is consistent with our previous research [15].Although there was no significant difference inanti-diabetics between the two groups during the three-month period, three in the a-LCD group and five in the LFD groupreduced the dosage of anti-diabetic drugs. After controlling the rate of change of anti-diabetics as a covariate, the HbA1c in the a-LCD group was still significantly lower than that in the LFD group, indicating that the hypoglycemic effect of LCD was better than that in the LFD group. The reasons for the potential benefit of a-LCD on HbA1c were shown in those studies [15,27].

4.2. *Effect of a-LCD on Weight and BMI*

Nuts have rich energy density and high fat [40], the greater fat availability may reduce gastric emptying rate to increase the satiety [41]. In this study, a-LCD decreased weight ($p < 0.05$) and BMI ($p < 0.05$) of patients with T2DM, further confirming the effectiveness of LCD in improving weight and BMI. The results are in agreement with the result of our previous study and the reason for the potential benefit of a-LCD on weight and BMI were shown in that study [15].

4.3. *Effect of a-LCD on Depression Score*

The impact of LCD on depression is controversial. Brinkworth et al. [42] used monounsaturated and polyunsaturated fat instead of carbohydrate to form LCD and assessed the effect of LCD on psychological mood state and well-being in obese patients with T2DM. The results found that the Beck Depression Inventory Score declined over time in theboth LCD and LFD groups ($p < 0.05$). Saslow et al. [43] assessed the effect of a 3-month LCD (lower their carbohydrate consumption and derive their remaining calories from fat) and a LFD on psychological outcomes in obesity/overweight patients with T2DM or pre-diabetes. No significant differences in depression scores were observed between the two groups ($p > 0.05$). In the current study, we found that a-LCD significantly decreased the depression score compared to LFD ($p < 0.01$) in patients with T2DM, which is not consistent with the findings in above-mentioned studies. The important reason for the inconsistent effect of LCD on depression may be due to the difference in the composition of the food for LCD. A major difference was that we used almond to replace carbohydrate. Almond as a commonly eaten nut, is a rich source of dietary fiber, polyphenols, and unsaturated fatty acids [44], that may be protective against the development of depression [45–47]. With regard to the association of nuts intake and mental health, most of studies showed the positive effect of nuts. In the PREDIMED trial, an RCT with the Mediterranean diet supplemented with nuts showed a 40% lower risk of depression in patients with T2DM (RR = 0.59, 95% CI 0.36–0.98) [18]. An RCT conducted by Pribis et al. [19] explored the effect of walnut consumption on mood in young adults and observed a significant medium effect size improvement in the Total Mood Disturbance Score (−27.5%, $p = 0.043$) in males. Another reason for the inconsistent results with other studies may be the different participants in their studies who were obese.

4.4. *Effect of a-LCD on Regulation of Gut Microbiota and GLP-1 Expression*

In our study, the a-LCD and LFD at 3 months increased Chao1 and PD index in the two groups, although there were no significantdifferences between the two groups. Increased microbiome diversity could promote greater stability of the microbiome in the long term, thereby contributing to functional resilience against extreme stress and perturbations [48].

Currently, there are no reports of gut microbiota in T2DM with depression, but there is evidence of significant differences between depressed patients and healthy people [49]. Jiang et al. [49] compared the composition between depressed patients with healthy people, and the result indicated that, at the phylum level, depressed patients had higher population of *Bacteroidetes*. After the intervention of the a-LCD, we observed the changes of the above-mentioned bacteria. At the phylum levels, *Bacteroidetes* decreased significantly in the a-LCD group. We also found that a-LCD for 3 months decreased the population of the pathogenic bacterium *Bacteroides*, which is consistent with the study of Dhillon et al. [50]. The above result show that a-LCD could regulate the gut bacteria and the improvement of depression score in the a-LCD may be through modulating of the microbiome-gut-brain.

A growing understanding of the microbiome-gut-brain connections is revealing the pathways by which food choices may affect depression [51], and GLP-1 is an important regulator of microbiota-gut-brain signaling in health and stress-related psychiatric illnesses [26]. Almonds are a rich source of fiber, unsaturated fats, and polyphenols, all nutrients that can favorably alter the gut microbiome [50] and its consumption increases the number of SCFAs-producing bacteria [23].

SCFAs in combination with GPR43 can promote the secretion of GLP-1 [25]. GLP-1, produced both in peripheral L-cells of the gastrointestinal tract and in the brain, is an anorexigenic peptide and treatment target for T2DM [26]. GLP-1 analog liraglutide has been recently reported to attenuate depressive behaviors via improving hippocampal plasticity in mice [52]. GLP-1 receptor agonists have also been shown to have neuroprotective effects both in diabetic [53] and depressed [54] mice. The study of Grant et al. [55] showed that a depression and anxiety score generally tends to improve in GLP-1 analog exenatide-treated T2DM patients and it could be used as an adjunctive therapy for depression in diabetes.

An important finding of the present study was that the a-LCD significantly increased the relative abundance of SCFAs-producing bacteria*Roseburis* [24] ($p < 0.01$, FDR < 0.01) and *Ruminococcus* [24]($p < 0.05$, FDR $= 0.073$), which is consistent with the study by Holscher et al. [56], where they found that almond consumption increased the *Roseburia* ($p < 0.05$). Compared to the baseline, SCFAs-producing bacteria *Roseburia* ($p < 0.05$, FDR $= 0.021$) and *Eubacterium* ($p < 0.01$, FDR $= 0.013$) were significantly increased in the a-LCD group. However, other studies found that almond consumption also increased the population of SCFAs-producing bacteria *Bifidobacterium* and *Lactobacillus* [23], although these were not consistent with our findings, which may be due to the differences in ethnicity [57].

Research has indicated that GLP-1 levels decrease significantly in the T2DM patients [58]. In our study, GLP-1 concentration decreased at the third month compared to the level of the baseline, although there were no statistical differences. However, it is worth noting that GLP-1 concentration in the LCD group was significantly higher than that in the LFD group in the third month ($p < 0.05$), indicating a-LCD maintained the GLP-1 secretion. An RCT randomly assigned a trial diet with 28 g almonds or without almonds and the result indicated that the rise in GLP-1 concentration at 30 min post-meal was due to the effect of almond ingestion for both non-diabetic and T2DM groups [59].Based on the results of this study, we speculate that the role of a-LCD in improving depression in patients with T2DM may be associated with it stimulating the growth of SCFAs-producing bacteria, then increasing SCFAs and GPR43 activation, further maintaining GLP-1 secretion. However, we did not observe the change in SCFAs and GPR43 activation due to the limited fund. In further study, the SCFAs and GPR43 activation should be explored.

5. Conclusions

Based on the findings of this study, the a-LCD may be an effective intervention for the improvement of both depression and glycometabolism in patients with T2MD. A-LCD significantly increased the SCFAs-producing bacteria and maintained the GLP-1 secretion. We speculate that a-LCD improving depression in T2DM patients may be associated with it stimulating the growth of SCFAs-producing bacteria, increasing SCFAs production and GPR43 activation, and further maintaining GLP-1 secretion. In futurestudies, the SCFAs and GPR43 activation should be further examined.

6. Limitations

There are several limitations of our study. One of the limitations is that the present study was conducted in a T2DM population with and without depression, which may limit the a-LCDeffect on depression. Further studies that examine the effects of a-LCD in patients with diabetes with clinical depression are required to understand the effectiveness of the current findings. We did not monitor the dynamic changes of depression over the three-month period; therefore, we could not find the earliest time point for improvement in depression. Due to the limitation of fund, the analysis method of gut microbiota needs to be improved in the further study.

This will be taken into consideration in future research.

Supplementary Materials:
Supplementary Table S1: ITT of glycated hemoglobin (%) between the two groups; Supplementary Table S2: ITT of depression scores between the two groups; Supplementary Figure S1: The Comparison of Chao 1 and PD

between the two groups (NS: no significant difference); Supplementary Figure S2: The Comparison of Chao 1 and PD within the groups (** $p< 0.05$; *** $p< 0.01$); Supplementary Figure S3: Comparison of beta-diversity of gut microbiota between two groups (A: Baseline; B: Third month); Supplementary Figure S4: Comparison of BetFa-diversity of gut microbiota within the group (A: a-LCD group; B: LFD group). The abscissa represents the first principal component, and the percentage represents the contribution value of the first principal component to the sample difference; the ordinate represents the second principal component, and the percentage represents the contribution value of the second principal component to the sample difference. Each point in the graph represents a sample, and the samples of the same group are represented by the same color.

Author Contributions: M.R. and H.Z. analyzed the data. M.R. wrote the initial draft, which was revised by O.O., X.W. and M.R., J.Q., A.H., Q.J., Q.F. collected the data. X.W. contributed most to the design of this research, and all of the other authors participated in the study design and quality control. Y.H. methodology ans supervision. M.R. and H.Z. contributed equally to this study. O.O. and X.W. are the corresponding authors. All authors have read and agreed to the published version of the manuscript.

Acknowledgments: We thank the patients with T2DM who volunteered to participate in this study. We also thank all of the staff in the Endocrine Division of the Second Affiliated Hospital of Soochow University—Xiaoyan Zhang, and Li Wang—who provided us with assistance so as to ensure that the study was conducted.

References

1. Cho, N.H.; Shaw, J.; Karuranga, S.; Huang, Y.; Fernandes, J.D.D.R.; Ohlrogge, A.; Malanda, B. IDF Diabetes Atlas: Global estimates of diabetes prevalence for 2017 and projections for 2045. *Diabetes Res. Clin. Pr.* **2018**, *138*, 271–281. [CrossRef]
2. Semenkovich, K.; Brown, M.E.; Svrakic, D.M.; Lustman, P.J. Depression in type 2 diabetes mellitus: Prevalence, impact, and treatment. *Drugs* **2015**, *75*, 577–587. [CrossRef] [PubMed]
3. Ali, S.; Stone, M.A.; Peters, J.L.; Davies, M.J.; Khunti, K. The prevalence of co-morbid depression in adults with Type 2 diabetes: A systematic review and meta-analysis. *Diabet. Med.* **2006**, *23*, 1165–1173. [CrossRef] [PubMed]
4. Anderson, R.J.; Freedland, K.E.; Clouse, R.E.; Lustman, P.J. The prevalence of comorbid depression in adults with diabetes: A meta-analysis. *Diabetes Care* **2001**, *24*, 1069–1078. [CrossRef] [PubMed]
5. Young-Hyman, D.; De Groot, M.; Hill-Briggs, F.; Gonzalez, J.S.; Hood, K.K.; Peyrot, M. Psychosocial Care for People With Diabetes: A Position Statement of the American Diabetes Association. *Diabetes Care* **2016**, *39*, 2126–2140. [CrossRef]
6. Global Guideline for Type 2 Diabetes: Recommendations for standard, comprehensive, and minimal care. *Diabet. Med.* **2006**, *23*, 579–593. [CrossRef] [PubMed]
7. Antoine, M.-H.; Gall, D.; Schiffmann, S.N.; Lebrun, P. Tricyclic antidepressant imipramine reduces the insulin secretory rate in islet cells of Wistar albino rats through a calcium antagonistic action. *Diabetologia* **2004**, *47*, 909–916. [CrossRef]
8. Society, C.D. Guidelines for the prevention and treatment of type 2 diabetes in China. *Chin. Med. J.* **2017**, *10*, 4–67.
9. Meng, Y.; Bai, H.; Wang, S.; Li, Z.; Wang, Q.; Chen, L. Efficacy of low carbohydrate diet for type 2 diabetes mellitus management: A systematic review and meta-analysis of randomized controlled trials. *Diabetes Res. Clin. Pract.* **2017**, *131*, 124–131. [CrossRef]
10. Hite, A.H.; Berkowitz, V.G.; Berkowitz, K. Low-carbohydrate diet review: Shifting the paradigm. *Nutr. Clin. Pract.* **2011**, *26*, 300–308. [CrossRef]
11. Evert, A.B.; Dennison, M.; Gardner, C.D.; Garvey, W.T.; Lau, K.H.K.; MacLeod, J.; Mitri, J.; Pereira, R.F.; Rawlings, K.; Robinson, S.; et al. Nutrition Therapy for Adults With Diabetes or Prediabetes: A Consensus Report. *Diabetes Care* **2019**, *42*, 731–754. [CrossRef] [PubMed]
12. Pellegrin, K.L.; O'Neil, P.M.; Stellefson, E.J.; Fossey, M.D.; Ballenger, J.C.; Cochrane, C.E.; Currey, H.S. Average daily nutrient intake and mood among obese women. *Nutr. Res.* **1998**, *7*, 18. [CrossRef]
13. Deijen, J.B.; Heemstra, M.L.; Orlebeke, J.F. Dietary effects on mood and performance. *J. Psychiatr. Res.* **1989**, *23*, 275–283. [CrossRef]
14. Rosenthal, N.E.; Genhart, M.J.; Caballero, B.; Jacobsen, F.M.; Skwerer, R.G.; Coursey, R.D.; Rogers, S.; Spring, B. Psychobiological effects of carbohydrate- and protein-rich meals in patients with seasonal affective disorder and normal controls. *Biol. Psychiatry* **1989**, *25*, 1029–1040. [CrossRef]

15. Wang, L.-L.; Wang, Q.; Hong, Y.; Ojo, O.; Jiang, Q.; Hou, Y.-Y.; Huang, Y.-H.; Wang, X. The Effect of Low-Carbohydrate Diet on Glycemic Control in Patients with Type 2 Diabetes Mellitus. *Nutrients* **2018**, *10*, 661. [CrossRef]
16. Pribis, P.; Shukitt-Hale, B. Cognition: The new frontier for nuts and berries. *Am. J. Clin. Nutr.* **2014**, *100* (Suppl. 1), 347S–352S. [CrossRef]
17. Mischoulon, D.; Nierenberg, A.; Schettler, P.J.; Kinkead, B.L.; Fehling, K.; Martinson, M.A.; Rapaport, M.H. A double-blind, randomized controlled clinical trial comparing eicosapentaenoic acid versus docosahexaenoic acid for depression. *J. Clin. Psychiatry* **2014**, *76*, 54–61. [CrossRef]
18. Sánchez-Villegas, A.; Martínez-González, M.A.; Estruch, R.; Salas-Salvadó, J.; Corella, D.; Covas, M.I.; Arós, F.; Romaguera, D.; Gomez-Gracia, E.; Lapetra, J.; et al. Mediterranean dietary pattern and depression: The PREDIMED randomized trial. *BMC Med.* **2013**, *11*, 208. [CrossRef]
19. Pribis, P. Effects of Walnut Consumption on Mood in Young Adults—A Randomized Controlled Trial. *Nutrients* **2016**, *8*, 668. [CrossRef]
20. Arab, L.; Guo, R.; Elashoff, D.A. Lower Depression Scores among Walnut Consumers in NHANES. *Nutrients* **2019**, *11*, 275. [CrossRef]
21. Su, Q.; Yu, B.; He, H.; Zhang, Q.; Meng, G.; Wu, H.; Du, H.; Liu, L.; Shi, H.; Xia, Y.; et al. NUT CONSUMPTION IS ASSOCIATED WITH DEPRESSIVE SYMPTOMS AMONG CHINESE ADULTS. *Depress. Anxiety* **2016**, *33*, 1065–1072. [CrossRef] [PubMed]
22. Mandalari, G.; Nueno-Palop, C.; Bisignano, G.; Wickham, M.S.J.; Narbad, A. Potential prebiotic properties of almond (Amygdalus communis L.) seeds. *Appl. Environ. Microbiol.* **2008**, *74*, 4264–4270. [CrossRef] [PubMed]
23. Liu, Z.; Lin, X.; Huang, G.; Zhang, W.; Rao, P.; Ni, L. Prebiotic effects of almonds and almond skins on intestinal microbiota in healthy adult humans. *Anaerobe* **2014**, *26*, 1–6. [CrossRef]
24. Dalile, B.; Van Oudenhove, L.; Vervliet, B.; Verbeke, K. The role of short-chain fatty acids in microbiota–gut–brain communication. *Nat. Rev. Gastroenterol. Hepatol.* **2019**, *16*, 461–478. [CrossRef] [PubMed]
25. Psichas, A.; Sleeth, M.L.; Murphy, K.G.; Brooks, L.; Bewick, G.A.; Hanyaloglu, A.C.; Ghatei, M.A.; Bloom, S.R.; Frost, G.S. The short chain fatty acid propionate stimulates GLP-1 and PYY secretion via free fatty acid receptor 2 in rodents. *Int. J. Obes.* **2014**, *39*, 424–429. [CrossRef]
26. Lach, G.; Schellekens, H.; Dinan, T.G.; Cryan, J.F. Anxiety, Depression, and the Microbiome: A Role for Gut Peptides. *Neurotherapeutics* **2017**, *15*, 36–59. [CrossRef] [PubMed]
27. Hou, Y.-Y.; Ojo, O.; Wang, L.-L.; Wang, Q.; Jiang, Q.; Shao, X.-Y.; Wang, X. A Randomized Controlled Trial to Compare the Effect of Peanuts and Almonds on the Cardio-Metabolic and Inflammatory Parameters in Patients with Type 2 Diabetes Mellitus. *Nutrients* **2018**, *10*, 1565. [CrossRef]
28. Asghari, G.; Ghorbani, Z.; Mirmiran, P.; Azizi, F. Nut consumption is associated with lower incidence of type 2 diabetes: The Tehran Lipid and Glucose Study. *Diabetes Metab.* **2017**, *43*, 18–24. [CrossRef]
29. Wade, A.T.; Davis, C.R.; Dyer, K.A.; Hodgson, J.M.; Woodman, R.J.; Keage, H.A.D.; Murphy, K.J. A Mediterranean diet supplemented with dairy foods improves mood and processing speed in an Australian sample: Results from the MedDairy randomized controlled trial. *Nutr. Neurosci.* **2020**, *23*, 646–658. [CrossRef]
30. Li, S.-C.; Liu, Y.-H.; Liu, J.-F.; Chang, W.-H.; Chen, C.-M. Almond consumption improved glycemic control and lipid profiles in patients with type 2 diabetes mellitus. *Metabolism* **2011**, *60*, 474–479. [CrossRef]
31. Galletly, C.; Moran, L.; Noakes, M.; Clifton, P.M.; Tomlinson, L.; Norman, R.J. Psychological benefits of a high-protein, low-carbohydrate diet in obese women with polycystic ovary syndrome—A pilot study. *Appetite* **2007**, *49*, 590–593. [CrossRef]
32. Collier, G.; O'Dea, K. The effect of coingestion of fat on the glucose, insulin, and gastric inhibitory polypeptide responses to carbohydrate and protein. *Am. J. Clin. Nutr.* **1983**, *37*, 941–944. [CrossRef]
33. Cook, K.F.; Jensen, S.E.; Schalet, B.D.; Beaumont, J.L.; Amtmann, D.; Czajkowski, S.; DeWalt, D.A.; Fries, J.F.; Pilkonis, P.A.; Reeve, B.B.; et al. PROMIS measures of pain, fatigue, negative affect, physical function, and social function demonstrated clinical validity across a range of chronic conditions. *J. Clin. Epidemiol.* **2016**, *73*, 89–102. [CrossRef]
34. Kuczynski, J.; Lauber, C.L.; Walters, W.A.; Parfrey, L.W.; Clemente, J.C.; Gevers, D.; Knight, R. Experimental and analytical tools for studying the human microbiome. *Nat. Rev. Genet.* **2011**, *13*, 47–58. [CrossRef]

35. Fadrosh, D.W.; Ma, B.; Gajer, P.; Sengamalay, N.; Ott, S.; Brotman, R.M.; Ravel, J. An improved dual-indexing approach for multiplexed 16S rRNA gene sequencing on the Illumina MiSeq platform. *Microbiome* **2014**, *2*, 6. [CrossRef]
36. Caporaso, J.G.; Kuczynski, J.; Stombaugh, J.; Bittinger, K.; Bushman, F.D.; Costello, E.K.; Fierer, N.; Peña, A.G.; Goodrich, J.K.; Gordon, J.I.; et al. QIIME allows analysis of high-throughput community sequencing data. *Nat. Methods* **2010**, *7*, 335–336. [CrossRef] [PubMed]
37. Quast, C.; Pruesse, E.; Yilmaz, P.; Gerken, J.; Schweer, T.; Yarza, P.; Peplies, J.; Glöckner, F.O. The SILVA ribosomal RNA gene database project: Improved data processing and web-based tools. *Nucleic Acids Res.* **2013**, *41*, D590–D596. [CrossRef]
38. Edgar, R.C. UPARSE: Highly accurate OTU sequences from microbial amplicon reads. *Nat. Methods* **2013**, *10*, 996–998. [CrossRef]
39. Nicolucci, A.C.; Hume, M.P.; Martínez, I.; Mayengbam, S.; Walter, J.; Reimer, R.A. Prebiotics Reduce Body Fat and Alter Intestinal Microbiota in Children Who Are Overweight or With Obesity. *Gastroenterology* **2017**, *153*, 711–722. [CrossRef]
40. Vadivel, V.; Kunyanga, C.N.; Biesalski, H.K. Health benefits of nut consumption with special reference to body weight control. *Nutrition* **2012**, *28*, 1089–1097. [CrossRef]
41. Tan, S.-Y.; Dhillon, J.; Mattes, R.D. A review of the effects of nuts on appetite, food intake, metabolism, and body weight. *Am. J. Clin. Nutr.* **2014**, *100* (Suppl. 1), 412S–422S. [CrossRef]
42. Brinkworth, G.D.; Luscombe-Marsh, N.D.; Thompson, C.H.; Noakes, M.; Buckley, J.D.; Wittert, G.; Wilson, C.J. Long-term effects of very low-carbohydrate and high-carbohydrate weight-loss diets on psychological health in obese adults with type 2 diabetes: Randomized controlled trial. *J. Intern. Med.* **2016**, *280*, 388–397. [CrossRef] [PubMed]
43. Saslow, L.R.; Kim, S.; Daubenmier, J.J.; Moskowitz, J.T.; Phinney, S.D.; Goldman, V.; Murphy, E.J.; Cox, R.M.; Morán, P.; Hecht, F.M. A randomized pilot trial of a moderate carbohydrate diet compared to a very low carbohydrate diet in overweight or obese individuals with type 2 diabetes mellitus or prediabetes. *PLoS ONE* **2014**, *9*, e91027. [CrossRef] [PubMed]
44. Sugizaki, C.S.A.; Naves, M.M.V. Potential Prebiotic Properties of Nuts and Edible Seeds and Their Relationship to Obesity. *Nutrients* **2018**, *10*, 1645. [CrossRef] [PubMed]
45. Swann, O.G.; Kilpatrick, M.; Breslin, M.; Oddy, W.H. Dietary fiber and its associations with depression and inflammation. *Nutr. Rev.* **2019**, *78*, 394–411. [CrossRef]
46. Sureda, A.; Tejada, S. Polyphenols and depression: From chemistry to medicine. *Curr. Pharm. Biotechnol.* **2015**, *16*, 259–264. [CrossRef] [PubMed]
47. Deacon, G.; Kettle, C.; Hayes, D.; Dennis, C.; Tucci, J. Omega 3 polyunsaturated fatty acids and the treatment of depression. *Crit. Rev. Food Sci. Nutr.* **2015**, *57*, 212–223. [CrossRef]
48. Yachi, S.; Loreau, M. Biodiversity and ecosystem productivity in a fluctuating environment: The insurance hypothesis. *Proc. Natl. Acad. Sci. USA* **1999**, *96*, 1463–1468. [CrossRef]
49. Jiang, H.; Ling, Z.; Zhang, Y.; Mao, H.; Ma, Z.; Yin, Y.; Wang, W.; Tang, W.; Tan, Z.; Shi, J.; et al. Altered fecal microbiota composition in patients with major depressive disorder. *Brain Behav. Immun.* **2015**, *48*, 186–194. [CrossRef]
50. Dhillon, J.; Li, Z.; Ortiz, R.M. Almond Snacking for 8 wk Increases Alpha-Diversity of the Gastrointestinal Microbiome and Decreases Bacteroides fragilis Abundance Compared with an Isocaloric Snack in College Freshmen. *Curr. Dev. Nutr.* **2019**, *3*, nzz079. [CrossRef]
51. Dash, S.; Clarke, G.; Berk, M.; Jacka, F.N. The gut microbiome and diet in psychiatry: Focus on depression. *Curr. Opin. Psychiatry* **2015**, *28*, 1–6. [CrossRef]
52. Weina, H.; Yuhu, N.; Christian, H.; Birong, L.; Feiyu, S.; Le, W. Liraglutide attenuates the depressive- and anxiety-like behaviour in the corticosterone induced depression model via improving hippocampal neural plasticity. *Brain Res.* **2018**, *1694*, 55–62. [CrossRef] [PubMed]
53. Gault, V.A.; Hölscher, C. GLP-1 receptor agonists show neuroprotective effects in animal models of diabetes. *Peptides* **2018** *100*, 101–107. [CrossRef]
54. Zhao, Y.; Li, H.; Fang, F.; Qin, T.; Xiao, W.; Wang, Z.; Ma, S.-P. Geniposide improves repeated restraint stress-induced depression-like behavior in mice by ameliorating neuronal apoptosis via regulating GLP-1R/AKT signaling pathway. *Neurosci. Lett.* **2018**, *676*, 19–26. [CrossRef] [PubMed]

55. Grant, P.; Lipscomb, D.; Quin, J. Psychological and quality of life changes in patients using GLP-1 analogues. *J. Diabetes Complicat.* **2011**, *25*, 244–246. [CrossRef] [PubMed]
56. Holscher, H.D.; Taylor, A.M.; Swanson, K.S.; Novotny, J.A.; Baer, D.J. Almond Consumption and Processing Affects the Composition of the Gastrointestinal Microbiota of Healthy Adult Men and Women: A Randomized Controlled Trial. *Nutrients* **2018**, *10*, 126. [CrossRef] [PubMed]
57. Nishijima, S.; Suda, W.; Oshima, K.; Kim, S.-W.; Hirose, Y.; Morita, H.; Hattori, M. The gut microbiome of healthy Japanese and its microbial and functional uniqueness. *DNA Res.* **2016**, *23*, 125–133. [CrossRef]
58. Senyigit, A.; Tabak, O.; Orhanoglu, T.; Karadag, A.; Ugurlu, S.; Uzun, H.; Konukoglu, D. Glucagon-like peptide-1 levels and dipeptidyl peptidase-4 activity in type 2 diabetes. *Clin. Investig. Med.* **2017**, *40*, E188–E199. [CrossRef]
59. Cohen, A.E.; Johnston, C.S. Almond ingestion at mealtime reduces postprandial glycemia and chronic ingestion reduces hemoglobin A1c in individuals with well-controlled type 2 diabetes mellitus. *Metabolism* **2011**, *60*, 1312–1317. [CrossRef]

2

Inadequate Vitamin C Status in Prediabetes and Type 2 Diabetes Mellitus: Associations with Glycaemic Control, Obesity and Smoking

Renée Wilson [1], Jinny Willis [2], Richard Gearry [1], Paula Skidmore [3], Elizabeth Fleming [3], Chris Frampton [1] and Anitra Carr [4,*]

1 Department of Medicine, University of Otago, Christchurch 8011, New Zealand; renee.wilson@postgrad.otago.ac.nz (R.W.); richard.gearry@otago.ac.nz (R.G.); chris.frampton@otago.ac.nz (C.F.)

2 Lipid and Diabetes Research Group, Canterbury District Health Board, Christchurch 8011, New Zealand; jinny.willis@cdhb.health.nz

3 Department of Human Nutrition, University of Otago, Dunedin 9016, New Zealand; paula.skidmore@otago.ac.nz (P.S.); liz.fleming@otago.ac.nz (E.F.)

4 Department of Pathology, University of Otago, Christchurch 8011, New Zealand

* Correspondence: anitra.carr@otago.ac.nz

Abstract: Vitamin C (ascorbate) is an essential micronutrient in humans, being required for a number of important biological functions via acting as an enzymatic cofactor and reducing agent. There is some evidence to suggest that people with type 2 diabetes mellitus (T2DM) have lower plasma vitamin C concentrations compared to those with normal glucose tolerance (NGT). The aim of this study was to investigate plasma vitamin C concentrations across the glycaemic spectrum and to explore correlations with indices of metabolic health. This is a cross-sectional observational pilot study in adults across the glycaemic spectrum from NGT to T2DM. Demographic and anthropometric data along with information on physical activity were collected and participants were asked to complete a four-day weighed food diary. Venous blood samples were collected and glycaemic indices, plasma vitamin C concentrations, hormone tests, lipid profiles, and high-sensitivity C-reactive protein (hs-CRP) were analysed. A total of 89 participants completed the study, including individuals with NGT ($n = 35$), prediabetes ($n = 25$), and T2DM managed by diet alone or on a regimen of Metformin only ($n = 29$). Plasma vitamin C concentrations were significantly lower in individuals with T2DM compared to those with NGT (41.2 μmol/L versus 57.4 μmol/L, $p < 0.05$) and a higher proportion of vitamin C deficiency (i.e. <11.0 μmol/L) was observed in both the prediabetes and T2DM groups. The results showed fasting glucose ($p = 0.001$), BMI ($p = 0.001$), smoking history ($p = 0.003$), and dietary vitamin C intake ($p = 0.032$) to be significant independent predictors of plasma vitamin C concentrations. In conclusion, these results suggest that adults with a history of smoking, prediabetes or T2DM, and/or obesity, have greater vitamin C requirements. Future research is required to investigate whether eating more vitamin C rich foods and/or taking vitamin C supplements may reduce the risk of progression to, and/or complications associated with, T2DM.

Keywords: vitamin C; glycaemic control; metabolic health; prediabetes; type 2 diabetes mellitus

---

1. Introduction

Type 2 diabetes mellitus (T2DM) is a complex disorder influenced by both genetic and environmental factors. It is characterized by chronic hyperglycemia, altered insulin secretion, and insulin resistance [1]. As in many Western countries, T2DM is associated with increased morbidity and mortality due to microvascular (e.g. retinopathy, nephropathy, and neuropathy) and macrovascular complications (e.g. myocardial infarction, peripheral vascular disease, and stroke) [1]. Diabetes is one of the largest global health emergencies with 415 million people between the ages of 20 and 70 worldwide estimated as having diabetes in 2015 and the prevalence is increasing [2]. T2DM accounts for at least 90% of all cases of diabetes [2]. In 2016, approximately 5% of New Zealanders were living with diabetes compared to an estimated 6.5% of people in the UK [3,4].

Research suggests that chronic low grade inflammation and oxidative stress plays a pivotal role in the development of insulin resistance and T2DM, as well as the related complications [5]. Vitamin C is an essential micronutrient with potent antioxidant properties [6]. Vitamin C can protect important biomolecules from oxidation through participating in oxidation-reduction reactions whereby it is readily oxidized to dehydroascorbic acid, which in turn is rapidly reduced back to ascorbate [7]. Vitamin C is naturally present in fruit and vegetables, is often added as a preservative to foods/beverages, and is also used as a dietary supplement [6]. As a result of being water-soluble, it has a relatively short half-life in the body due to rapid renal clearance and a regular and adequate intake is required to prevent deficiency.

Previous research suggests that people with T2DM have lower plasma vitamin C concentrations than those with normal glucose control [8–10]. There are several proposed mechanisms including: (1) increased ascorbate excretion in those with microalbuminuria, (2) blood glucose may compete with vitamin C for uptake into cells due to its structural similarity to the oxidised form (dehydroascorbic acid), and (3) increased oxidative stress may deplete antioxidant stores [8]. Recent research has indicated that the glucose-dependent inhibition of dehydroascorbic acid uptake into erythrocytes may contribute to enhanced erythrocyte fragility and could potentially contribute to complications such as diabetic microvascular angiopathy [11].

As dietary vitamin C contributes to plasma vitamin C concentrations, potential differences in the intake between those with normal glucose control and T2DM must also be considered. A prospective study of 48,850 men revealed that while the baseline consumption of fruit and vegetables was similar, men who developed T2DM increased their consumption of fruit and vegetables by 1.6 serves/week compared to an increase of 0.7 serves/week in those who remained diabetes free [12]. Therefore, it seems that people with T2DM are altering their diet in an attempt to manage their blood sugar. Indeed, clinical advice to those newly-diagnosed with T2DM focuses on improving the diet. However, the dietary changes appear to be small and, furthermore, those with T2DM appear to have a similar intake of fruit and vegetables to those without T2DM [12].

The lower plasma vitamin C concentrations reported in people with T2DM has led to a growing interest in the role that vitamin C may afford against the development of T2DM and associated complications. A prospective survey of the Dutch and Finnish cohorts within the Seven Countries Study revealed an inverse association between dietary vitamin C intake and glucose intolerance, suggesting that antioxidants such as vitamin C may play a protective role against the development of impaired glucose tolerance and T2DM [13]. Further, the European Prospective Investigation of Cancer (EPIC)-Norfolk Study of some 21,000 individuals ascertained 735 cases of T2DM after a 12 year follow-up, and demonstrated a strong inverse association between plasma vitamin C concentration and T2DM risk [14].

However, studies investigating plasma vitamin C and glycaemic control have often failed to account for factors such as smoking status and dietary vitamin C intake, which are known to impact plasma vitamin C concentrations. When dietary intake is taken into account there are conflicting results, with one study showing a low plasma vitamin C concentration in people with diabetes consuming a similar amount of dietary vitamin C to those without diabetes [15], compared to another study that reported no differences in serum vitamin C concentrations in people grouped by T2DM status after adjustment for dietary vitamin C intake [16]. Therefore, the objective of this study was to determine the association between plasma vitamin C status and glycaemic control accounting for vitamin C intake in adults.

2. Materials and Methods

2.1. Study Participants

This study was approved by the New Zealand Central Health and Disability Ethics Committee (consent no. 14/CEN/34). Written informed consent was obtained from all participants. Individuals aged $\geq$ 18 years meeting the inclusion criteria detailed below were recruited from General Practice, Prediabetes and Diabetes Services, Retinal Screening Services, Pharmacies, and from local advertisements. Fasting glucose cut-off values for normal glucose tolerance (NGT), prediabetes, and T2DM were based on the American Diabetes Association (ADA) criteria [1]. Those taking Metformin were also included in the T2DM group. A total of 101 individuals underwent a screening questionnaire to ascertain the eligibility for the study. Ninety participants were enrolled and 89 participants completed the study. One participant was excluded due to incomplete sample collection.

2.2. Study Design

This was a cross-sectional observational pilot study that was part of a wider study on the gut microbiota and glycaemic control. At their study appointment, participants completed demographic and physical activity questionnaires. Anthropometric data were collected including the body mass index (BMI), waist and hip circumference, and bioelectrical impedance. The completed four-day weighed food diary was reviewed and additional information was added if necessary. A venous blood sample was also collected after an overnight fast and the blood pressure was measured.

2.2.1. Inclusion Criteria

Individuals aged $\geq$18 years with: NGT (fasting glucose $\leq$5.5 mmol/L) (n = 35), prediabetes (fasting glucose $\geq$5.6 mmol/L) (n = 25), T2DM taking no diabetes medication (fasting glucose $\geq$7.0 mmol/L) or on a regimen of Metformin only (n = 29).

2.2.2. Exclusion Criteria

Individuals unable to give informed consent, those who had taken antibiotics in the last month, those with a medical history of significant gastrointestinal disease e.g. inflammatory bowel disease, those who had undergone a previous bowel resection, and individuals taking diabetes medication other than Metformin.

2.3. Demographic Information

Participants recorded their date of birth, sex, ethnicity, qualification, and smoking status. They also recorded information on current medication and supplement use.

2.4. Anthropometric Measures

Weight (kg). Participants were asked to remove their footwear and heavy outer clothing such as jackets and were weighed to the nearest 0.1 kg on calibrated Tanita scales (Model BWB-800A, Tanita Corporation, Tokyo, Japan).

Height (m). Measured once to the nearest mm using calibrated height measures.

BMI (kg/m^2). Widely accepted as an appropriate population-level indicator of excess body fat [17]. BMI is calculated by weight in kilograms divided by height in metres squared.

Waist circumference and the waist-to-hip ratio are alternative anthropometric measures that also indicate whether excess body fat is centrally or peripherally located.

Waist circumference (cm). The World Health Organisation (WHO) STEPwise Approach to Surveillance (STEPS) protocol for measuring the waist circumference was used. The measurement was made at the approximate midpoint between the lower margin of the last palpable rib and the top of the iliac crest [18]. The tightness of the tape was controlled by using a Gulick II Measuring tape

(Model 67020, Country Technology Inc, Gays Mills, Wisconsin, WI, USA). Two to three measures were recorded and if the difference between the measurements exceeded 1.5 cm, a third measure was taken. The measures for each participant were averaged.

Hip circumference (cm). Measured to the nearest mm around the widest portion of the buttocks with the tape parallel to the floor using a Gulick II Measuring tape, as described above.

Waist-to-hip ratio. Calculated by dividing the waist circumference by the hip measurement.

Fat mass (%). Measured using the BIA 450 Bioimpedance Analyser (Biodynamics Corporation, Seattle, Washington, DC, USA). Patient assessments were conducted using a connection between the individual's wrist and ankle and the analyser using standard ECG sensor pad electrodes (CONMED Corporation, Utica, New York, NY, USA).

Blood Pressure. Measured using an automated blood pressure monitor (Bp TRU, BTM-300, Omron Healthcare Co., Ltd, Muko, Kyoto, Japan). The measurement was repeated if the results were outside the normal range. If there was an obvious outlier, this result was removed and the other results were averaged.

2.5. *Blood Parameters*

Venous blood samples were collected after a 12–hour fast.

Glycated haemoglobin (HbA1c). Determined in EDTA blood by standard methods (Bio-rad Variant HPLC, Bio-Rad, Hercules, California, CA, USA) at an International Accreditation New Zealand (IANZ) laboratory.

Glucose. Fasting glucose was measured in blood collected in fluoride oxalate venoject tubes by standard methods (Glucose Hexokinase Enzymatic Assay, Abbott c series analyser, Abbott Park, Illinois, USA) at an IANZ laboratory.

Lipid parameters. Total cholesterol (TC), HDL-cholesterol (HDL), LDL-cholesterol (LDL), and triglycerides (TG) were determined in lithium heparin blood by standard methods (Abbott c series analyser, Abbott Park, Illinois, IL, USA) at an IANZ laboratory.

High-sensitivity C-reactive protein (hs-CRP). The inflammatory marker hs-CRP was measured using end-point nephelometry at an IANZ laboratory.

Plasma vitamin C and hormones. EDTA blood was collected and centrifuged for 15 min at 1500 g at 4 °C. The plasma was stored −80 °C prior to analysis.

2.5.1. Plasma Vitamin C

Stored plasma was rapidly thawed, and acidified with perchloric acid and a metal chelator (DTPA) to precipitate the protein and stabilise the ascorbate [19]. Following centrifugation, the supernatant was treated with a reducing agent (TCEP) to recover any ascorbate that had become oxidised during the processing and storage of the samples [20]. The vitamin C concentration of the processed samples was determined using high performance liquid chromatography (HPLC) with electrochemical detection in the Department of Pathology, University of Otago Christchurch, as described previously [19].

2.5.2. Plasma Ghrelin, Leptin, and Adiponectin

Plasma hormones were determined by the Christchurch Heart Institute, Department of Medicine, University of Otago, Christchurch.

Plasma ghrelin was measured by an in-house radioimmunoassay (RIA) following extraction from plasma using Sep Pak C_{18} cartridges, as described previously [21]. The assay recognises the total circulating ghrelin (i.e. both octanoyl and non-octanoyl forms). The cross reactivities of other peptides in the assay, including vasointestinal peptide, prolactin, galanin, growth hormone releasing hormone, neuropeptide Y, brain natriuretic peptide, atrial natriuretic peptide, endothelin-1, and angiotensin II were all less than 0.03%. The RIA had a mean detection limit of 10.8 ± 0.8 pmol/L and mean ED_{50} of 136.2 ± 10.0 pmol/L over 23 consecutive assays.

Plasma leptin and adiponectin were measured using commercial enzyme-linked immunosorbent assays (ELISA) from BioVendor (Brno, Czech Republic), Research and Diagnostic products (RD191001100 Human Leptin ELISA and RD191023100 Human Adiponectin ELISA) according to the manufacturer's instructions.

2.5.3. Plasma Insulin

Plasma insulin was measured using the Roche Cobas e411 method in an IANZ laboratory. After storage at −80 °C, thawed plasma was pre-treated using 25% polyethylene glycol to precipitate any unwanted antibodies.

2.6. Dietary Intake of Vitamin C, Macronutrients, and Fibre

Participants completed a four day (non-consecutive) weighed food diary (including one weekend day) prior to their study visit. Participants received training using the Salter digital scales and on how to record the data, either at home or in the clinic, prior to the diary being completed. Once completed, the diary was also reviewed at their second study visit to add any missing information if necessary. The food diaries were entered into the nutrient analysis programme Kai-culator (version 1.08d, Department of Human Nutrition, University of Otago, Dunedin, New Zealand). Kai-culator uses the 2014 version of the New Zealand food composition database "NZ FOODfiles". The methodology for entering the diaries was developed by a dietitian and data entry was undertaken by an experienced dietitian and an experienced nutritionist who cross-checked each other's data and were overseen by an experienced nutritionist and dietitian. A further 16% of the diaries were checked again for accuracy. The Acceptable Macronutrient Distribution Ranges (AMDR) are the recommendations for the balance of protein, fat, and carbohydrate in the diet with respect to the relative contribution to dietary energy [22]. Total daily vitamin C, energy, and fibre were calculated, along with the percent energy values for fat, carbohydrate, and protein. Participants were asked to record the name of dietary supplements taken within the last month, the amount per dose, the frequency, when they started taking the supplement, and when their last dose was.

2.7. Physical Activity

Participants completed the self-administered short form version of the International Physical Activity Questionnaire (IPAQ). The questionnaire asks about physical activity over the previous seven days.

2.8. Statistical Analyses

Standard descriptive statistics including means, standard deviations, frequencies, and percentages as appropriate were used to summarise the demographic, anthropometric, and laboratory results across participants grouped by fasting glucose and T2DM treatment. Four of the laboratory measures (hs-CRP, Ghrelin, Leptin, and Adiponectin) showed a strong positive skew and were therefore $\log_e$ transformed prior to analyses. These variables are described using geometric means and 95% confidence intervals. Associations between the clinical characteristics of the cohorts grouped by fasting glucose (including those treated with Metformin) were tested using one way analysis of variance (ANOVA) and chi-squared tests as appropriate. Where significant associations were identified, these were further explored with pair-wise comparisons amongst the fasting glucose groups. The univariate associations between plasma vitamin C and demographic, anthropometric, and laboratory measures were tested using Pearson's Correlations coefficients and one way ANOVA. Significant predictors identified from these univariate analyses were then combined in a multiple regression analysis to identify significant independent associations with plasma vitamin C. The two-tailed p-value < 0.05 was taken to indicate statistical significance. All statistical analyses were undertaken using SPSS (version 24.0, IBM Corp., Armonk, New York, NY, USA).

3. Results

3.1. Participant Characteristics

The NGT group was slightly younger than the prediabetes and T2DM groups and there were more females in the NGT group and less in the T2DM group. The majority of participants were European and there were a mix of qualifications, as would be expected given the age of the participants (Table 1). There were no significant differences in physical activity between the study groups although those in the NGT and prediabetes groups had reported slightly higher levels of activity than those with T2DM.

Table 1. General characteristics of participants classified as having normal glucose tolerance (NGT) (n = 35), prediabetes (n = 25), and T2DM (n = 29).

Characteristics	NGT	Prediabetes	T2DM	Total
Age * (years)	55 ± 13 [a]	63 ± 9 [b]	61 ± 11 [b]	59 ± 11
Sex *				
Female % (n)	74 (26) [a]	52 (13) [ab]	35 (10) [b]	55% (49)
Male % (n)	26 (9)	48 (12)	66 (19)	45% (40)
Ethnicity				
European % (n)	86 (30)	88 (22)	97 (28)	90% (80)
Maori % (n)	9 (3)	4 (1)	3 (1)	6% (5)
Pacific Island % (n)	0 (0)	4 (1)	0 (0)	1% (1)
Asian % (n)	3 (1)	4 (1)	0 (0)	2% (2)
Other % (n)	3 (1)	0 (0)	0 (0)	1% (1)
Qualification				
No Qualification % (n)	96 (3)	20 (5)	25 (7)	17% (15)
Secondary School % (n)	20 (7)	24 (6)	32 (9)	25% (22)
Post-Secondary Certificate, Diploma or Trade Diploma % (n)	43 (15)	20 (5)	25 (7)	31% (27)
University % (n)	27 (10)	36 (9)	18 (5)	27% (24)
Physical Activity (MET min/week)	1723 ± 1687	2496 ± 3671	1320 ± 1490	1772 ± 2327
Anthropometry				
Weight * (kg)	76 ± 18 [a]	89 ± 19 [b]	96 ± 20 [b]	86 ± 21
BMI * (kg/m^2)	28 ± 6 [a]	30 ± 7 [ab]	33 ± 6 [b]	30 ± 7
Fat Mass (%)	32 ± 8	33 ± 8	35 ± 7	33 ± 8
Waist Circumference * (cm)	89 ± 16 [a]	99 ± 14 [b]	110 ± 15 [c]	99 ± 17
Waist-to-Hip Ratio *	0.9 ± 0.1 [a]	0.9 ± 0.1 [b]	1.0 ± 0.1 [b]	0.9 ± 0.1
Blood Pressure Diastolic (mmHg)	78 ± 9	83 ± 8	79 ± 9	80 ± 9
Blood Pressure Systolic * (mmHg)	125 ± 14 [a]	132 ± 14 [ab]	135 ± 15 [b]	130 ± 15
Smoking Status				
Current Smoker % (n)	7 (2)	5 (1)	3 (1)	5% (4)
Ex-smoker % (n)	28 (8)	439 (9)	38 (11)	35% (28)
Non-smoker % (n)	66 (19)	52 (11)	59 (17)	60% (47)

Values represented as mean ± SD unless stated otherwise. *All p values from ANOVA tests. Groups sharing a common subscript letter denotes the study groups that do not differ significantly from each other at the 0.05 level based on characteristics from Post Hoc analysis. Note: There was missing data from one participant for qualification (1 × T2DM), 12 participants for physical activity (7 × NGT and 5 × prediabetes), five participants for waist-to-hip ratio (2 × NGT and 3 × prediabetes), nine participants for blood pressure measures (4 × NGT and 5 × prediabetes), and 10 participants did not provide smoking status data (6 × NGT, 4 × prediabetes).

The mean BMI for the NGT and prediabetes groups reflects the international BMI cut-off points for overweight (25.00–29.99 kg/m^2) and the T2DM group were obese (≥30.00 kg/m^2). The waist circumference and waist-to-hip ratio increased across the groups from NGT to T2DM along with fat mass (%), as would be expected given that obesity is a risk factor for T2DM.

3.2. Metabolic and Inflammatory Plasma Biomarkers

Glycaemic measures (fasting glucose and HbA1c), used as the basis for defining prediabetes and T2DM, increased from NGT to T2DM as expected and differed significantly between the study groups ($p < 0.05$, Table 2). Although fasting glucose was used as the basis for classifying participants in the analysis, the mean HbA1c of 35 mmol/mol for the NGT group and 40 mmol/mol for the prediabetes group were consistent with the New Zealand guidelines for the classification of diabetes based on HbA1c [23]. The mean HbA1c of 47 mmol/mol for the T2DM group is lower than the current threshold for the diagnosis of diabetes in New Zealand (50 mmol/mol) using this measure because some of the individuals in this category were treated with the biguanide oral hypoglycaemic drug, Metformin. Fasting and postprandial glucose were likely reduced in these treated individuals. The mean HbA1c for all participants was 41 mmol/mol (Table 2). While hs-CRP was inversely associated with glycaemic control, this was not significant.

Table 2. Laboratory measures of participants classified as having normal glucose tolerance (NGT) (n = 35), prediabetes (n = 25), and T2DM (n = 29).

Laboratory Measures	NGT	Prediabetes	T2DM	Total
Fasting Glucose * (mmol/L)	5.0 ± 0.4 [a]	6.2 ± 0.4 [b]	7.2 ± 1.3 [c]	6.0 ± 1.2
HbA1c * (mmol/mol)	35 ± 4 [a]	40 ± 5 [b]	47 ± 9 [c]	41 ± 8
hs-CRP (mg/L) Mean (95% CI)	1.2 (0.9–1.6)	1.6 (1.0–2.3)	2.1 (1.4–2.8)	1.6 (1.31.9)
Total Cholesterol * (mmol/L)	5.3 ± 0.9 [a]	5.9 ± 1.2 [a]	4.3 ± 1.1 [b]	5.0 ± 1.1
Cholesterol HDL * (mmol/L)	1.5 ± 0.4 [a]	1.3 ± 0.3 [b]	1.1 ± 0.2 [b]	1.3 ± 0.3
Cholesterol LDL * (Calc) (mmol/L)	3.4 ± 0.8 [a]	3.3 ± 1.0 [a]	2.5 ± 1.0 [b]	3.1 ± 1.0
Triglycerides * (mmol/L)	1.1 ± 0.4 [a]	1.3 ± 0.7 [ab]	1.4 ± 0.6 [b]	1.3 ± 0.6
Cholesterol (total/HDL) (ratio)	3.8 ± 0.8	4.2 ± 0.8	3.9 ± 1.1	4.0 ± 0.9
Fasting Insulin * (pmol/L)	53 ± 37 [a]	89 ± 53 [b]	95 ± 48 [b]	77 ± 49
Ghrelin * (pmol/L) Mean (95% CI)	171 (142–207) [a]	111 (88–140) [b]	112 (91–139) [b]	132 (117–150)
Leptin (ng/mL) Mean (95% CI)	27 (20–38)	33 (20–54)	33 (23–47)	31 (25–38)
Adiponectin * (μg/mL) Mean (95% CI)	11 (9–13) [a]	9 (7–11) [a]	7 (6–8) [b]	9 (8–10)
Plasma vitamin C * (μmol/L)	57 ± 14 [a]	48 ± 16 [b]	41 ± 18 [b]	49 ± 17

Values represented as mean ± SD unless stated otherwise. *All p values from ANOVA tests. Groups sharing a common subscript letter denotes the study groups that do not differ significantly from each other at the 0.05 level based on characteristics from Post Hoc analysis. Log conversion was carried out for Ghrelin, Leptin, Adiponectin, and hs-CRP. Note: There was missing data from three participants for plasma vitamin C (2 × NGT and 1 × prediabetes).

The average fasting insulin concentrations were consistent with the glycaemic measures and were significantly higher in the T2DM group compared to the NGT group. The increasing BMI across the groups was associated with the increase in leptin concentrations, and the reduction in ghrelin concentrations.

Total, HDL, and LDL cholesterol decreased from the NGT to the T2DM group, which may reflect the use of lipid lowering medications which are routinely used in individuals with T2DM.

There was a slight increase in TG across the groups, with the average for each group remaining below the recommended cut-off in New Zealand (<1.7 mmol/L). There were no significant differences in the total cholesterol/HDL ratio between groups, and each group was below the recommended cut-off in New Zealand of 4.5.

3.3. Dietary Intake of Vitamin C, Macronutrients, and Fibre

There were no significant differences in macronutrient intake and dietary vitamin C intake across the groups (Table 3). The AMDR range for protein is 15–25% of total energy, total fat 20−35% of total energy, and carbohydrate 45–65% of total energy [22]. All study groups had slightly higher average total fat intakes and slightly lower CHO intakes than recommended, but the average protein intake for all groups fell within the recommended range.

The adequate intake (AI) for dietary fibre in New Zealand and Australia is set at the median for dietary fibre intake recorded in the 1995 National Nutrition Survey of Australia (ABS 1998) and the 1997 National Nutrition Survey of New Zealand (MOH 1999) [22]. The AI is 25 g for women and 30 g for men. Although fibre intake is not reported by sex in Table 1, the average daily fibre intake for each group of 24 g, 25 g, and 27 g for the NGT, prediabetes, and T2DM groups, respectively, was similar to recommendations.

Six participants reported taking a high dose vitamin C supplement (≥500 mg vitamin C). The plasma vitamin C concentration of five of these participants ranged from 36–59 μmol/L, which reflects inadequate to adequate plasma vitamin C concentrations and suggests that they didn't take the supplement close to their study appointment. The other participant had a plasma vitamin C concentration of 74 µmol/L, which is a saturating concentration, but they also had an average dietary vitamin C intake of 194 mg/day and so this high plasma concentration could be explained by their dietary intake as 200 mg/day will saturate plasma [19].

Table 3. Dietary intake of participants classified as having normal glucose tolerance (NGT) ($n = 35$), prediabetes ($n = 25$), and T2DM ($n = 29$).

Total Daily Dietary intake	NGT	Prediabetes	T2DM	Total
Energy (KJ)	8192 ± 2336	8430 ± 2260	8033 ± 2416	8204 ± 2321
Fibre (g)	24 ± 9	25 ± 8	27 ± 9	25 ± 9
Protein (% of Energy)	17 ± 3	18 ± 4	17 ± 3	17 ± 3
Fat (% of Energy)	37 ± 6	39 ± 8	36 ± 7	37 ± 7
Carbohydrate (% of Energy)	44 ± 6	40 ± 8	44 ± 8	43 ± 7
Dietary Vitamin C Intake (mg)	103 ± 76	94 ± 58	101 ± 61	100 ± 66

Values represented as mean ± SD unless stated otherwise. Note: There was missing data from one participant for dietary information (1 × prediabetes). There were no significant differences between the study groups for any of the dietary intake measures.

3.4. Plasma Vitamin C Status and Dietary Vitamin C Intakes

A significant decrease in the mean plasma vitamin C concentration was observed between the NGT (57.4 µmol/L) and the prediabetes group (48.2 µmol/L) ($p = 0.035$) and the T2DM (41.2 µmol/L) group ($p < 0.001$) (Table 2). Furthermore, there was a much higher proportion of individuals with prediabetes and T2DM with deficient (4% and 3% respectively), marginal (14% in T2DM group), and inadequate (58% in prediabetes and 52% in T2DM group) plasma vitamin C concentrations, compared with the NGT group (3% marginal and 21% inadequate) (Figure 1).

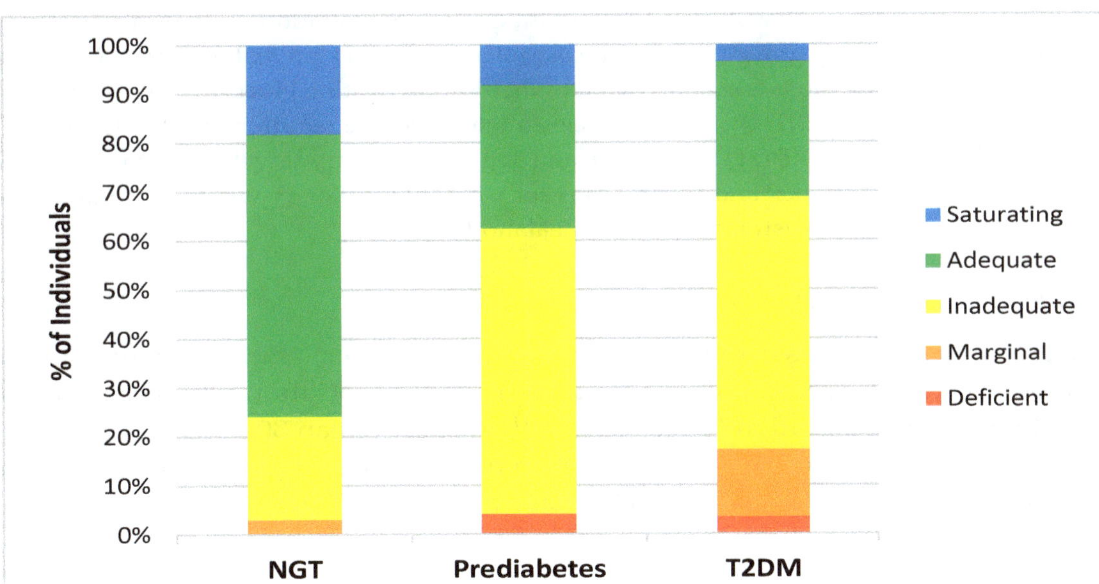

Figure 1. Plasma vitamin C status of individuals within study groups. Percentage of individuals from each study group [normal glucose tolerance (NGT), prediabetes, and type 2 diabetes mellitus (T2DM), including those taking no diabetes medication (fasting glucose ≥ 7.0 mmol/L or on a regimen of Metformin only (T2DM)], classified as having saturating (>70 µmol/L), adequate (51.0–69.9 µmol/L), inadequate (24.0–50.9 µmol/L), marginal (11.0–23.9 µmol/L), and deficient (<11.0 µmol/L) plasma vitamin C concentrations [24].

Although plasma vitamin C decreased from NGT to T2DM, there were no significant differences in dietary vitamin C concentrations between study groups determined from the four day weighed food diaries (Table 3). The majority of participants met the New Zealand recommended dietary intake

(RDI) of 45 mg/day (Figure 2). Furthermore, there were no participants in the T2DM group that had intakes below the New Zealand estimated average requirement (EAR) (30 mg/day). At the group level, it appears that most participants had an adequate fruit and vegetable intake to meet the recommended vitamin C intakes. However, few participants were reaching the New Zealand Ministry of Health's suggested dietary targets (SDT) to reduce chronic disease risk, i.e. 220 mg/day for men and 190 mg/d for women (Figure 2).

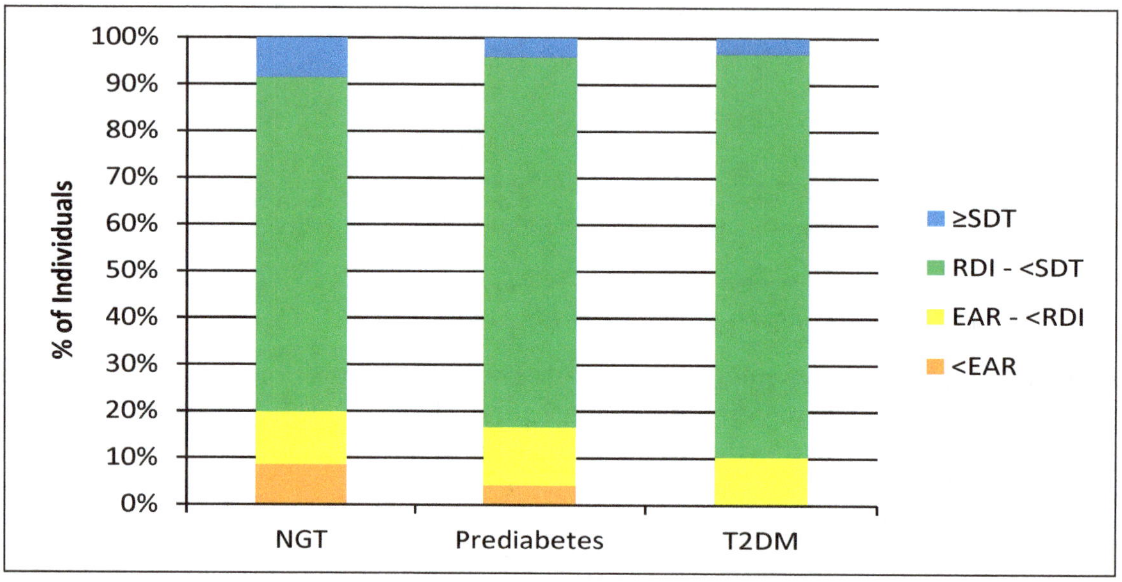

Figure 2. Individuals meeting New Zealand dietary intake recommendations for vitamin C. Percentage of individuals from each study group [normal glucose tolerance (NGT), prediabetes, and type 2 diabetes mellitus (T2DM), including those taking no diabetes medication (fasting glucose ≥7.0 mmol/L or on a regimen of Metformin only (T2DM)], meeting the estimated average requirement (EAR) (30 mg/day), recommended dietary intake (RDI) (45 mg/day), and suggested dietary target (SDT) to reduce chronic disease risk (220 mg/day for men and 190 mg/day for women) for dietary vitamin C intake using the nutrient reference values for Australia and New Zealand [22].

3.5. Plasma Vitamin C Correlations

There were no significant associations between age, gender, ethnicity, education level, and plasma vitamin C concentrations. There was a significant association between smoking history and plasma vitamin C concentration ($p = 0.035$), with current (mean 30.9 µmol/L) and ex-smokers (mean 47.3 µmol/L) having lower concentrations than non-smokers (mean 52.6 µmol/L). There was a significant linear association between vitamin C intake and plasma vitamin C concentration ($r = 0.353$, $p = 0.001$).

The three anthropometric measures (BMI, fat mass, and waist-to-hip ratio) were all significantly negatively associated with plasma vitamin C ($p < 0.05$) when conducting univariate analyses. When these three variables were included in a multiple regression, only BMI was independently negatively associated with plasma vitamin C ($p < 0.001$). Laboratory measurements (HbA1c, fasting glucose, TG, total chol/HDL chol, insulin, and hs-CRP) were negatively associated with plasma vitamin C ($p < 0.05$) and HDL chol and ghrelin were positively associated with plasma vitamin C ($p < 0.05$) in the univariate anlaysis (Table 4). When these variables were included in a multiple regression, only hs-CRP and fasting glucose were independently negatively associated with plasma vitamin C ($p < 0.05$).

A final multiple regression showed fasting glucose ($p = 0.001$), BMI ($p = 0.001$) and smoking history ($p = 0.003$) to be significant independent predictors of plasma vitamin C. Fasting glucose and BMI were negatively associated with plasma vitamin C, and current and ex-smokers had reduced plasma vitamin C concentrations compared to non-smokers. There was a strong positive association between hs-CRP concentrations and BMI ($r = 0.618$, $p < 0.001$). Accordingly, hs-CRP does not feature as an independent predictor of plasma vitamin C. Including dietary vitamin C intake in the above model (Table 5) showed that this was a significant independent predictor ($p = 0.032$) of plasma vitamin C concentrations, and BMI, fasting glucose, and smoking history remained as significant independent predictors ($R^2 = 0.43$).

Table 4. Pearson correlations of plasma vitamin C, glycaemic indices, hormones, lipids, high sensitivity C-reactive protein, and anthropometric measures.

Measure	Pearson Correlation
Fasting Glucose (mmol/L)	−0.411 ***
HbA1c (mmol/mol)	−0.334 ***
Total Cholesterol (mmol/L)	0.093
Triglycerides (mmol/L)	−0.322 **
Cholesterol (HDL)	0.295 **
Cholesterol (total/HDL)	−0.214 *
Cholesterol (LDL) calculated	0.086
Insulin (pmol/L)	−0.353 **
hs-CRP (mg/L)	−0.333 **
Ghrelin (pmol/L)	0.295 **
Leptin (ng/mL)	−0.183
Adiponectin (ng/mL)	0.202
BMI (kg/m2)	−0.446 ***
Waist-to-Hip Ratio	−0.274 *
Fat Mass (%)	−0.295 **

*** correlations significant at 0.001 level (2-tailed); ** correlations significant at the 0.01 level (2-tailed); * correlations significant at the 0.05 level (2-tailed).

Table 5. Multiple regression analysis showing significant associations with plasma vitamin C concentrations.

Measure	B	Lower 95% CI	Upper 95% CI	*p* Value
BMI	−0.9	−1.4	−0.4	0.001
Current Smoker	−21.9	−35.8	−7.9	0.003
Ex-Smoker	−4.9	−11.2	1.5	0.128
Fasting Glucose	−4.4	−7.1	−1.8	0.001
Dietary vitamin C	0.05	0.01	0.10	0.032

B: coefficient from the multiple linear regression model.

4. Discussion

4.1. Predictors of Plasma Vitamin C

This study showed fasting glucose, BMI, smoking history, and dietary vitamin C intake to be significant independent predictors of plasma vitamin C concentrations. The inverse association between fasting glucose and plasma vitamin C concentration shown in this study is in agreement with earlier studies [8–10]. In addition, the mean plasma vitamin C concentration was significantly lower in the prediabetes group (compared to the NGT group, suggesting that a reduction in plasma vitamin C concentration occurs in parallel with the decline in glucose tolerance during the progression to T2DM. It has been proposed that the uptake of dehydroascorbic acid, the oxidized form of vitamin C, by the glucose transporters (GLUTs), could be competitively inhibited by elevated blood glucose levels [25]. This could contribute to complications such as diabetic microvascular angiopathy due to erythrocyte fragility, as erythrocytes lack the sodium-dependent vitamin C transporters (SVCTs) and are dependent on the GLUTs for the uptake of vitamin C [11]. Our study also found plasma vitamin C concentration to be inversely related to BMI, which concurs with previous research [26]. Individuals with a higher weight are prone to vitamin C inadequacy and are known to require higher intakes of vitamin C in order to reach adequate plasma concentrations [27,28].

Oxidative stress is defined as a significant imbalance between the production of reactive oxygen species (ROS) and antioxidant defenses, and leads to alterations in signalling pathways and to potential tissue damage [29]. ROS activate nuclear factor κB (NFκB), a pro-inflammatory transcription factor, triggering a signalling cascade that leads to the continued synthesis of oxidative species and low-grade chronic inflammation [29]. High-sensitivity CRP, produced by the liver, reflects the presence of inflammation in the body. The concentration of hs-CRP increased with the deterioration of glycaemic control and increase in BMI. This result is consistent with the evidence suggesting that obesity can lead to chronic activation of the innate immune system and low-grade systemic inflammation and oxidative stress, which have been implicated in the development of insulin resistance and T2DM [5,30,31]. Hyperglycaemia, increased plasma concentrations of free fatty acids (FFAs), and hyperinsulinaemia have all been linked to an increased production of ROS [29,31]. Our data showed an inverse relationship between hs-CRP and plasma vitamin C. It is therefore hypothesized that lower plasma vitamin C in those with higher BMI, prediabetes, and T2DM reflects the depletion of the vitamin due to its antioxidant and anti-inflammatory activities.

Consistent with the role of vitamin C as an antioxidant, our data showed a significant inverse relationship between plasma vitamin C concentration and smoking status, with ex- and current-smokers having lower plasma vitamin C concentrations than non-smokers, which is consistent with previous research [32,33]. It has long been recognised that smokers and passive smokers have a lower vitamin C status than non-smokers partly due to poor dietary habits, but also due to the oxidizing properties of tobacco smoke, resulting in an increased turnover of vitamin C [34].

As expected, dietary vitamin C was found to be a predictor for plasma vitamin C concentration. However, when the dietary intake of the vitamin was corrected for by covariate analysis fasting glucose, BMI and smoking status remained as significant independent predictors of plasma vitamin C concentration. That is, the associations observed were not solely explained by differences in dietary intake. This result is at odds with one study that reported no differences in serum vitamin C concentrations in people grouped by diabetes status after adjustment for dietary vitamin C intake [16].

4.2. Metabolic Hormones

The average fasting insulin concentrations were consistent with the glycaemic measures and were significantly higher in the T2DM group compared to the NGT group. A higher fasting insulin concentration indicates insulin resistance, a well-known contributor to impaired glucose tolerance and T2DM. Leptin and ghrelin are two hormones that have a major influence on energy balance [35]. Leptin is a mediator of long-term regulation of energy balance, suppressing food intake and thereby inducing weight loss. Ghrelin, on the other hand, is a fast-acting hormone, seemingly playing a role in meal initiation. In obese patients, the circulating concentration of leptin is increased, whereas surprisingly, ghrelin is decreased [35]. It is now established that obese patients are leptin-resistant [35]. Indeed, in this study, the increasing BMI across the groups was associated with an increase in leptin concentrations and a reduction in ghrelin concentrations. There was an inverse relationship between insulin and leptin and plasma vitamin C, and a positive relationship between ghrelin and plasma vitamin C; however, these hormones were also associated with fasting glucose and were thus not included as independent predictors of plasma vitamin C.

4.3. Clinical Significance

As hyperglycemia is associated with increased oxidative stress, a role for antioxidants such as vitamin C in the prevention of T2DM and/or the reduction of complications is a reasonable proposition. Indeed, a recent meta-analysis of 15 randomized control trials (RCTs) investigating vitamin C supplementation and insulin resistance and biomarkers of glycaemic control (fasting glucose, HbA1c) found that doses of ≥200 mg/day vitamin C significantly reduced glucose concentrations in patients with T2DM, particularly if the intervention was for more than 30 days and in older individuals [36]. Furthermore, a recent 12 month RCT found that treating those with T2DM with both Metformin and vitamin C was more effective at reducing HbA1c and risk factors for diabetes-related long-term complications than treating with Metformin alone [37].

Although T2DM is not traditionally considered a risk factor for vitamin C deficiency, our research indicates that those with prediabetes or T2DM are more likely to have inadequate or deficient plasma vitamin C concentrations. This did not appear to be due to a lower dietary vitamin C intake, so dietary advice needs to emphasise the importance of consuming high vitamin C foods, aiming for an intake of at least 200 mg/day [22]. This is particularly relevant in light of the associated T2DM risk factors of higher BMI and smoking status, both of which impact vitamin C status. Further research into the possibility of a higher RDI for vitamin C for those with prediabetes and T2DM is warranted, in line with what has been recommended in some countries for smokers [38].

4.4. Study Strengths and Limitations

Our study used robust methodology for dietary intake, plasma vitamin C, and statistical analysis, and accounted for other factors that are known to impact plasma vitamin C concentration such as smoking status, dietary vitamin C intake, and supplement use. The participants with T2DM were clinically well defined and were either not treated with diabetes medication or treated with a single oral hypoglycaemic agent only (Metformin). Those taking Metformin were included in the overall analysis. When the Metformin treated cases were excluded, the correlation between fasting glucose and plasma vitamin C concentrations was similar in direction and magnitude ($n = 64$, $r = -0.477$, $p < 0.001$) to the entire cohort ($n = 86$, $r = -0.411$, $p = 0.001$). Further, the current norm is for Metformin treatment to be initiated at diagnosis, rather than after the failure of diet and lifestyle changes to optimize glucose control. As such, it will become increasingly difficult to recruit treatment-naïve individuals with T2DM to studies.

T2DM has been shown to increase the urinary excretion of vitamin C, leading to reduced plasma vitamin C concentrations in a rodent model [39]. Whether this also occurs in humans is unknown. In addition, the duration of T2DM was not reported. Indeed, many individuals have undiagnosed T2DM for a significant period of time prior to formal diagnosis, making it very difficult to interpret data on the duration of the disease. There are always limitations around the self-reporting of dietary data and supplement use, and the study cohort was relatively small with 89 participants. Our study had only one measure of plasma vitamin C per participant and so future research should ideally incorporate repeated samples to account for any temporal fluctuations. There was a limitation around the lack of detail with regards to vitamin C supplement use; however, only six participants reported taking high dose vitamin C supplements and the use was sporadic.

5. Conclusions

Our cross-sectional observational study has identified a moderate inverse relationship between plasma vitamin C and both fasting glucose and BMI in adult subjects across the glycaemic spectrum. The relationship can be explained by the depletion of vitamin C due to oxidative stress and inflammation resulting from dysglycaemia, overweight/obesity, and smoking, rather than lower dietary intakes. Further research is required to determine whether those with an increased dietary intake through fruit and vegetables and/or vitamin C supplementation have a decreased risk of progression to T2DM and/or complications associated with the metabolic syndrome and T2DM.

Acknowledgments: We would like to thank all participants for volunteering their time to take part in the study, Sharon Berry for helping take blood samples, and Angie Anderson and Lizzie Jones for food diary data entry. Rénee Wilson, Jinny Willis, Richard Gearry, and Paula Skidmore are the recipients of a Zespri International Ltd. grant. Anitra Carr is the recipient of a Health Research Council of New Zealand Sir Charles Hercus Health Research Fellowship.

Author Contributions: R.W. conducted participant recruitment and interviews; R.W., P.S., and L.F. completed the dietary analysis, A.C. vitamin C analysis, and C.F. statistical analysis; R.W., A.C., and J.W. undertook the conception and writing of the paper; R.G. and P.S. edited the paper.

References

1. American Diabetes Association. Diagnosis and classification of diabetes mellitus. *Diabetes Care* **2014**, *37*, S81–S90.
2. International Diabetes Federation. IDF diabetes atlas 2015. Available online: http://www.diabetesatlas.org. (accessed on 5 June 2017).
3. Ministry of Health. Virtual diabetes register 2017. Available online: http://www.health.govt.nz/our-work/diseases-and-conditions/diabetes/about-diabetes/virtual-diabetes-register-vdr. (accessed on 11 June 2017).
4. Primary Care Domain NHS Digital. Quality and outcomes framework-prevalence, achievements and exceptions report 2016. Available online: http://www.content.digital.nhs.uk/catalogue/PUB22266 (accessed on 25 June 2017).
5. McArdle, M.; Finucane, O.; Connaughton, R.; McMorrow, A.; Roche, H. Mechanisms of obesity-induced inflammation and insulin resistance: insights into the emerging role of nutritional strategies. *Front. Endocrinol. (Lausanne)* **2013**, *4*, 1–23. [CrossRef] [PubMed]
6. Carr, A.C.; Frei, B. Toward a new recommended dietary allowance for vitamin C based on antioxidant and health effects in humans. *Am. J. Clin. Nutr.* **1999**, *69*, 1086–1107. [PubMed]
7. Carr, A.; Frei, B. Does vitamin C act as a pro-oxidant under physiological conditions? *FASEB J.* **1999**, *13*, 1007–1024. [PubMed]
8. Will, J.C.; Byers, T. Does diabetes mellitus increase the requirement for vitamin C? *Nutr. Rev.* **1996**, *54*, 193–202. [CrossRef] [PubMed]
9. Sargeant, L.; Wareham, N.; Bingham, S.; Day, N. Vitamin C and hyperglycemia in the European prospective investigation into cancer-Norfolk (EPIC-Norfolk) study: A population-based study. *Diabetes Care.* **2000**, *23*, 726–732. [CrossRef] [PubMed]
10. Kositsawat, J.; Freeman, V.L. Vitamin C and A1c relationship in the National Health and Nutrition Examination Survey (NHANES) 2003–2006. *J. Am. Coll. Nutr.* **2011**, *30*, 477–483. [CrossRef] [PubMed]
11. Tu, H.; Li, H.; Wang, Y.; Niyyati, M.; Wang, Y.; Leshin, J.; Levine, M. Low red blood cell vitamin C concentrations induce red blood cell fragility: A link to diabetes via glucose, glucose transporters, and dehydroascorbic Acid. *EBioMedicine* **2015**, *2*, 1735–1750. [CrossRef] [PubMed]
12. Olofsson, C.; Discacciati, A.; Akesson, A.; Orsini, N.; Brismar, K.; Wolk, A. Changes in fruit, vegetable and juice consumption after the diagnosis of type 2 diabetes: A prospective study in men. *Br. J. Nutr.* **2017**, *117*, 712–719. [CrossRef] [PubMed]
13. Feskens, E.J.M.; Virtanen, S.M.; Räsänen, L.; Tuomilehto, J.; Stengård, J.; Pekkanen, J.; Nissinen, A.; Kromhout, D. Dietary factors determining diabetes and impaired glucose tolerance: A 20-year follow-up of the Finnish and Dutch cohorts of the Seven Countries Study. *Diabetes Care.* **1995**, *18*, 1104–1112. [CrossRef] [PubMed]
14. Harding, A.H.; Wareham, N.J.; Bingham, S.A.; Khaw, K.; Luben, R.; Welch, A.; Forouhi, N.G. Plasma vitamin C level, fruit and vegetable consumption, and the risk of new-onset type 2 diabetes mellitus: The European prospective investigation of cancer-Norfolk prospective study. *Arch. Intern. Med.* **2008**, *168*, 1493. [CrossRef] [PubMed]
15. Som, S.; Basu, S.; Mukherjee, D.; Deb, S.; Choudhury, P.R.; Mukherjee, S.; Chatterjee, S.N.; Chatterjee, I.B. Ascorbic acid metabolism in diabetes mellitus. *Metabolism* **1981**, *30*, 572–577. [CrossRef]
16. Will, J.; Ford, E.; Bowman, B. Serum vitamin C concentrations and diabetes: Findings from the third National Health and Nutrition Examination Survey, 1988–1994. *Am. J. Clin. Nutr.* **1999**, *70*, 49–52. [PubMed]
17. World Health Organization. Obesity: Preventing and managing the global epidemic. Report of a WHO consultation. 2000. Available online: http://www.who.int/nutrition/publications/obesity/WHO_TRS_894/en/ (accessed on 10 June 2017).
18. World Health Organization. Section 5: Collecting step 2 data: Physical measurements 2017. Available online: http://www.who.int/chp/steps/Part3_Section5.pdf?ua=1 (accessed on 19 June 2017).

19. Carr, A.C.; Pullar, J.M.; Moran, S.; Vissers, M.C. Bioavailability of vitamin C from kiwifruit in non-smoking males: Determination of 'healthy' and 'optimal' intakes. *J. Nutr. Sci.* **2012**, *1*, e14. [CrossRef] [PubMed]
20. Sato, Y.; Uchiki, T.; Iwama, M.; Kishimoto, Y.; Takahashi, R.; Ishigami, A. Determination of dehydroascorbic acid in mouse tissues and plasma by using tris(2-carboxyethyl)phosphine hydrochloride as reductant in metaphosphoric acid/ethylenediaminetetraacetic acid solution. *Biol. Pharm. Bull.* **2010**, *33*, 364–369. [CrossRef] [PubMed]
21. Bang, A.S.; Soule, S.G.; Yandle, T.G.; Richards, A.M.; Pemberton, C.J. Characterisation of proghrelin peptides in mammalian tissue and plasma. *J. Endocrinol.* **2007**, *192*, 313–323. [CrossRef] [PubMed]
22. National Health and Medical Research Council. Nutrient Reference Values for Australia and New Zealand Including Recommended Dietary Intakes Canberra: ACT: National Health and Medical Research Council. 2006. Available online: https://www.nhmrc.gov.au/_files_nhmrc/file/publications/17122_nhmrc_nrv_update-dietary_intakes-web.pdf (accessed on 12 June 2017).
23. New Zealand Society for the Study of Diabetes. NZSSD position statement on the diagnosis of, and screening for, type 2 diabetes 2011. Available online: http://www.nzssd.org.nz/HbA1c/1.%20NZSSD%20position%20statement%20on%20screening%20for%20type%202%20diabetes%20final%20Sept%202011.pdf (accessed on 20 June 2017).
24. Lykkesfeldt, J.; Poulsen, H.E. Is vitamin C supplementation beneficial? Lessons learned from randomised controlled trials. *Br. J. Nutr.* **2010**, *103*, 1251–1259. [CrossRef] [PubMed]
25. Girgis, C.; Christie-David, D.; Gunton, J. Effects of vitamins C and D in type 2 diabetes mellitus. *Nutr. Diet. Suppl.* **2015**, *7*, 21–28. [CrossRef]
26. Johnston, C.S.; Beezhold, B.L.; Mostow, B.; Swan, P.D. Plasma vitamin C is inversely related to body mass index and waist circumference but not to plasma adiponectin in nonsmoking adults. *J. Nutr.* **2007**, *137*, 1757–1762. [PubMed]
27. Block, G.; Mangels, A.R.; Patterson, B.H.; Levander, O.A.; Norkus, E.P.; Taylor, P.R. Body weight and prior depletion affect plasma ascorbate levels attained on identical Vitamin C intake: A controlled-diet study. *J. Am. Coll. Nutr.* **1999**, *18*, 628–637. [CrossRef] [PubMed]
28. Carr, A.C.; Pullar, J.M.; Bozonet, S.M.; Vissers, M.C. Marginal ascorbate status (hypovitaminosis C) results in an attenuated response to vitamin C supplementation. *Nutrients* **2016**, *8*, 341. [CrossRef] [PubMed]
29. Lamb, R.E.; Goldstein, B.J. Modulating an oxidative-inflammatory cascade: Potential new treatment strategy for improving glucose metabolism, insulin resistance, and vascular function. *Int. J. Clin. Pract.* **2008**, *62*, 1087–1095. [CrossRef] [PubMed]
30. Calle, M.C.; Fernandez, M.L. Inflammation and type 2 diabetes. *Diabetes Metab.* **2012**, *38*, 183–191. [CrossRef] [PubMed]
31. Garcia-Bailo, B.; El-Sohemy, A.; Haddad, P.S.; Arora, P.; Benzaied, F.; Karmali, M.; Badawi, A. Vitamins D, C, and E in the prevention of type 2 diabetes mellitus: Modulation of inflammation and oxidative stress. *Biologics* **2011**, *5*, 7–19. [PubMed]
32. Schectman, G.; Byrd, J.; Gruchow, H. The influence of smoking on vitamin C status in adults. *Am. J. Public Health* **1989**, *79*, 158. [CrossRef] [PubMed]
33. Pfeiffer, C.M.; Sternberg, M.R.; Schleicher, R.L.; Rybak, M.E. Dietary supplement use and smoking are important correlates of biomarkers of water-soluble vitamin status after adjusting for sociodemographic and lifestyle variables in a representative sample of U.S. adults. *J. Nutr.* **2013**, *143*, 957S–965S. [CrossRef] [PubMed]
34. Lykkesfeldt, J.; Michels, A.J.; Frei, B. Vitamin C. *Adv. Nutr.* **2014**, *5*, 16–18. [CrossRef] [PubMed]
35. Klok, M.D.; Jakobsdottir, S.; Drent, M.L. The role of leptin and ghrelin in the regulation of food intake and body weight in humans: A review. *Obes. Rev.* **2007**, *8*, 21–34. [CrossRef] [PubMed]
36. Ashor, A.W.; Werner, A.D.; Lara, J.; Willis, N.D.; Mathers, J.C.; Siervo, M. Effects of vitamin C supplementation on glycaemic control: a systematic review and meta-analysis of randomised controlled trials. *Eur. J. Clin. Nutr.* **2017**. [CrossRef] [PubMed]
37. Gillani, S.W.; Sulaiman, S.A.S.; Abdul, M.I.M.; Baig, M.R. Combined effect of metformin with ascorbic acid versus acetyl salicylic acid on diabetes-related cardiovascular complication a 12-month single blind multicenter randomized control trial. *Cardiovasc. Diabetol.* **2017**, *16*, 103. [CrossRef] [PubMed]

38. Institute of Medicine, Panel on Dietary Antioxidants Related Compounds. *Dietary Reference Intakes for Vitamin C, Vitamin E, Selenium, and Carotenoids: A Report of the Panel on Dietary Antioxidants and Related Compounds, Subcommittees on Upper Reference Levels of Nutrients and of Interpretation and Use of Dietary Reference Intakes, and the Standing Committee on the Scientific Evaluation of Dietary Reference Intakes, Food and Nutrition Board, Institute of Medicine*; National Academy Press: Washington, DC, USA, 2000.
39. Zebrowski, E.J.; Bhatnagar, P.K. Urinary excretion pattern of ascorbic acid in streptozotocin diabetic and insulin treated rats. *Pharmacol. Res. Commun.* **1979**, *11*, 95–103. [CrossRef]

3

Dietary Protein Consumption and the Risk of Type 2 Diabetes

Shuang Tian [1,2], Qian Xu [2], Ruyue Jiang [2], Tianshu Han [2], Changhao Sun [2,*] and Lixin Na [2,*]

1 Nutrition Department, Longgang Hospital of Traditional Chinese Medicine, Shenzhen 518000, Guangdong, China; 18504541023@163.com

2 National Discipline, Department of Nutrition and Food Hygiene, School of Public Health Harbin Medical University, Harbin 150081, China; XUQIAN9188@163.com (Q.X.); jruyue@163.com (R.J.); snowcalendar@126.com (T.H.)

* Correspondence: changhaosun2002@163.com (C.S.); nalixin2003@163.com (L.N.)

Abstract: Recently, some studies have focused on the relationship between dietary protein intake and the risk of type 2 diabetes mellitus (T2DM), but the conclusions have been inconsistent. Therefore, in this paper, a systematic review and meta-analysis of cohort studies regarding protein consumption and T2DM risk are conducted in order to present the association between them. We searched the PubMed and Embase databases for cohort studies on dietary protein, high-protein food consumption and risk of T2DM, up to July 2017. A summary of relative risks was compiled by the fixed-effect model or random-effect model. Eleven cohort studies regarded protein intake and T2DM (52,637 cases among 483,174 participants). The summary RR and 95% CI (Confidence Interval) of T2DM was 1.12 (1.08–1.17) in all subjects, 1.13 (1.04–1.24) in men, and 1.09 (1.04–1.15) in women for total protein; 1.14 (1.09–1.19) in all subjects, 1.23 (1.09–1.38) in men, and 1.11 (1.03–1.19) in women for animal protein; 0.96 (0.88–1.06) in all subjects, 0.98 (0.72–1.34) in men, and 0.92 (0.86–0.98) in women for plant protein. We also compared the association between different food sources of protein and the risk of T2DM. The summary RR (Relative Risk) and 95% CI of T2DM was 1.22 (1.09–1.36) for red meat, 1.39 (1.29–1.49) for processed meat, 1.03 (0.89–1.17) for fish, 1.03 (0.64–1.67) for egg, 0.89 (0.84–0.94) for total dairy products, 0.87 (0.78–0.96) for whole milk, 0.83 (0.70–0.98) for yogurt, 0.74 (0.59–0.93) in women for soy. This meta-analysis shows that total protein and animal protein could increase the risk of T2DM in both males and females, and plant protein decreases the risk of T2DM in females. The association between high-protein food types and T2DM are also different. Red meat and processed meat are risk factors of T2DM, and soy, dairy and dairy products are the protective factors of T2DM. Egg and fish intake are not associated with a decreased risk of T2DM. This research indicates the type of dietary protein and food sources of protein that should be considered for the prevention of diabetes.

Keywords: protein; diabetes; systematic review; meta-analysis

---

1. Introduction

Type 2 diabetes is rapidly increasing in the world. Ninety percent of patients with diabetes have type 2 diabetes [1]. Type 2 diabetes patients are at increased risk of cardiovascular disease, neuropathies, nephropathies, gangrene, and leg ulcers [2]. From the date of diagnosis, patients with T2DM have to face at least eight years of economic burden [3].

Evidence suggests that dietary factors may influence the risk of T2DM [4]. Many previous studies have focused on dietary macronutrient intake associated with diabetes risk [5,6], but the main content of those studies was carbohydrates and fats. Recently, some studies focused on the relationship between dietary protein intake and the risk of T2DM. High-protein diets have shown beneficial effects on glucose homeostasis in some short–term trials [7,8]. Subsequent longitudinal studies have evaluated the associations between dietary protein intake and risk of T2DM as well as the type of dietary protein and risk of T2DM.A study focusing on the Mediterranean islands showed that animal protein consumption was associated with a higher prevalence of diabetes among the elderly, and a recommended range of protein from plant sources appears was seen to be considerably protective [9]. Some other publications have also reported an increased risk of T2DM with a high intake of total protein [10–14] and animal protein [10,13–15], and a decreased risk of T2DM with a high intake of plant protein [14,15]. However, there have been no reports that how an association between T2DM and total protein [15–18], animal protein [16–18] and plant protein intake or a high risk of T2DM with a high intake of plant protein [10,13].The association between dietary protein and T2DM is still debated.

In the present study, we conducted a systematic review and meta-analysis of cohort studies to clarify the association of protein consumption with risk of T2DM. In order to provide a better dietary instruction for the lay public, we also conducted a systematic review and meta-analysis of cohort studies to study the association between different kinds of high-protein food and the risk of T2DM.

2. Materials and Methods

2.1. Search Strategy

We searched relevant studies from the Embase and PubMed electronic databases from their starting dates to July 2017.

Protein: search items included: 'dietary protein' or 'protein intake' or 'plant protein' or 'animal protein' or 'food' and 'diabetes' or 'diabetes mellitus' or 'T2DM' and 'population' or 'human'.

Meat: search items included: 'red meat' or 'processed meat' or 'food' and 'diabetes' or 'diabetes mellitus' or 'T2DM' and 'population' or 'human'.

Fish: search items included: 'fish' or 'seafood' or 'food' and 'diabetes' or 'diabetes mellitus' or 'T2DM' and 'population' or 'human'.

Egg: search items included: 'egg' or 'food' and 'diabetes' or 'diabetes mellitus' or 'T2DM' and 'population' or 'human'.

Dairy: search items included: 'dairy' or 'milk' or 'dairy product' or 'yogurt' or 'food' and 'diabetes' or 'diabetes mellitus' or 'T2DM' and 'population' or 'human'.

Soy: search items included: 'soy' or 'legume' or 'soy product' or 'food' and 'diabetes' or 'diabetes mellitus' or 'T2DM' and 'population' or 'human'.

Eligible studies are selected by further manual scanning of all included studies and relevant reference lists.

2.2. Study Selection

All included studies should match the following criteria:(1) the study must have a cohort design; (2) the endpoint of the study was the incidence or mortality of the T2DM; (3) the study had to report risk ratios and the results had to be within a 95% CI in the paper (if this not clear, we requested this information from the authors); and (4) the study had to show the participants' intake of dietary protein or other high-protein foods such as meat, fish, egg, dairy, soy.

2.3. Data Extraction

We extracted the following information from each publication we selected: first the author of the publication, publication year, the country where the study was conducted, the number of the samples and cases, T2DM diagnosis and criteria, the year the study began and finished, the years of follow-up, the methods of diet exposure assessment, the RRs and 95% CI, and the adjustment factors (Tables S1–S12).

2.4. Statistical Methods

We used effect models to calculate the summary RRs and 95% confidence to compare the highest dietary protein consumption with the lowest dietary protein consumption [19]. Two-sided $p < 0.05$ was considered statistically significant. The black square in the forest plots represents the weight contribution of every study. In order to evaluate the extent of variability, the I^2-test statistic was adapted to estimate the heterogeneity [20].When $I^2 < 50\%$ and $p > 0.05$, there was no heterogeneity; we used the fixed-effect model. The random-effect model was selected when $I^2 > 50\%$ or $p < 0.05$. We used the Egger linear regression test and Begg rank correlation test to search for publication bias. When $p > 0.05$, there was no publication bias. Comprehensive Meta-Analysis V2 was employed for data analysis.

3. Results

3.1. Dietary Protein Intake and Risk of T2DM

We included 11 cohort studies in the analysis (Figure 1, Tables S1 and S2). Six of the studies were from the Unite States, three from Europe, one from Asia, one from Melboume, one from Finland.

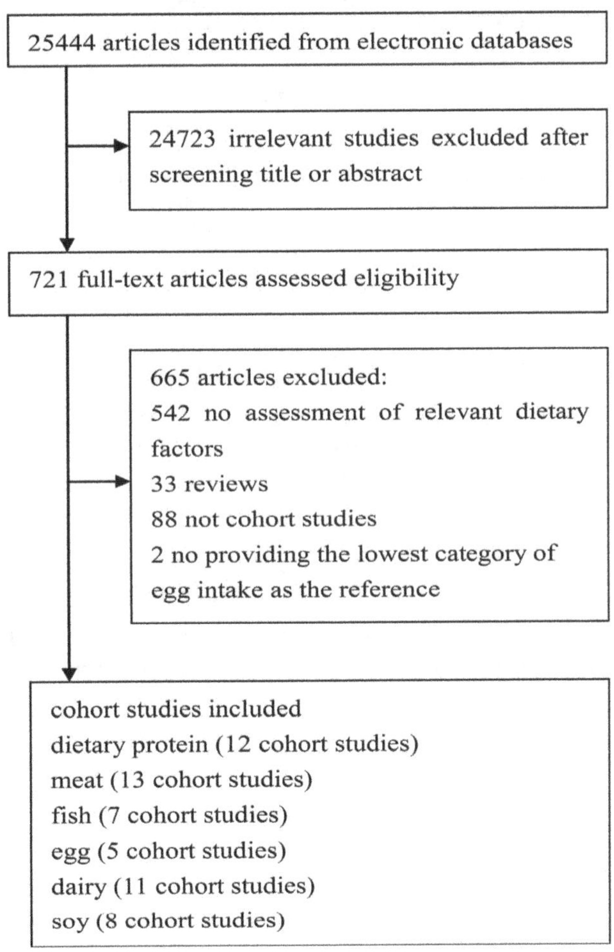

Figure 1. Flow chart for study selection.

Total Protein Eleven cohort studies [10–18] researched the association between total protein intake and the risk of T2DM, included 52,637 cases among 483,174 participants. The summary RR and 95% CI for high vs. low values of all studies was 1.12 (1.08–1.17) (Figure 2a), ($I^2 = 18.72$, $p = 0.25$) in all subjects, 1.13 (1.04–1.24) (Figure 2b) ($I^2 = 11.78$, $p = 0.34$) in men, and 1.09(1.04–1.15) (Figure 2c) ($I^2 = 43.39$, $p = 0.10$) in women.

	Study name	Risk ratio	Lower limit	Upper limit	Z-Value	p-Value
a	Monique. 2014(m) [10]	1.040	0.828	1.307	0.337	0.736
	Monique. 2014(w) [10]	1.370	1.054	1.780	2.355	0.019
	Ulrika. 2013(m) [11]	1.210	0.978	1.497	1.755	0.079
	Ulrika. 2013(w) [11]	1.300	1.030	1.640	2.211	0.027
	Tiinker. 2011 [12]	1.160	1.051	1.281	2.937	0.003
	Sluijs. 2010 [13]	1.160	1.064	1.265	3.366	0.001
	Malik. 2016(1) [14]	1.040	0.959	1.128	0.943	0.346
	Malik. 2016(2) [14]	1.030	0.921	1.152	0.519	0.604
	Malik. 2016(3) [14]	1.180	1.040	1.339	2.560	0.010
	Weo. 2013 [15]	1.280	0.898	1.825	1.364	0.173
	Akiko. 2015(m) [16]	1.360	0.867	2.133	1.339	0.181
	Akiko. 2015(w) [16]	0.870	0.549	1.378	-0.593	0.553
	Xiawen. 2017 [17]	1.230	0.965	1.568	1.671	0.095
	Virtanen. 2017 [18]	0.910	0.621	1.333	-0.484	0.628
	Overall(I^2=18.72, P=0.25)	1.121	1.078	1.166	5.687	0.000
b	Monique. 2014 [10]	1.040	0.828	1.307	0.337	0.736
	Ulrika. 2013 [11]	1.210	0.978	1.497	1.755	0.079
	Malik. 2016 [14]	1.180	1.040	1.339	2.560	0.010
	Akiko. 2015 [16]	1.360	0.867	2.133	1.339	0.181
	Virtanen. 2017 [18]	0.910	0.697	1.188	-0.694	0.488
	Overall(I^2=11.78, P=0.34)	1.134	1.036	1.242	2.736	0.006
c	Monique. 2014 [10]	1.370	1.054	1.780	2.355	0.019
	Ulrika. 2013 [11]	1.300	1.030	1.640	2.211	0.027
	Tinker. 2011 [12]	1.160	1.051	1.281	2.937	0.003
	Mailk. 2016 (1) [14]	1.040	0.959	1.128	0.943	0.346
	Mailk. 2016 (2) [14]	1.030	0.921	1.152	0.519	0.604
	Weo. 2013 [15]	1.280	0.898	1.825	1.364	0.173
	Akiko. 2015 [16]	0.870	0.549	1.378	-0.593	0.553
	Overall(I^2=43.39, P=0.10)	1.094	1.040	1.152	3.440	0.001

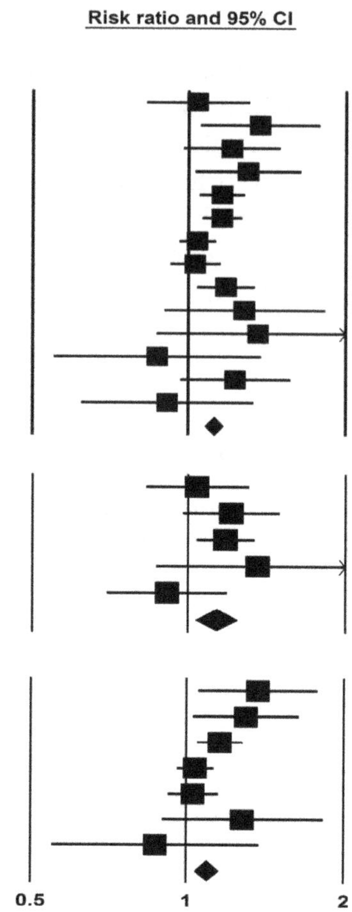

Figure 2. Total protein and type 2 diabetes relative risks(RRs) for (**a**) the highest vs. the lowest intake in all subjects and (**b**) the highest vs. the lowest intake in men (**c**) the highest vs. the lowest intake in women. The RR of each study is represented by a square, 95% CI are represented by the horizontal lines, and the diamond represents the estimate and its 95% CI.

Animal Protein Nine cohort studies [10,13–18] researched the association between animal protein intake and the risk of T2DM. This included 31,557 cases among 380,689 participants. The summary RR and 95% CI for high vs. low values of all studies was 1.14 (1.09–1.19) (Figure 3a), (I^2 = 43.39, p = 0.30) in all subjects, 1.23 (1.09–1.38) (Figure 3b), (I^2 = 0.00, p = 0.44) in men, and 1.11 (1.03–1.19) (Figure 3c), (I^2 = 32.04, p = 0.21) in women.

Plant Protein Nine cohort studies [10,13–18] researched the association between plant protein and the risk of T2DM, included 31,817 cases among 381,879 participants. The summary RR and 95% CI for high vs. low values of all studies was 0.96 (0.88–1.06) (Figure 4a), (I^2 = 59.01, p = 0.07) in all subjects. We used a sensitivity analysis to exclude the most influential studies: the summary RR and 95% CI ranged from 0.92 (0.87–0.98) when the European men's study [10] was excluded to 0.98 (0.87–1.10) when the USA men's study [14] was excluded. The heterogeneity was partly because of the European men's study [10] and when we excluded this study, there was moderate heterogeneity (I^2 = 14.85, p = 0.31). The summary RR and 95% CI was 0.98 (0.72–1.34) (Figure 4b) (I^2 = 78.57, p = 0.003) in men. A sensitivity analysis was used to exclude the most influential studies: the summary RR and 95% CI ranged from 0.88 (0.76–1.02) when the European study [10] was excluded to 1.07 (0.75–1.52) when the Finnish men's study [18] was excluded. The heterogeneity in men still existed after sensitivity analysis, partly because there were only four cohort studies about the association between plant protein intake and the risk of T2DM in men. The summary RR and 95% CI was 0.92 (0.86–0.97) (Figure 4c) (I^2 = 45.72, p = 0.12) in women.

	Study name	Risk ratio	Lower limit	Upper limit	Z-Value	p-Value
a	Monique. 2014(m) [10]	1.010	0.712	1.433	0.056	0.956
	Monique. 2014(w) [10]	1.380	1.006	1.893	1.998	0.046
	Sluijs. 2010 [13]	1.130	1.043	1.224	3.001	0.003
	Malik. 2016(1) [14]	1.060	0.969	1.159	1.277	0.202
	Malik. 2016(2) [14]	1.110	0.983	1.254	1.681	0.093
	Malik. 2016(3) [14]	1.270	1.107	1.457	3.418	0.001
	Weo. 2013 [15]	1.490	1.027	2.163	2.098	0.036
	Akiko. 2015(m) [16]	1.460	0.940	2.269	1.683	0.092
	Akiko 2015(w) [16]	1.370	0.822	2.284	1.207	0.228
	Xiaowei. 2017 [17]	1.290	0.993	1.675	1.909	0.056
	Virtanen. 2017 [18]	1.040	0.706	1.532	0.199	0.843
	Overall(I^2=43.39, P=0.30)	1.139	1.087	1.193	5.453	0.000
b	Monique. 2014 [10]	1.010	0.712	1.433	0.056	0.956
	Malik. 2016 [14]	1.270	1.107	1.457	3.418	0.001
	Akiko. 2015 [16]	1.460	0.940	2.269	1.683	0.092
	Virtanen. 2017 [18]	1.040	0.706	1.532	0.199	0.843
	Overall(I^2=0.00, P=0.44)	1.228	1.092	1.380	3.440	0.001
c	Monique. 2014 [10]	1.380	1.006	1.893	1.998	0.046
	Malik. 2016(1) [14]	1.060	0.969	1.159	1.277	0.202
	Malik. 2016(2) [14]	1.110	0.983	1.254	1.681	0.093
	Weo. 2013 [15]	1.490	1.027	2.163	2.098	0.036
	Akiko. 2015 [16]	1.370	0.822	2.284	1.207	0.228
	Overall(I^2=32.04, P=0.21)	1.107	1.033	1.185	2.902	0.004

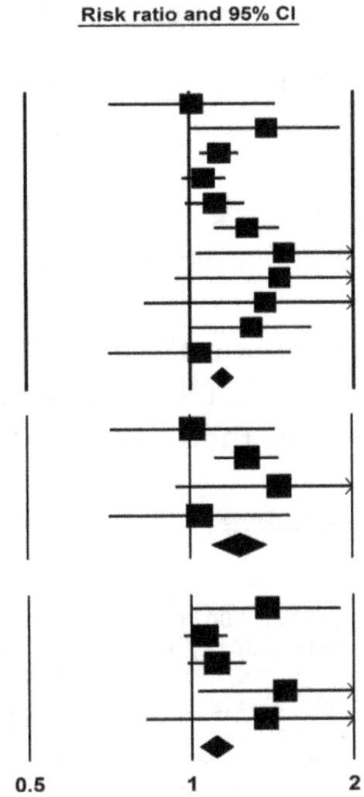

Figure 3. Animal protein and type 2 diabetes RRs for (**a**) the highest vs. the lowest intake in all subjects and (**b**) the highest vs. the lowest intake in men (**c**) the highest vs. the lowest intake in women. The RR of each study is represented by a square, 95% CI are represented by the horizontal lines, and the diamond represents the estimate and its 95% CI.

	Study name	Risk ratio	Lower limit	Upper limit	Z-Value	p-Value
a	Monique. 2014(m) [10]	1.500	1.163	1.935	3.122	0.002
	Monique. 2014(w) [10]	1.240	0.913	1.685	1.375	0.169
	Sluijs. 2010 [13]	1.040	0.834	1.297	0.349	0.727
	Malik. 2016(1) [14]	0.890	0.813	0.974	-2.534	0.011
	Malik. 2016(2) [14]	0.950	0.851	1.061	-0.911	0.362
	Malik. 2016(3) [14]	0.910	0.842	0.983	-2.398	0.016
	Weo. 2013 [15]	0.690	0.495	0.961	-2.195	0.028
	Akiko. 2015(m) [16]	0.880	0.598	1.295	-0.648	0.517
	Akiko. 2015(w) [16]	0.910	0.612	1.354	-0.465	0.642
	Xiawen. 2017 [17]	1.020	0.731	1.423	0.117	0.907
	Virtanen. 2017 [18]	0.700	0.453	1.082	-1.604	0.109
	Overall(I^2=59.01, P=0.07)	0.962	0.877	1.056	-0.810	0.418
b	Monique. 2014 [10]	1.500	1.163	1.935	3.122	0.002
	Malik. 2016 [14]	0.910	0.772	1.073	-1.124	0.261
	Akiko. 2015 [16]	0.880	0.598	1.295	-0.648	0.517
	Virtanen. 2017 [18]	0.700	0.453	1.082	-1.604	0.109
	Overall(I^2=78.57, P=0.003)	0.982	0.720	1.339	-0.114	0.909
c	Monique. 2014 [10]	1.240	0.913	1.685	1.375	0.169
	Malik. 2016(1) [14]	0.890	0.813	0.974	-2.534	0.011
	Malik. 2016(2) [14]	0.950	0.851	1.061	-0.911	0.362
	Weo. 2013 [15]	0.690	0.495	0.961	-2.195	0.028
	Akiko. 2015 [16]	0.910	0.612	1.354	-0.465	0.642
	Overall(I^2=45.72, P=0.12)	0.916	0.858	0.978	-2.609	0.009

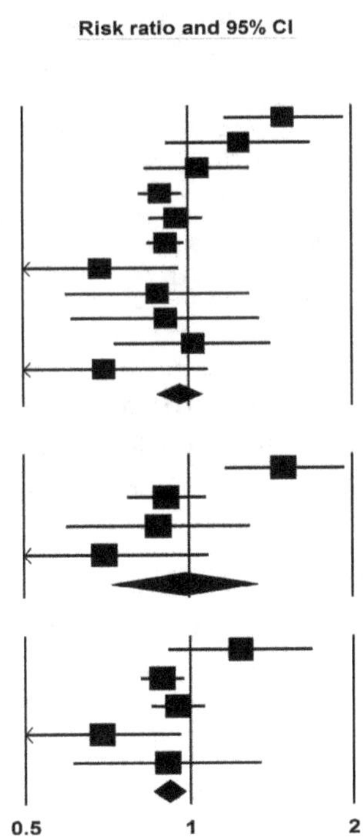

Figure 4. Plant protein and type 2 diabetes RRs for (**a**) the highest vs. the lowest intake in all subjects and (**b**) the highest vs. the lowest intake in men (**c**) the highest vs. the lowest intake in women. The RR of each study is represented by a square, 95% CI are represented by the horizontal lines, and the diamond represents the estimate and its 95% CI.

3.2. High-Protein Food and Risk of T2DM

We also conducted a systematic review and meta-analysis of cohort studies to clarify the association with high dietary protein food consumption and the risk of T2DM.

Red Meat Thirteen cohort studies [6,18,21–31] researched the association between red meat consumption and the risk of T2DM (Figure 1, Tables S3 and S4).The summary RR and 95% CI for high vs. low red meat consumption was 1.22 (1.09–1.36) (Figure 5a) (I^2 = 51.11, p = 0.01). We used a sensitivity analysis to exclude the most influential studies: the summary RR and 95% CI ranged from1.20 (1.07–1.35) when the U.S. Study [24] was excluded to 1.26 (1.15–1.38) when the Chinese study [25] was excluded. The heterogeneity was partly because of the Chinese study [25], and when we excluded this study, there was moderate heterogeneity (I^2 = 27.68, p = 0.17).

	Study name	Risk ratio	Lower limit	Upper limit	Z-Value	p-Value
a	Van Dam. 2002 [6]	1.050	0.849	1.299	0.450	0.653
	Virtanen. 2017 [18]	1.080	0.776	1.503	0.457	0.648
	Hodge. 2007 [21]	1.170	0.830	1.650	0.896	0.370
	Fung. 2004 [22]	1.360	1.183	1.564	4.317	0.000
	Schulze. 2003 [23]	1.440	0.921	2.252	1.598	0.110
	Song. 2004 [24]	1.250	0.938	1.666	1.522	0.128
	Villegas. 2006 [25]	0.940	0.789	1.119	-0.695	0.487
	Simmons. 2007 [26]	2.260	1.099	4.647	2.217	0.027
	Lee . 2004 [27]	1.190	0.973	1.455	1.696	0.090
	Schulze. 2007 [28]	1.640	1.229	2.188	3.361	0.001
	Montonen. 2005 [29]	0.990	0.718	1.366	-0.061	0.951
	Sanchis. 2016 [30]	1.850	1.032	3.316	2.066	0.039
	Vang. 2008 [31]	1.270	1.057	1.526	2.553	0.011
	Overall(I²=51.10, P=0.01)	1.221	1.099	1.357	3.706	0.000
b	Van Dam. 2002 [6]	1.460	1.143	1.865	3.030	0.002
	Virtanen. 2017 [18]	1.070	0.772	1.483	0.406	0.685
	Hodge. 2007 [21]	1.110	0.790	1.560	0.601	0.548
	Fung. 2004 [22]	1.600	1.391	1.841	6.569	0.000
	Schulze. 2003 [23]	1.820	1.341	2.471	3.838	0.000
	Song. 2004 [24]	1.380	1.112	1.713	2.922	0.003
	Villegas. 2006 [25]	1.180	1.001	1.391	1.970	0.049
	Simmons. 2007 [26]	2.950	1.390	6.260	2.818	0.005
	Montonen. 2005 [29]	1.220	0.888	1.676	1.227	0.220
	Sanchis. 2016 [30]	1.260	0.881	1.802	1.266	0.206
	Vang. 2008 [31]	1.380	1.048	1.817	2.295	0.022
	Overall(I²=49.32, P=0.03)	1.386	1.288	1.491	8.752	0.000

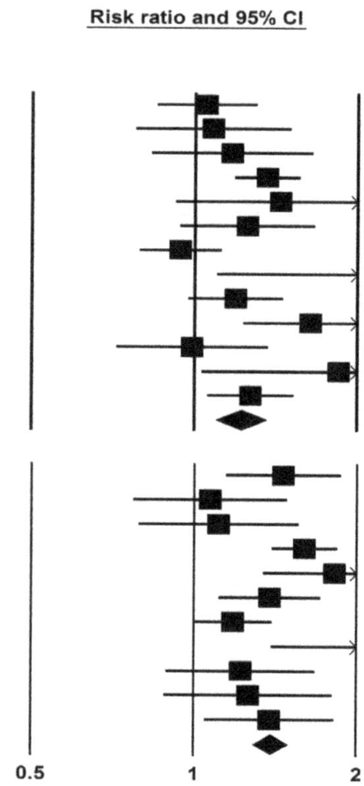

Figure 5. (**a**) Red meat (**b**) processed meat and type 2 diabetes RRs for the highest vs. the lowest intake in all subjects. The RR of each study is represented by a square, 95% CI are represented by the horizontal lines, and the diamond represents the estimate and its 95% CI.

Processed Meat Eleven cohort studies [6,18,21–26,29–31] researched the association between processed meat consumption and the risk of T2DM (Figure 1, Tables S3 and S4), the summary RR and 95% CI for high vs. low of processed meat consumption was 1.39 (1.29–1.49) (Figure 5b) (I^2 = 49.32, p = 0.03).

Fish Nine cohort studies [18,29,32–38] researched the association between fish consumption and the risk of T2DM (Figure 1, Tables S5 and S6), the summary RR and 95% CI for high vs. low values of fish consumption was 1.03 (0.89–1.17) (Figure 6) (I^2 = 79.71, p < 0.001). We used a sensitivity analysis to exclude the most influential studies: the summary RR ranged from0.99 (0.89–1.10) when the American study [33] was excluded to 1.50 (0.92–1.20) when the Japanese study [35] was excluded. The heterogeneity was partly because of the Japanese study [35], and when we excluded this study, there was moderate heterogeneity (I^2 = 79.41, p < 0.001).

Study name	Risk ratio	Lower limit	Upper limit	Z-Value	p-Value
Virtanen. 2017 [18]	0.840	0.622	1.134	-1.139	0.255
Montonen. 2005 [29]	1.080	0.802	1.454	0.507	0.612
Wallin,A. 2015 [32]	1.000	0.849	1.178	0.000	1.000
Djousse. 2011 [33]	1.490	1.303	1.704	5.827	0.000
Villegas,R. 2011(m) [34]	0.860	0.757	0.977	-2.325	0.020
Villegas,R. 2011(w) [34]	0.920	0.730	1.160	-0.706	0.480
Nanri,A. 2011(m) [35]	0.730	0.536	0.994	-2.001	0.045
Nanri,A. 2011(w) [35]	1.010	0.687	1.484	0.051	0.960
Geertruida,J. 2009 [36]	1.050	0.799	1.379	0.351	0.726
Patel,P.S. 2009 [37]	0.750	0.583	0.965	-2.238	0.025
Kaushik. 2009(1) [38]	1.290	1.055	1.577	2.481	0.013
Kaushik. 2009(2) [38]	1.320	0.996	1.750	1.930	0.054
Kaushik. 2009(3) [38]	1.160	0.957	1.406	1.513	0.130
Overall(I^2=79.71, P<0.001)	1.025	0.897	1.172	0.363	0.717

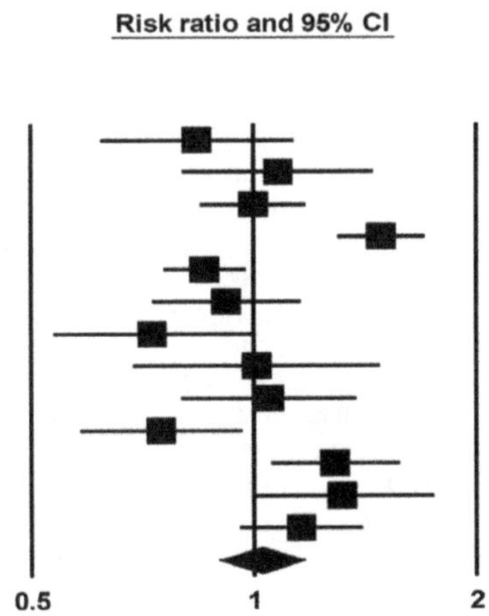

Figure 6. Fish and type 2 diabetes RRs for the highest vs. the lowest intake in all subjects. The RR of each study is represented by a square, 95% CI are represented by the horizontal lines, and the diamond represents the estimate and its 95% CI.

Egg Five cohort studies [18,39–42] researched the association between egg consumption and the risk of T2DM (Figure 1, Tables S7 and S8), the summary RR and 95% CI for high vs. low of egg consumption was 1.03 (0.64–1.67) (Figure 7) (I^2 = 91.12, $p < 0.001$). We used a sensitivity analysis to exclude the most influential studies: the summary RR ranged from 0.97 (0.49–1.88) when the Lithuanian study [39] was excluded to 1.57 (1.30–1.89) when the Finnish study [42] was excluded. The heterogeneity was partly because of the Finnish study [42], and when we excluded this study, there was moderate heterogeneity (I^2 = 69.43, p = 0.06).

Study name	Risk ratio	Lower limit	Upper limit	Z-Value	p-Value
Virtanen. 2017 [18]	0.740	0.487	1.124	-1.413	0.158
Djousse.2009(m) [39]	1.580	1.246	2.004	3.775	0.000
Djousse.2009(w) [39]	1.770	1.285	2.439	3.492	0.000
Djousse.2010(m) [40]	1.810	0.773	4.237	1.367	0.172
Djousse.2010(w) [40]	0.380	0.103	1.407	-1.449	0.147
Djousse.2016 [41]	1.520	1.171	1.972	3.150	0.002
Virtanen.2015 [42]	0.380	0.271	0.532	-5.624	0.000
Overall(I^2=91.12, P<0.0001)	1.030	0.636	1.669	0.121	0.904

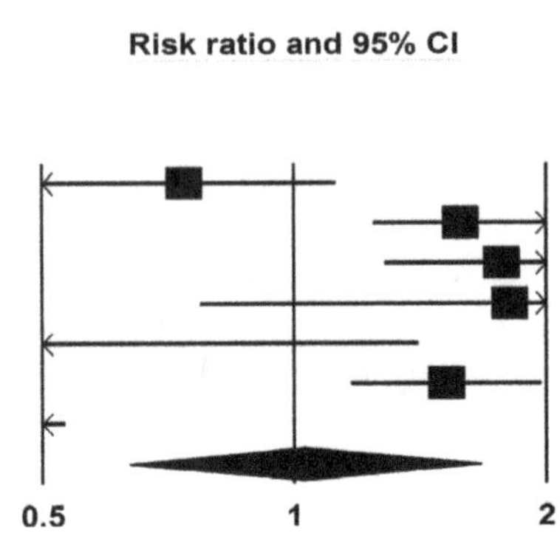

Figure 7. Egg and type 2 diabetes RRs for the highest vs. the lowest intake in all subjects. The RR of each study is represented by a square, 95% CI are represented by the horizontal lines, and the diamond represents the estimate and its 95% CI.

TotalDairyProduct Consumption Eleven cohort studies [18,43–52] researched the association between total dairy product consumption and the risk of T2DM (Figure 1, Tables S9 and S10), the summary RR and 95% CI for high vs. low total dairy product consumption was 0.89 (0.84–0.94) (Figure 8a) (I^2 = 48.81, p = 0.03).

	Study name	Risk ratio	Lower limit	Upper limit	Z-Value	p-Value
a	Virtanen. 2017 [18]	1.350	0.952	1.914	1.684	0.092
	Grantham. 2013(m) [43]	0.530	0.291	0.964	-2.079	0.038
	Grantham. 2013(w) [43]	0.860	0.505	1.465	-0.555	0.579
	Choi,HK.2005(m) [44]	0.770	0.622	0.953	-2.401	0.016
	Liu S.2006(w) [45]	0.790	0.667	0.936	-2.729	0.006
	Van Dam2008(w) [46]	0.930	0.751	1.152	-0.666	0.506
	Diaz-Lopez. 2016 [47]	0.680	0.471	0.982	-2.057	0.040
	Karen L.2011(w) [48]	0.930	0.831	1.041	-1.261	0.207
	Kirii,K2009(m) [49]	1.180	0.896	1.554	1.180	0.238
	Kirii,K2009(w) [49]	0.710	0.512	0.984	-2.056	0.040
	Ewood.2007(m) [50]	0.570	0.200	1.627	-1.050	0.294
	Talaei. 2017 [51]	0.900	0.828	0.978	-2.486	0.013
	Overall(I^2=48.81, P=0.03)	0.889	0.843	0.938	-4.284	0.000
b	Virtanen. 2017 [18]	0.950	0.700	1.290	-0.329	0.742
	Grantham. 2013(m) [43]	0.570	0.319	1.018	-1.901	0.057
	Grantham. 2013(w) [43]	0.670	0.400	1.121	-1.525	0.127
	Grantham. 2013(m2) [43]	1.430	0.832	2.457	1.295	0.195
	Grantham. 2013(w2) [43]	0.890	0.451	1.755	-0.336	0.737
	Choi. 2015(m) [44]	0.730	0.594	0.897	-3.001	0.003
	Choi. 2005(m2) [44]	0.970	0.779	1.208	-0.272	0.786
	Liu S. 2006(w) [45]	0.790	0.671	0.931	-2.818	0.005
	Liu S. 2006(m2) [45]	1.050	0.885	1.246	0.558	0.577
	Van Dam. 2008(w) [46]	0.870	0.758	0.998	-1.989	0.047
	Van Dam. 2008(m2) [46]	1.030	0.882	1.203	0.374	0.709
	Diaz-Lopez. 2016 [47]	0.650	0.450	0.939	-2.292	0.022
	Karen L. 2011(w) [48]	0.650	0.440	0.960	-2.164	0.030
	Overall(I^2=52.20, P=0.01)	0.866	0.780	0.961	-2.706	0.007
c	Virtanen. 2017 [18]	1.130	0.851	1.501	0.843	0.399
	Grantham. 2013(m) [43]	1.020	0.557	1.869	0.064	0.949
	Grantham. 2013(w) [43]	1.230	0.741	2.042	0.800	0.424
	Liu S. 2006 [45]	0.820	0.697	0.965	-2.385	0.017
	Diaz-Lopez. 2016 [47]	0.600	0.419	0.859	-2.794	0.005
	Karen L. 2011(w) [48]	0.460	0.311	0.681	-3.875	0.000
	Kirii. 2009(m) [49]	1.010	0.750	1.360	0.066	0.948
	Kirii. 2009(w) [49]	0.770	0.584	1.016	-1.847	0.065
	Choi. 2005(m) [51]	0.830	0.655	1.052	-1.542	0.123
	Overall(I^2=62.06, P=0.007)	0.830	0.703	0.981	-2.185	0.029

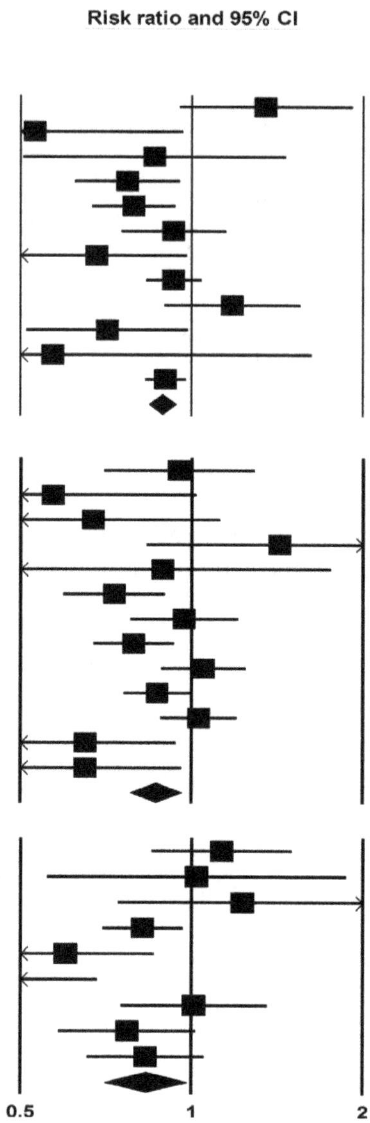

Figure 8. (**a**) Total dairy products (**b**) whole milk (**c**) yogurt and type 2 diabetes RRs for the highest vs. the lowest intake in all subjects. The RR of each study is represented by a square, 95% CI are represented by the horizontal lines, and the diamond represents the estimate and its 95% CI.

Whole Milk Seven cohort studies [18,43–48] researched the association between whole milk consumption and risk of T2DM (Figure 1, Tables S9 and S10), the summary RR and 95% CI for high vs. low of fat dairy consumption was 0.87 (0.78–0.96) (Figure 8b) (I^2 = 52.20, p = 0.01). We used a sensitivity analysis to exclude the most influential studies: the summary RR ranged from 0.85 (0.76–0.94) when the American study [46] was excluded to 0.89 (0.80–0.99) when the Japanese study [44] was excluded. The heterogeneity was partly because of the American study [46], and when we excluded this study, there was moderate heterogeneity (I^2 = 46.87, p = 0.04).

Yogurt Seven cohort studies [18,43,44,47–49] researched the association between yogurt consumption and the risk of T2DM (Figure 1, Tables S9 and S10).The summary RR for high vs. low yogurt consumption was 0.83 (0.70–0.98) (Figure 8c) (I^2 = 62.06, p = 0.01). We used a sensitivity analysis to exclude the most influential studies: the summary RR ranged from 0.81 (0.67–0.97) when the Japanese study [49] was excluded to 0.88 (0.76–1.00) when USA study [48] was excluded. The heterogeneity was partly because of the Japanese study [49], and when we excluded this study there was moderate heterogeneity (I^2 = 40.61, p = 0.11).

Soy Eight cohort studies [52–57] researched the association between legume consumption and the risk of T2DM (Figure 1, Tables S11 and S12), the summary RR for high vs. low soy consumption was 0.87 (0.74–1.01) (Figure 9a) (I^2 = 86.57, $p < 0.01$). We used a sensitivity analysis to exclude the most influential studies: the summary RR ranged from0.82 (0.68–0.98) when the American study [56] was excluded to 0.93 (0.81–1.06) when the Chinese study [53] was excluded. The heterogeneity was partly because of the American study [56], and when we excluded this study, there was moderate heterogeneity (I^2 = 69.34, $p < 0.01$). However, the summary RR for high vs. low soy was 0.74 (0.59–0.93) (Figure 9b), (I^2 = 82.09, $p < 0.001$) in women. We used a sensitivity analysis to exclude the most influential studies: the summary RR ranged from0.66 (0.49–0.90) when the American study [57] was excluded to 0.81 (0.65–1.00) when the Chinese study [54] was excluded. The heterogeneity was partly because of the American study [57], and when we excluded this study, there was moderate heterogeneity (I^2 = 0.00, $p = 0.67$).

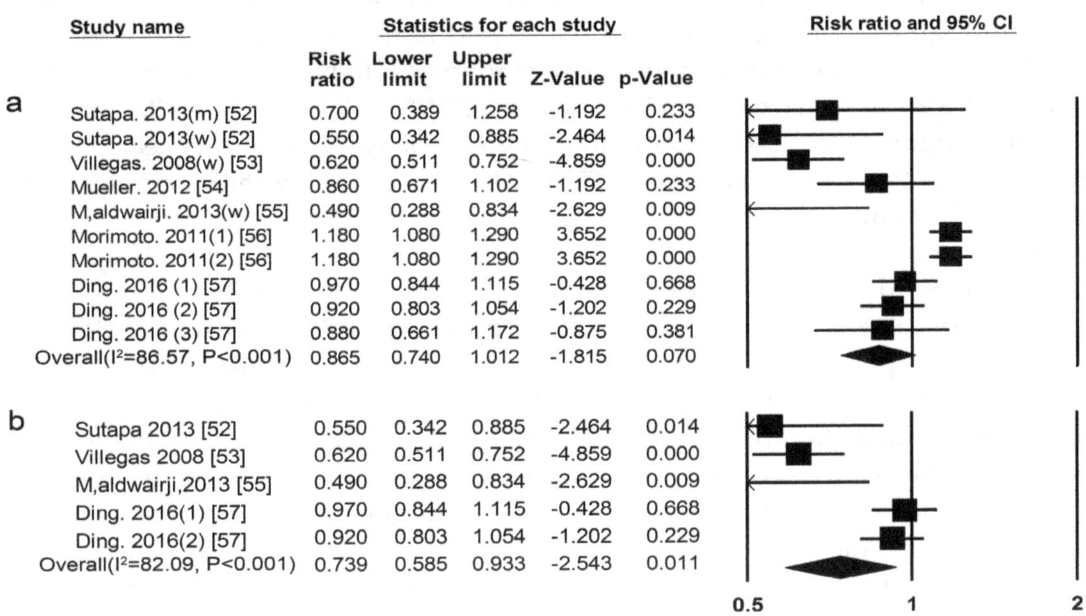

Figure 9. Soy and type 2 diabetes RRs for (**a**) the highest vs. the lowest intake in all subjects and (**b**) the highest vs. the lowest intake in women. The RR of each study is represented by a square, 95% CI are represented by the horizontal lines, and the diamond represents the estimate and its 95% CI.

3.3. Publication Bias

No significant publication bias was detected in the Begg-Mazumdar's test and Egger's test of our meta-analyses, provided in Table 1.

Table 1. Public bias and meta-analysis.

Proteins and Foods Sources	Begg-Mazumdar's Test	Egger's Test
Total protein (all)	0.74	0.38
Total protein (men)	0.46	0.74
Total protein (women)	0.55	0.33
Animal protein (all)	0.64	0.07
Animal protein (men)	0.73	0.57
Animal protein (women)	0.22	0.10
Plant protein (all)	0.76	0.50
Plant protein (men)	0.73	0.90
Plant protein (women)	0.81	0.91

Table 1. *Cont.*

Proteins and Foods Sources	Begg-Mazumdar's Test	Egger's Test
Red meat	0.30	0.33
Processed meat	0.88	0.99
Fish	0.58	0.43
Total dairy product	0.45	0.43
Whole milk	0.67	0.35
Yogurt	0.92	0.99
Egg	0.23	0.50
Soy	0.46	0.13

4. Discussion

According to the results of this meta-analysis, the intake of total protein and animal protein was associated with a high risk of T2DM both in males and females. The intake of plant protein was associated with low risk of T2DM in females, but not in males. In high animal protein food, red meat, and processed meat were associated with a high risk of T2DM in all subjects, while total dairy products, low-fat dairy, and yogurt were associated with a low risk of T2DM in all subjects, and egg and fish were not associated with a decreased risk of T2DM. In high plant protein food, soy was associated with a low risk of T2DM in females.

Higher intake of dietary protein is often associated with lifestyles, including physical activity, body weight, smoking, drinking. For example, we already know that overweight and obesity are risk factors for T2DM, and a meta-analysis showed that each unit increase of BMI would increase the risk for T2DM by approximately 20% [58]. In our meta-analysis, most studies were adjusted for known influencing factors, including age, BMI (Body Mass Index), smoking, physical activity, alcohol consumption, energy intake, family history of T2DM and menopausal status (among women).

The statistical power of the results could be significantly increased as the number of studies and the sample size increase, but it could also lead to heterogeneity. Some heterogeneity was due to different participants' characteristics and regions, and different dietary assessment methods. Thus, heterogeneity is usually used to explain the study characteristics and is difficult to interpret. In our study, the heterogeneities of total protein and animal protein were in the acceptable range, but the heterogeneity of plant protein was outside of the range. We found that the European study [10] contributed to the heterogeneity. When this study was excluded, the heterogeneities of both the overall and subgroup analyses were much lower. The reason that the European study [10] had inconsistent results compared with other studies was not clear, but it could partly be due to the participants in this study having a lower plant protein intake than other studies [13–18]. For red meat and processed meat, we found that the Chinese study [25] contributed to the heterogeneity. When this study is excluded, the heterogeneities were much lower. The reason that the Chinese study [25] had inconsistent results may be due to the participants in this study having a lower meat intake than other participants [6,18,21–24,26–31]. For fish, we found that the Japanese study [35] contributed to the heterogeneity, but the heterogeneity was not moderate when it was excluded, which means the association between fish and T2DM needs further refinement. For egg, we found that the Finnish study [42] contributed to the heterogeneity. When this study is excluded, the heterogeneity was much lower. The reason why the Finnish study [42] had inconsistent results compared with other studies was not clear, but it could partly be due to the participants in this study being older than the other studies [18,39–41]. For whole milk, we found that the American study [46] contributed to the heterogeneity, and the heterogeneity was moderate when it was excluded. The reason why the American study [46] had heterogeneity may be due to the milk intake of black women in America being different from the participants of other studies' [18,43–45,47,48]. For yogurt, the Japanese study [49] contributed to the heterogeneity. The reason why the Japanese study [49] had inconsistent results was not clear, but it could partly be due to the female participants in this study being older than other studies [18,43,44,47,48].

As meta-analysis is based on published studies, the publication bias affect is inevitable. It is particularly important to evaluate publication bias. In our meta-analysis, we used the Egger linear regression test and Begg rank correlation test to determine publication bias, and we found that there was no publication bias in our study.

Dietary protein and amino acids are involved in the modulations of insulin sensitivity and glucose metabolism. However, the results from human studies were still inconsistent. Some studies showed that high intake of dietary protein had negative effects on glucose homeostasis by facilitating insulin resistance and increasing gluconeogenesis [7,59,60]. Amino acid signaling may facilitate insulin resistance, by activation of the mammalian target of rapamycin (mTOR), a nutrient sensor that operates a detrimental feedback loop toward insulin receptor substrate 1 signaling [61–64]. Moreover, amino acids may also inhibit glucose uptake through phosphorylation of downstream factors of the insulin signaling cascade by the translation initiation factor serine-kinase-6-1 [63,65]. On the other hand, in vivo and in vitro studies also demonstrated that amino acids play a beneficial role in glucose homeostasis by modulating insulin action on hepatic glucose production and muscle glucose transport, secretion of glucagon and insulin, as well as various tissues gene and protein expression [64,66]. One of the possible mechanisms that might explain this was that higher protein reduced the amount of carbohydrate intake under isoenergy conditions and thus a smaller amount of glucose was absorbed after ingestion of the meals, with the consequence of a reduced store of glycogen and, thus, a decrease in glycogenolysis rate [67,68]. The other possible causal mechanism was amino acids stimulating the insulin secretion to intervene in the glucose metabolism and serve as substrates for gluconeogenesis; thus, increased gluconeogenesis could stimulate insulin secretion, which might prevent hyperglycemia [69].Additionally, some scientists think that different qualities rather than quantities of proteins play a more important role in insulin resistance [69]. Our study supported the hypothesis that animal proteins caused a high risk of T2DM in males and females, and plant proteins were protection factors of T2DM in females. We can find some support for this from the literature. The abundance in certain amino acids are different between animal proteins and plant proteins. This may contribute to the different effects between them on the risk of T2DM. Typically, plant protein contains lower levels of the branched chain amino acids leucine, isoleucine and valine and of the sulfur amino acid methionine as compared with animal proteins [70]. Branched chain amino acids and higher methionine intake have been associated with insulin resistance and type 2 diabetes [71,72]. In addition, dietary glycine is also mainly consumed from animal-based foods and some cohort studies have shown that glycine was positively associated with T2DM, and hypertension [72,73]. On the other hand, dietary glutamic acid, an amino acid that is mainly consumed from plant protein was found to be inversely associated with risks of hypertension and arterial stiffness [73,74]. So far, three intervention studies have compared the effects of animal protein with plant protein meals on glycaemic variables in people with T2DM, but they were obtained from three different results [75–77]. This should be further investigated in future studies.

From the current literature available, the inconsistency in association between plant protein and T2DM was probably due to gender difference. The negative association between plant protein or soy and T2DM was observed mainly in women, while most of the studies in men found null results. Therefore, results from all subjects without considering gender difference were different and the proportion of women in the study may influence the results. However, the exact mechanism is unclear.

In order to further refine and compare the association between different food sources of protein and T2DM, and facilitate dietary guidance, we have analyzed the relationship between different high-protein food and the risk of type 2 diabetes. We found that different high-protein foods play different roles in T2DM, even if they are all animal-based foods. Our results indicated that the intake of red meat and processed meat are risk factors for T2DM. They are also positively associated with weight gain [78], stroke [79], coronary heart disease [80] and mortality [81].First, the increased meat protein may increase iron load, which was associated with the increased risk of T2DM [82]. Moreover, the other nutrients in red and processed meat, including nitrites and advanced glycation end products, were also thought to mediate the association between meat intake and the risk of T2DM [83].The relationship between egg consumption and T2DM was not clear. Some studies have shown that egg intake was associated with a lower risk of T2DM [42].Some research showed that egg consumption was positively associated with the risk of T2DM in our study [39,84,85], and this result was supported by the AHA dietary guidelines which advise restricted egg consumption in adults for preventing cardiometabolic diseases [86–88].We found that total dairy products, whole milk, and yogurt intake were protective factors for T2DM. Some studies showed that milk proteins, like whey protein, may enhance satiety and reduce risk factors for T2DM [89]. The calcium and vitamin D in milk and its products may also contribute to its beneficial effects on T2DM [90].In our study, fish consumption was not associated with decreased risk of T2DM. This result may partly relate on the increase in plasma selenium level with the increment of fish intake, which may increase the risk of diabetes [91,92].The relationship between fish intake and the risk of T2DM needs further refinement. For high plant protein-based foods, there was a negative association between soy consumption and the risk of T2DM in this study. Soy protein may inhibit insulin secretion from pancreatic β cells or inhibit lipogenesis and enhance lipolysis in the adipose and liver to reduce adiposity [93].This protective effect may also be associated with biologically active ingredients such as phytoestrogen in soybeans [94].

Our meta-analysis also had limitations. First, publications into our research were adjusted for BMI, but some studies had measurement errors because of self-reporting of height and weight, resulting in the BMI relying on self-reporting, which could lead to confounding results. Second, some important factors that influence T2DM such as fiber, lipids, and carbohydrates, were only adjusted in some of these studies, which may also lead to confounding results. Additionally, limitations might be due to temporal bias. Studies with longer follow-up might beless influenced by temporal bias. In our studies, the follow-up period of each research study was different, so the temporal bias might impact the association between dietary protein intake and the risk of T2DM.

5. Conclusions

In summary, we found that total protein and animal protein consumption were the risk factors for T2DM, and plant protein was the protective factor for T2DM in women, but not in men. We also found that different high-protein foods have a different effect on T2DM risk, even if they all belong to animal proteins. These results underline the significance of taking into account what kind of dietary protein and food sources of protein are recommended for the prevention of diabetes.

Supplementary Materials:
Table S1: Characteristics of participants and follow-up in included studies of protein consumption in relation to the risk of T2DM, Table S2: Prospective cohort studies of protein consumption and type 2 diabetes, Table S3: Characteristics of participants and follow-up in included studies of meat consumption in relation to the risk of T2DM, Table S4: Prospective cohort studies of meat consumption and type 2 diabetes, Table S5: Characteristics of participants and follow-up in included studies of fish consumption in relation to the risk of T2DM, Table S6: Prospective cohort studies of fish consumption and type 2 diabetes, Table S7: Characteristics of participants and follow-up in included studies of egg consumption in relation to risk of T2DM, Table S8:Prospective cohort studies of egg consumption and type 2 diabetes, Table S9: Characteristics of participants and follow-up in included studies of dairy consumption in relation to the risk of T2DM, Table S10: Prospective cohort studies of dairy consumption and type 2 diabetes, Table S11: Characteristics of participants and follow-up in included studies of soy consumption in relation to the risk of T2DM, Table S12: Prospective cohort studies of soy consumption and type 2 diabetes.

Acknowledgments: This work was supported by funds from the National Natural Science Foundation of China (81202188, 81130049) and by the Wu Lian De Grant of Harbin Medical University (WLD-QN1406).

Author Contributions: Shuang Tian analyzed the data, and wrote the manuscript. Qian Xu, Ruyue Jiang and Tianshu Han supervised the analysis, reviewed the manuscript, and contributed to the discussion. Lixin Na and Changhao Sun developed the study design, acquired funding and administrated the project.

References

1. Guariguata, L.; Whiting, D.R.; Hambleton, I.; Beagley, J.; Linnenkamp, U.; Shaw, J.E. Globalestimates of diabetes prevalence for 2013 and projections for 2035. *Diabetes Res. Clin. Pract.* **2014**, *103*, 137–149. [CrossRef] [PubMed]
2. American Diabetes Association. Standards of medical care in diabetes—2006. *Diabetes Care* **2006**, *29* (Suppl. 1), S4–S42.
3. Nichols, G.A.; Glauber, H.S.; Brown, J.B. Type 2 diabetes: Incremental medical care costs during the 8 years preceding diagnosis. *Diabetes Care* **2002**, *23*, 1654–1659. [CrossRef]
4. Tuomilehto, J.; Lindström, J.; Eriksson, J.G.; Valle, T.T.; Hämäläinen, H.; Ilanne-Parikka, P.; Keinänen-Kiukaanniemi, S.; Laakso, M.; Louheranta, A.; Rastas, M.; et al. Prevention of: Type 2 diabetes mellitus by changes in lifestyle among subjects with impaired glucose tolerance. *N. Engl. J. Med.* **2011**, *344*, 1343–1350. [CrossRef] [PubMed]
5. Schulze, M.B.; Schulz, M.; Heidemann, C.; Schienkiewitz, A.; Hoffmann, K.; Boeing, H. Carbohydrate intake and incidence of type 2 diabetes in the European Prospective Investigation into Cancer and Nutrition (EPIC)-Potsdam Study. *Br. J. Nutr.* **2008**, *99*, 1107–1116. [CrossRef] [PubMed]
6. Van Dam, R.M.; Willett, W.C.; Rimm, E.B.; Stampfer, M.J.; Hu, F.B. Dietary fat and meat intake in relation to risk of type 2 diabetes in men. *Diabetes Care* **2002**, *25*, 417–424. [CrossRef] [PubMed]
7. Weickert, M.O.; Roden, M.; Isken, F.; Hoffmann, D.; Nowotny, P.; Osterhoff, M.; Blaut, M.; Alpert, C.; Gögebakan, Ö.; Bumke-Vogt, C.; et al. Effects of supplemented isoenergetic diets differing in cereal fiber and protein content on insulin sensitivity in overweight humans. *Am. J. Nutr.* **2011**, *94*, 459–471. [CrossRef] [PubMed]
8. Nuttal, F.Q.; Schweim, K.; Hoover, H.; Gannon, M.C. Effect of the LoBAG30 diet on blood glucose control in people with type 2 diabetes. *Br. J. Nutr.* **2008**, *99*, 511–519. [CrossRef] [PubMed]
9. Pounis, G.D.; Tyrovolas, S.; Antonopoulou, M.; Zeimbekis, A.; Anastasiou, F.; Bountziouka, V.; Metallinos, G.; Gotsis, E.; Lioliou, E.; Polychronopoulos, E.; et al. Long-term animal-protein consumption is associated with an increased prevalence of diabetes among the elderly: The Mediterranean islands (MEDIS) study. *Diabetes Metab.* **2010**, *36*, 484–490. [CrossRef] [PubMed]
10. Van Nielen, M.; Feskens, E.J.; Mensink, M.; Sluijs, I.; Molina, E.; Amiano, P.; Ardanaz, E.; Balkau, B.; Beulens, J.W.; Boeing, H.; et al. Dietary protein intake and incidence of type 2 diabetes in Europe: The EPIC-InterAct Case-Cohort Study. *Diabetes Care* **2014**, *37*, 1854–1862. [CrossRef] [PubMed]
11. Ericson, U.; Sonestedt, E.; Gullberg, B.; Hellstrand, S.; Hindy, G.; Wirfalt, E.; Orho, M. High intakes of protein and processed meat associate with increased incidence of type 2 diabetes. *Br. J. Nutr.* **2013**, *109*, 1143–1153. [CrossRef] [PubMed]
12. Tinker, L.F.; Sarto, G.E.; Howard, B.V.; Huang, Y.; Neuhouser, M.L.; Mossavar-Rahmani, Y.; Beasley, J.M.; Margolis, K.L.; Eaton, C.B.; Phillips, L.S.; et al. Biomarker-calibrated dietary energy and protein intake associations with diabetes risk among postmenopausal women from the Women's Health Initiative. *Am. J. Clin. Nutr.* **2011**, *94*, 1600–1606. [CrossRef] [PubMed]
13. Sluijs, I.; Beulens, J.W.; Spijkerman, A.M.; Grobbee, D.E.; van der Schouw, Y.T. Dietary intake of total, animal, and vegetable protein and risk of type 2 diabetes in the European Prospective Investigation into Cancer and Nutrition(EPIC)-NL study. *Diabetes Care* **2010**, *33*, 43–48. [CrossRef] [PubMed]
14. Malik, V.; Li, Y.; Tobias, D.; Pan, A.; Hu, F. Dietary protein intake and risk of type 2 diabetes in U.S. men and women. *Am. J. Epidemiol.* **2016**, *183*, 715–728. [CrossRef] [PubMed]
15. Bao, W.; Bowers, K.; Tobias, D.; Hu, F.; Zhang, C. Prepregnancy dietary protein intake, major dietary protein sources, and the risk of gestational diabetes mellitus: A Prospective cohort study. *Diabetes Care* **2013**, *36*, 2001–2008. [CrossRef] [PubMed]
16. Nanri, A.; Mizoue, T.; Kurotani, K.; Goto, A.; Oba, S.; Noda, M.; Sawada, N.; Tsugane, S. Low-carbohydrate diet and type 2 diabetes risk in Japanese men and women: The Japan Public Health Center-Based Prospective Study. *PLoS ONE* **2015**, *10*, e0118377. [CrossRef] [PubMed]
17. Shang, X.; Scott, D.; Hodge, A.M.; English, D.R.; Giles, G.G.; Ebeling, P.R.; Sanders, K.M. Dietary protein intake and risk of type 2 diabetes: Results from Melboune Collaborative Cohort study and a meta-analysis of prospective studies. *Am. J. Clin. Nutr.* **2016**, *104*, 1352–1365. [CrossRef] [PubMed]

18. Virtanen, H.E.; Koskinen, T.T.; Voutilainen, S.; Mursu, J.; Tuomainen, T.P.; Kokko, P.; Virtanen, J.K. Intake of different dietary proteins and risk of type 2 diabetes in men: The Kuopio Ischaemic Heart Disease Risk Factor Study. *Br. J. Nutr.* **2017**, *117*, 882–893. [CrossRef] [PubMed]
19. Der Simonian, R.; Laird, N. Meta-analysis in clinical trials. *Control Clin. Trials* **1986**, *7*, 177–188. [CrossRef]
20. Higgins, J.P.; Thompson, S.G. Quantifying heterogeneity in a meta-analysis. *Stat. Med.* **2002**, *21*, 1539–1558. [CrossRef] [PubMed]
21. Hodge, A.M.; English, D.R.; O'Dea, K.; Giles, G.G. Dietary patterns and diabetes incidence in the Melbourne Collaborative Cohort Study. *Am. J. Epidemiol.* **2007**, *165*, 603–610. [CrossRef] [PubMed]
22. Fung, T.T.; Schulze, M.; Manson, J.E.; Willett, W.C.; Hu, F.B. Dietary patterns, meat intake, and the risk of type 2 diabetes in women. *Arch. Intern. Med.* **2004**, *164*, 2235–2240. [CrossRef] [PubMed]
23. Schulze, M.B.; Manson, J.E.; Willett, W.C.; Hu, F.B. Processed meat intake and incidence of type 2 diabetes in younger and middle-aged women. *Diabetologia* **2003**, *46*, 1465–1473. [CrossRef] [PubMed]
24. Song, Y.; Manson, J.E.; Buring, J.E.; Liu, S. A prospective study of red meat consumption and type 2 diabetes in middle-aged and elderly women: The women's health study. *Diabetes Care* **2004**, *27*, 2108–2115. [CrossRef] [PubMed]
25. Villegas, R.; Shu, X.O.; Gao, Y.T.; Yang, G.; Cai, H.; Li, H.; Zheng, W. The association of meat intake and the risk of type 2 diabetes may be modified by body weight. *Int. J. Med. Sci.* **2006**, *3*, 152–159. [CrossRef] [PubMed]
26. Simmons, R.K.; Harding, A.H.; Wareham, N.J.; Griffin, S.J. Do simple questions about diet and physical activity help to identify those at risk of type 2 diabetes? *Diabet. Med.* **2007**, *24*, 830–835. [CrossRef] [PubMed]
27. Lee, D.H.; Folsom, A.R.; Jacobs, D.R., Jr. Dietary iron intake and type 2 diabetes incidence in postmenopausal women: The Iowa Women's Health Study. *Diabetologia* **2004**, *47*, 185–194. [CrossRef] [PubMed]
28. Schulze, M.B.; Hoffmann, K.; Boeing, H.; Linseisen, J.; Rohrmann, S.; Möhlig, M.; Pfeiffer, A.F.; Spranger, J.; Thamer, C.; Häring, H.U.; et al. An accurate risk score based on anthropometric, dietary, and lifestyle factors to predict the development of type 2 diabetes. *Diabetes Care* **2007**, *30*, 510–515. [CrossRef] [PubMed]
29. Montonen, J.; Jarvinen, R.; Heliovaara, M.; Reunanen, A.; Aromaa, A.; Knekt, P. Food consumption and the incidence of type II diabetes mellitus. *Eur. J. Clin. Nutr.* **2005**, *59*, 441–448. [CrossRef] [PubMed]
30. Mari-Sanchis, A.; Gea, A.; Basterra-Gortari, F.J.; Martinez-Gonzalez, M.A.; Beunza, J.J.; Bes-Rastrollo, M. Meat consumption and risk of developing type 2 diabetes in the SUN Project: A highly educated middle-class population. *PLoS ONE* **2016**, *11*, e0157990. [CrossRef] [PubMed]
31. Vang, A.; Singh, P.N.; Lee, J.W.; Haddad, E.H.; Brinegar, C.H. Meats, processed meats, obesity, weight gain and occurrence of diabetes among adults: Findings from adventist health studies. *Ann. Nutr. Metab.* **2008**, *52*, 96–104. [CrossRef] [PubMed]
32. Wallin, A.; Di Giuseppe, D.; Orsini, N.; Åkesson, A.; Forouhi, N.G.; Wolk, A. Fish consumption and frying of fish in relation to type 2 diabetes incidence: A prospective cohort study of Swedish men. *Eur. J. Nutr.* **2017**, *56*, 843–852. [CrossRef] [PubMed]
33. Djoussé, L.; Gaziano, J.M.; Buring, J.E.; Lee, I.M. Dietary omega-3 fatty acids and fish consumption and risk of type 2 diabetes. *Am. J. Clin. Nutr.* **2011**, *93*, 140–150. [CrossRef] [PubMed]
34. Villegas, R.; Xiang, Y.; Elasy, T.; Li, H.; Yang, G.; Cai, H.; Ye, F.; Gao, Y.; Shyr, Y.; Zheng, W.; et al. Fish, shellfish, and long-chain *n*-3 fatty acid consumption and risk of incident type 2 diabetes in middle-aged Chinese men and women. *Am. J. Clin. Nutr.* **2011**, *94*, 543–551. [CrossRef] [PubMed]
35. Nanri, A.; Mizoue, T.; Noda, M.; Takahashi, Y.; Poudel, T.; Kato, M.; Oba, S.; Inoue, M.; Tsugane, S. Fish intake and type 2 diabetes in Japanese men and women: The Japan Public Health Center-based Prospective Study. *Am. J. Clin. Nutr.* **2011**, *94*, 884–891. [CrossRef] [PubMed]
36. Geertruida, J.; Ballegooijen, A.; Kuijsten, A.; Sijbrands, E.; Rooij, F.; Geleijnse, J.; Hofman, A.; Witteman, J.; Fesken, E. Eating fish and risk of type 2 diabetes: A population-based, prospective follow-up study. *Diabetes Care* **2009**, *32*, 2021–2026.
37. Patel, P.; Sharp, S.; Luben, R.; Khaw, K.; Bingham, S.; Wareham, N.; Forouhi, N. Association between type of dietary fish and seafood intake and the risk of incident type 2 diabetes: The European prospective investigation of cancer (EPIC)-Norfolk cohort study. *Diabetes Care* **2009**, *32*, 1857–1863. [CrossRef] [PubMed]
38. Kaushik, M.; Mozaffarian, D.; Spiegelman, D.; Manson, J.E.; Willett, W.C.; Hu, F.B. Long chain omega-3 fatty acids, fish intake, and the risk of type 2 diabetes mellitus. *Am. J. Clin. Nutr.* **2009**, *90*, 613–620. [CrossRef] [PubMed]

39. Djousse, L.; Gaziano, J.M.; Buring, J.E.; Lee, I.M. Egg consumption and risk of type 2 diabetes in men and women. *Diabetes Care* **2009**, *32*, 295–300. [CrossRef] [PubMed]
40. Djoussé, L.; Kamineni, A.; Nelson, T.L.; Carnethon, M.; Mozaffarian, D.; Siscovick, D.; Mukamal, K.J. Egg consumption and risk of type 2 diabetes in older adults. *Am. J. Clin. Nutr.* **2010**, *92*, 422–427. [CrossRef] [PubMed]
41. Djousse, L.; Petrone, A.; Hickson, D.; Talegawkar, S.; Dubbert, P.; Taylor, H.; Tucker, K. Egg consumption and risk of type 2 diabetes among African Americans: The Jackson Heart Study. *Clin. Nutr.* **2016**, *53*, 679–684. [CrossRef] [PubMed]
42. Virtanen, J.; Mursu, J.; Tuomainen, T.; Virtanen, H.; Voutilainen, S. Egg consumption and risk of incident type 2 diabetes in men: The Kuopio Ischaemic Heart Disease Risk Factor Study. *Am. J. Clin. Nutr.* **2015**, *101*, 1088–1096. [CrossRef] [PubMed]
43. Grantham, N.; Magliano, D.; Hodge, A.; Jowett, J.; Meikle, P.; shaw, J. The association between dairy food intake and the incidence of diabetes in Australia: The Australian Diabetes Obesity and Lifestyle Study (AusDiab). *Public Health Nutr.* **2013**, *16*, 339–345. [CrossRef] [PubMed]
44. Choi, H.K.; Willett, W.C.; Stampfer, M.J.; Rimm, E.; Hu, F.B. Dairy consumption and risk of type 2 diabetes mellitus in men: A prospective study. *Arch. Intern. Med.* **2005**, *165*, 997–1003. [CrossRef] [PubMed]
45. Liu, S.; Choi, H.K.; Ford, E.; Song, Y.; Klevak, A.; Buring, J.E.; Manson, J.E. A prospective study of dairy intake and the risk of type 2 diabetes in women. *Diabetes Care* **2006**, *29*, 1579–1584. [CrossRef] [PubMed]
46. Van Dam, R.M.; Hu, F.B.; Rosenberg, L.; Krishnan, S.; Palmer, J.R. Dietary calcium and magnesium, major food sources, and risk of type 2 diabetes in U.S. black women. *Diabetes Care* **2006**, *29*, 2238–2243. [CrossRef] [PubMed]
47. Díaz-López, A.; Bulló, M.; Martínez-González, M.A.; Corella, D.; Estruch, R.; Fitó, M.; Gómez-Gracia, E.; Fiol, M.; de la Corte, F.J.G.; Ros, E.; et al. Dairy product consumption and risk of type 2 diabetes in an elderly Spanish Mediterranean population at high cardiovascular risk. *Eur. J. Nutr.* **2016**, *55*, 349–360. [CrossRef] [PubMed]
48. Margolis, K.L.; Wei, F.; de Boer, I.H.; Howard, B.V.; Liu, S.; Manson, J.E.; Mossavar-Rahmani, Y.; Phillips, L.S.; Shikany, J.M.; Tinker, L.F. A diet high in low-fat dairy products lowers diabetes risk in postmenopausal women. *J. Nutr.* **2011**, *141*, 1969–1974. [CrossRef] [PubMed]
49. Kirii, K.; Mizoue, T.; Iso, H.; Takahashi, Y.; Kato, M.; Inoue, M.; Noda, M.; Tsugane, S.; Japan Public Health Center-based Prospective Study Group. Calcium, vitamin D and dairy intake in relation to type 2 diabetes risk in a Japanese cohort. *Diabetologia* **2009**, *52*, 2542–2550. [CrossRef] [PubMed]
50. Elwood, P.C.; Pickering, J.E.; Fehily, A.M. Milk and dairy consumption, diabetes and the metabolic syndrome: The Caerphilly prospective study. *J. Epidemiol. Community Health* **2007**, *61*, 695–698. [CrossRef] [PubMed]
51. Talaei, M.; Pan, A.; Yuan, J.M.; Koh, W.P. Dairy intake and risk of type 2 diabetes. *Clin. Nutr.* **2017**, *17*, 1–7. [CrossRef] [PubMed]
52. Sutapa, A.; Shah, E. Association between legume intake and self-reported diabetes among adult men and women in India. *BMC Public Health* **2013**, *13*, 706.
53. Villegas, R.; Gao, Y.; Yang, G.; Li, H.; Elasy, T.; Zheng, W.; Shu, X. Legume and soy food intake and the incidence of type 2 diabetes in the Shanghai Women's Health Study. *Am. J. Clin. Nutr.* **2008**, *87*, 162–167. [PubMed]
54. Mueller, N.; Odegaard, A.; Gross, M.; Koh, W.; Yu, M.; Yuan, J.; Pereira, M. Soy intake and risk of type 2 diabetes in Chinese Singaporeans. *Eur. J. Nutr.* **2012**, *51*, 1033–1040. [CrossRef] [PubMed]
55. Aldwairji, M.; Orfila, C.; Burley, V.J. Legume intake and risk of type 2 diabetes in British women. *Proc. Nutr. Soc.* **2013**, *72*, E275. [CrossRef]
56. Morimoto, Y.; Steinbrecher, A.; Kolonel, L.; Maskarinec, G. Soy consumption is not protective against diabetes in Hawaii: The Multiethnic Cohort. *Eur. J. Clin. Nutr.* **2011**, *65*, 279–282. [CrossRef] [PubMed]
57. Ding, M.; Pan, A.; Manson, J.E.; Willett, W.C.; Malik, V.; Rosner, B.; Giovannucci, E.; Hu, F.B.; Sun, Q. Consumption of soy foods and isoflavones and risk of type 2diabetes: A pooled analysis of three U.S. cohorts. *Eur. J. Clin. Nutr.* **2016**, *70*, 1381–1387. [CrossRef] [PubMed]
58. Hartemink, N.; Boshuizen, H.C.; Nagelkerke, N.J.; Jacobs, M.A.; van Houwelingen, H.C. Combining risk estimates from observational studies with different exposure cutpoints: A meta-analysis on body mass index and diabetes type 2. *Am. J. Epidemiol.* **2006**, *163*, 1042–1052. [CrossRef] [PubMed]

59. Linn, T.; Geyer, R.; Prassek, S.; Laube, H. Effect of dietary protein intake on insulin secretion and glucose metabolism in insulin-dependent diabetes mellitus. *J Clin. Endocrinol. Metab.* **1996**, *81*, 3938–3943. [PubMed]
60. Linn, T.; Santosa, B.; Grönemeyer, D.; Aygen, S.; Scholz, N.; Busch, M.; Bretzel, R.G. Effect of long-term dietary protein intake on glucose metabolism in humans. *Diabetologia* **2000**, *43*, 1257–1265. [CrossRef] [PubMed]
61. Patti, M.E.; Brambilla, E.; Luzi, L.; Landaker, E.J.; Kahn, C.R. Bidirectional modulation of insulin action by amino acids. *J. Clin. Investig.* **1998**, *101*, 1519–1529. [CrossRef] [PubMed]
62. Takano, A.; Usui, I.; Haruta, T.; Kawahara, J.; Uno, T.; Iwata, M.; Kobayashi, M. Mammalian target of rapamycin pathway regulates insulin signaling via subcellular redistribution of insulin receptor substrate 1 and integrates nutritional signals and metabolic signals of insulin. *Mol. Cell. Biol.* **2001**, *21*, 5050–5062. [CrossRef] [PubMed]
63. Tremblay, F.; Krebs, M.; Dombrowski, L.; Brehm, A.; Bernroider, E.; Roth, E.; Nowotny, P.; Waldhäusl, W.; Marette, A.; Roden, M. Overactivation of S6 kinase 1 as a cause of human insulin resistance during increased amino acid availability. *Diabetes* **2005**, *54*, 2674–2684. [CrossRef] [PubMed]
64. Tremblay, F.; Marette, A. Amino acid and insulin signaling via the mTOR/p70 S6 kinase pathway. A negative feedback mechanism leading to insulin resistance in skeletal muscle cells. *J. Biol. Chem.* **2001**, *276*, 38052–38060. [PubMed]
65. Um, S.H.; D'Alessio, D.; Thomas, G. Nutrient overload, insulin resistance, and ribosomal protein S6 kinase 1, S6K1. *Cell Metab.* **2006**, *3*, 393–402. [CrossRef] [PubMed]
66. Gulve, E.A.; Cartee, G.D.; Holloszy, J.O. Prolonged incubation of skeletal muscle in vitro: Prevention of increases in glucose transport. *Am. J. Physiol.* **1991**, *261*, 154–160.
67. Gannon, M.C.; Nuttall, F.Q. Effect of a high-protein, low-carbohydrate diet on blood glucose control in people with type 2 diabetes. *Diabetes* **2004**, *53*, 2375–2382. [CrossRef] [PubMed]
68. Nuttall, F.Q.; Gannon, M.C. Metabolic response of people with type 2 diabetes to a high-protein diet. *Nutr. Metab.* **2004**, *1*. [CrossRef] [PubMed]
69. Tremblay, F.; Lavigne, C.; Jacques, H.; Marette, A. Role of dietary proteins and amino acids in the pathogenesis of insulin resistance. *Annu. Rev. Nutr.* **2007**, *27*, 293–310. [CrossRef] [PubMed]
70. Richter, C.K.; Skulas-Ray, A.C.; Champagne, C.M.; Kris-Etherton, P.M. Plantprotein and animal proteins: Do they differentially affect cardiovascular disease risk? *Adv. Nutr.* **2015**, *6*, 712–728. [CrossRef] [PubMed]
71. Newgard, C.B. Interplay between lipids and branched-chain amino acids in development of insulin resistance. *Cell Metab.* **2012**, *15*, 606–614. [CrossRef] [PubMed]
72. Wittenbecher, C.; Muhlenbruch, K.; Kroger, J.; Jacobs, S.; Kuxhaus, O.; Floegel, A.; Fritsche, A.; Pischon, T.; Prehn, C.; Adamski, J.; et al. Amino acids, lipid metabolites, and ferritin as potential mediators linking red meat consumption to type 2 diabetes. *Am. J. Clin. Nutr.* **2015**, *101*, 1241–1250. [CrossRef] [PubMed]
73. Stamler, J.; Brown, I.J.; Daviglus, M.L.; Chan, Q.; Miura, K.; Okuda, N.; Ueshima, H.; Zhao, L.; Elliott, P. Dietary glycine and blood pressure: The international study on macro/micronutrients and blood pressure. *Am. J. Clin. Nutr.* **2013**, *98*, 136–145. [CrossRef] [PubMed]
74. Jennings, A.; MacGregor, A.; Welch, A.; Chowienczyk, P.; Spector, T.; Cassidy, A. Amino acid intakes are inversely associated with arterial stiffness and central blood pressure in women. *J. Nutr.* **2015**, *145*, 2130–2138. [CrossRef] [PubMed]
75. Azadbakht, L.; Atabak, S.; Esmaillzadeh, A. Soy protein intake, cardiorenal indices, and C-reactive protein in type 2 diabetes with nephropathy: A longitudinal randomized clinical trial. *Diabetes Care* **2008**, *31*, 648–654. [CrossRef] [PubMed]
76. Wheeler, M.L.; Fineberg, S.E.; Fineberg, N.S.; Gibson, R.G.; Hackward, L.L. Animal versus plant protein meals in individuals with type 2 diabetesand microalbuminuria: Effects on renal, glycemic, and lipid parameters. *Diabetes Care* **2002**, *25*, 1277–1282. [CrossRef] [PubMed]
77. Sucher, S.; Markova, M.; Hornemann, S.; Pivovarova, O.; Rudovich, N.; Thomann, R.; Schneeweiss, R.; Rohn, S.; Pfeiffer, A.F. Compar ison of the effects of diets high in animal or plantprotein on metaboli c and cardiov ascular markers in type 2diabetes: A randomize clinical trial. *Diabetes Obes. Metab.* **2017**, *19*, 944–952. [CrossRef] [PubMed]
78. Mozaffarian, D.; Hao, T.; Rimm, E.B.; Willett, W.C.; Hu, F.B. Changes in diet and lifestyle and long-term weight gain in women and men. *N. Engl. J. Med.* **2011**, *364*, 2392–2404. [CrossRef] [PubMed]

79. Bernstein, A.M.; Pan, A.; Rexrode, K.M.; Stampfer, M.; Hu, F.B.; Mozaffarian, D.; Willett, W.C. Dietary protein sources and the risk of stroke in men and women. *Stroke* **2012**, *43*, 637–644. [CrossRef] [PubMed]
80. Bernstein, A.M.; Sun, Q.; Hu, F.B.; Stampfer, M.J.; Manson, J.E.; Willett, W.C. Major dietary protein sources and risk of coronary heart disease in women. *Circulation* **2010**, *122*, 876–883. [CrossRef] [PubMed]
81. Pan, A.; Sun, Q.; Bernstein, A.M.; Schulze, M.B.; Manson, J.E.; Stampfer, M.J.; Willett, W.C.; Hu, F.B. Red meat consumption and mortality: Results from 2 prospective cohort studies. *Arch. Intern. Med.* **2012**, *172*, 555–563. [PubMed]
82. Pan, A.; Sun, Q.; Bernstein, A.M.; Schulze, M.B.; Manson, J.E.; Willett, W.C.; Hu, F.B. Red meat consumption and risk of type 2 diabetes: 3 cohorts of U.S. adults and an updated meta-analysis. *Am. J. Clin. Nutr.* **2011**, *94*, 1088–1096. [CrossRef] [PubMed]
83. Forouhi, N.G.; Harding, A.H.; Allison, M.; Sandhu, M.S.; Welch, A.; Luben, R.; Bingham, S.; Khaw, K.T.; Wareham, N.J. Elevated serum ferritin levels predict new-onset type 2 diabetes: Results from the EPIC-Norfolk prospective study. *Diabetologia* **2007**, *50*, 949–956. [CrossRef] [PubMed]
84. Shi, Z.; Yuan, B.; Zhang, C.; Zhou, M.; Holmboe-Ottesen, G. Egg consumption and the risk of diabetes in adults, Jiangsu, China. *Nutrition* **2011**, *27*, 194–198. [CrossRef] [PubMed]
85. Radzeviciene, L.; Ostrauskas, R. Egg consumption and the risk of type 2 diabetes mellitus: A case-control study. *Public Health Nutr.* **2012**, *15*, 1437–1441. [CrossRef] [PubMed]
86. Expert Panel on Detection, Evaluation, and Treatment of High Blood Cholesterol in Adults. Executive summary of the third report of the National Cholesterol Education Program (NCEP) Expert Panel on detection, evaluation, and treatment of high blood cholesterol in adults (Adult Treatment Panel III). *JAMA* **2001**, *285*, 2486–2497.
87. Grundy, S.; Becker, D.; Clark, L.T.; Cooper, R.S.; Denke, M.A.; Howard, J.; Hunninghake, D.B.; Illingworth, D.R.; Luepker, R.V.; McBride, P.; et al. Third report of the National Cholesterol Education Program (NCEP) Expert Panel on detection, evaluation, and treatment of high blood cholesterol in adults (Adult Treatment Panel III) Final Report. *Circulation* **2002**, *106*, 3143.
88. Krauss, R.M.; Deckelbaum, R.J.; Ernst, N.; Fisher, E.; Howard, B.V.; Knopp, R.H.; Kotchen, T.; Lichtenstein, A.H.; McGill, H.C.; Pearson, T.A.; et al. Dietary guidelines for healthy American adults. A statement for health professionals from the Nutrition Committee, American heart association. *Circulation* **1996**, *94*, 1795–1800. [CrossRef] [PubMed]
89. Luhovyy, B.L.; Akhavan, T.; Anderson, G.H. Whey proteins in the regulation of food intake and satiety. *J. Am. Coll. Nutr.* **2007**, *26*, 704S–712S. [CrossRef] [PubMed]
90. Kuroda, M.; Sakaue, H. Role of vitamin D and calciumin obesity and type 2 diabetes. *Clin. Calcium* **2016**, *26*, 349–354. [PubMed]
91. Berr, C.; Akbaraly, T.; Arnaud, J.; Hininger, I.; Roussel, A.M.; Gateau, P.B. Increased selenium intake in elderly high fish consumers may account for health benefits previously ascribed to omega-3 fatty acids. *J. Nutr. Health Aging* **2009**, *13*, 14–18. [CrossRef] [PubMed]
92. Bleys, J.; Navas-Acien, A.; Guallar, E. Serum selenium and diabetes in U.S. adults. *Diabetes Care* **2007**, *30*, 829–834. [CrossRef] [PubMed]
93. Bhathena, S.J.; Velasquez, M.T. Beneficial role of dietary phytoestrogens in obesity and diabetes. *Am. J. Clin. Nutr.* **2002**, *76*, 1191–1201. [PubMed]
94. Jayagopal, V.; Albertazzi, P.; Kilpatrick, E.S.; Howarth, E.M.; Jennings, P.E.; Hepburn, D.A.; Atkin, S.L. Beneficial effects of soy phytoestrogen intake in postmenopausal women with type 2 diabetes. *Diabetes Care* **2002**, *25*, 1709–1714. [CrossRef] [PubMed]

4

Dose-Response Relationship between Dietary Magnesium Intake and Risk of Type 2 Diabetes Mellitus

Xin Fang [1,*,†], Hedong Han [2,†], Mei Li [3], Chun Liang [3], Zhongjie Fan [4], Jan Aaseth [5,6], Jia He [2,*], Scott Montgomery [7,8,9] and Yang Cao [1,7]

[1] Unit of Biostatistics, Institute of Environmental Medicine, Karolinska Institutet, Stockholm 17177, Sweden; yang.cao@ki.se
[2] Department of Health Statistics, Second Military Medical University, Shanghai 200433, China; he_dong1102@126.com
[3] Department of Cardiology, Shanghai Changzheng Hospital, Second Military Medical University, Shanghai 200003, China; happyxiaoant@126.com (M.L.); chunliangliang@hotmail.com (C.L.)
[4] Department of Cardiology, Peking Union Medical College Hospital, Peking Union Medical College, Chinese Academy of Medical Sciences, Beijing 100730, China; Fan@pumch.cn
[5] Faculty of Public Health, Hedmark University of Applied Sciences, Elverum 2411, Norway; jaol-aas@online.no
[6] Innlandet Hospital Trust, Kongsvinger Hospital Division, Kongsvinger 2226, Norway
[7] Clinical Epidemiology and Biostatistics, School of Medical Sciences, Örebro University, Örebro 70182, Sweden; scott.montgomery@regionorebrolan.se
[8] Clinical Epidemiology Unit, Karolinska University Hospital, Karolinska Institutet, Stockholm 17177, Sweden
[9] Department of Epidemiology and Public Health, University College London, London WC1E 6BT, UK
* Correspondence: xin.fang@ki.se (X.F.); hejia63@yeah.net (J.H.)

† These authors contributed equally to this work.

Abstract: The epidemiological evidence for a dose-response relationship between magnesium intake and risk of type 2 diabetes mellitus (T2D) is sparse. The aim of the study was to summarize the evidence for the association of dietary magnesium intake with risk of T2D and evaluate the dose-response relationship. We conducted a systematic review and meta-analysis of prospective cohort studies that reported dietary magnesium intake and risk of incident T2D. We identified relevant studies by searching major scientific literature databases and grey literature resources from their inception to February 2016. We included cohort studies that provided risk ratios, i.e., relative risks (RRs), odds ratios (ORs) or hazard ratios (HRs), for T2D. Linear dose-response relationships were assessed using random-effects meta-regression. Potential nonlinear associations were evaluated using restricted cubic splines. A total of 25 studies met the eligibility criteria. These studies comprised 637,922 individuals including 26,828 with a T2D diagnosis. Compared with the lowest magnesium consumption group in the population, the risk of T2D was reduced by 17% across all the studies; 19% in women and 16% in men. A statistically significant linear dose-response relationship was found between incremental magnesium intake and T2D risk. After adjusting for age and body mass index, the risk of T2D incidence was reduced by 8%–13% for per 100 mg/day increment in dietary magnesium intake. There was no evidence to support a nonlinear dose-response relationship between dietary magnesium intake and T2D risk. The combined data supports a role for magnesium in reducing risk of T2D, with a statistically significant linear dose-response pattern within the reference dose range of dietary intake among Asian and US populations. The evidence from Europe and black people is limited and more prospective studies are needed for the two subgroups.

Keywords: magnesium; dietary intake; type 2 diabetes; prospective study; cohort study; meta-analysis

1. Introduction

Type 2 diabetes mellitus (T2D) represents a growing public health burden across the world and is a leading cause of death. In 2013, an estimated 340 million people worldwide had T2D and this number is expected to increase to 400 million or more by 2030 [1,2]. Obesity and diet are widely believed to play an important role in the development of T2D [3,4]. Magnesium is the most abundant divalent intracellular cation, the second most abundant cellular ion next to potassium and the fourth cation in general in the human body. Of the 21–28 g of magnesium present in the adult human body, 99% is distributed in the intracellular compartment, and only 1% in the extracellular fluid [5]. Magnesium has received considerable interest for its potential in improving insulin sensitivity and preventing diabetes [6–9]. T2D is often accompanied by altered magnesium status. An increased prevalence of magnesium deficit has been identified in T2D patients, especially in those with poorly controlled glycemic profiles, longer duration of disease and the presence of micro- and macro-vascular chronic complications [10–12]. A number of prospective cohort studies of magnesium intake and diabetes incidence have been conducted [7,13–24] and statistically significant negative associations between magnesium intake and risk of T2D were reported in previous meta-analyses [25–27]. However, these meta-analyses did not examine whether the association was confounded by other established risk factors such as being overweight and other factors highly associated with magnesium intake, such as amount of cereal fiber, and whether the relationship is linear.

During the past few years, the number of studies on this topic has increased. With mounting evidence, we conducted a meta-analysis of prospective cohort studies for the following purpose: (1) to update the epidemiological evidence on the association between magnesium intake and T2D risk; (2) to evaluate the association according to characteristics of study designs and population; and (3) to examine the linear and nonlinear dose-response pattern of magnesium intake and T2D risk.

2. Materials and Methods

The protocol for this systematic review was registered in the PROSPERO database of prospectively registered systematic reviews in February 2016 (www.crd.york.ac.uk/PROSPERO; CRD42016033519). The completed review conforms to the standard criteria PRISMA (Preferred Reporting Items for Systematic Reviews and Meta-Analysis) and MOOSE (Meta-analysis of Observational Studies in Epidemiology) [28,29].

2.1. Data Sources and Searches

We conducted a systematic review for all population-based studies that evaluated the association of magnesium intake with T2D. We searched Pubmed (http://www.ncbi.nlm.nih.gov/), Web of Science (http://webofscience.com/), ScienceDirect (http://www.sciencedirect.com/) and China Knowledge Resource Integrated Database (http://oversea.cnki.net/kns55/default.aspx) and the Cochrane Library (http://www.cochranelibrary.com/) from their inception to 29 February, 2016. The later cut-off date to 30 June 2016 was subsequently revised to include the latest published studies. To avoid publication bias, we also used the National Library of Medicine Gateway (https://gateway.nlm.nih.gov/), Virtual Health Library (http://pesquisa.bvsalud.org/portal/), the System for Information on Grey Literature in Europe (http://www.opengrey.eu/), the National Academic Research and Collaborations Information System (http://www.narcis.nl/?Language=en) and Grey Literature Report (www.greylit.org) to find potential unpublished relevant studies. Key search terms included magnesium intake, type 2 diabetes, diabetes mellitus, prospective study, longitudinal study, cohort study, and nested case-control study, combined with incidence or risk. These searches were supplemented by hand-searching of the reference lists of identified research articles or relevant reviews. No language restrictions were imposed.

2.2. *Inclusion Criteria*

We only included original research in this meta-analysis. Reviews, editorials, commentaries and letters were not eligible. All population-based cohort studies (including nested case-control studies) were included if they fulfilled the following criteria: (1) had a prospective study design; (2) the doses of magnesium intake (dietary and supplemental) were reported; (3) the endpoint of interest was incidence of T2D; (4) the risk ratio was reported such as relative risk (RR), odds ratio (OR) or hazard ratio (HR), as well as the associated 95% confidence interval (CI) or other data to estimate the variance or accuracy (standard deviation or standard error) were reported; (5) the risk assessment had to be adjusted for potential confounding factors or by other forms of standardization (if applicable). For multiple studies using the same population, only the study with the largest number of events or with adjustment for additional potential confounders was included. Studies were excluded if they: (1) focused on the populations with disrupted mineral homeostasis (such as patients with heart failure or kidney disease); (2) were narrative reviews, editorial papers, methodological papers, experimental studies, case control or cross-sectional; (3) assessed type 1 diabetes; (4) identified a dietary pattern that did not fit into healthy or unhealthy dietary pattern categories; (5) evaluated magnesium only in drinking water or had no reliable magnesium estimates. For included studies only in abstract form, we tried to contact authors to obtain the necessary estimates or risks and relevant accuracy.

2.3. *Quality Assessment and Data Extraction*

Computerized bibliographic searches of pre-determined literature databases used an optimized version of the Cochrane Collaboration search strategy [30]. Three investigators (X.F., C.L. and M.L.) screened all the identified titles and abstracts for relevance ($n = 2858$). Full papers were downloaded for all the abstracts judged potentially relevant ($n = 60$). No new studies were identified among the cited references of all included articles. Of 60 full-text articles reviewed independently, we excluded 35 studies for the following reasons: they were not prospective studies ($n = 14$); outcomes were not T2D ($n = 9$); did not report dietary magnesium ($n = 7$); did not assess the risk ($n = 3$); or duplicated another study ($n = 1$). All papers identified through the screening process were assessed for relevance independently by two investigators (C.L. and M.L.) using standardized study assessment and a sorting form. The studies were evaluated and scored based on the guidelines adapted from the tools for assessing quality and susceptibility to bias in observational studies in epidemiology [31]. Inter-rater agreement was substantial (Cohen $\kappa > 0.6$) [32]. No studies were excluded by the quality assessment. In total, 25 studies met the inclusion criteria and were included in the meta-analysis.

Full papers were obtained for all abstracts judged potentially relevant. Data extraction was conducted independently by two investigators (X.F. and M.L.) with the use of a standardized electronic form in Microsoft Excel. The following data were extracted from each study: first author's surname; study design; location; year the study started, finished and was published; age; sex; ethnicity; sample size (number of those with T2D and the total number of participants); diseases present at baseline (hypertension or hypercholesterolemia, etc.); magnesium intake modes (dietary or supplemental) and dose; as well as covariates adjusted for in the multivariable analysis. For magnesium intake, data on assessment method used (food frequency questionnaire, dietary recall, other) and whether the data were energy-adjusted (yes, no) were obtained. For each study, the median magnesium intake for each quantile (tertile, quartile or quintile) of magnesium intake was assigned as the representative dose. When the median intake per quantile was not provided, we assigned the midpoint of lower and upper boundaries in each quantile as the average intake. If the lower or upper boundary for the lowest or highest quantile, respectively, was not reported, we assumed that the boundary has the same amplitude as the closest quantile. The increment of dietary magnesium intake was calculated as the difference between the representative dose of the higher quantiles and the representative dose of the control quantile.

For each dose quantile, we extracted RR, OR or HR with their measure of uncertainty (standard error) or variance (95% CI). Risk estimates for continuous exposure were also extracted. If estimates were presented for more than one multivariate model, we only extracted estimates from the model maximally adjusted for potential confounding variables to ensure a conservative conclusion. Because there are studies based on the same cohort but conducted at different times, they shared the T2D patients. When we calculated the total participants and T2D cases, we only used the studies with the largest numbers.

2.4. Statistical Analysis

We used OR and HR as RR in our pooled analysis because when event rates are small, the OR, HR and RR approximate one another [33]. We estimated a pooled risk with 95% CI for a 100 mg/day increase in daily magnesium intake for the studies. To maximize all the data for calculating the pooled dose-response, the restricted maximum likelihood (REML) approach proposed by Harbord [34], which provides improved estimation of the between-study variance, was used to compute the linear trend of the log transformed risk estimates across magnesium intake doses. We also performed subgroup analysis by level of magnesium intake increment, sex, geographic area and adjustment.

The Higgins's I^2 statistic, a quantitative measure of inconsistency, was calculated to evaluate the statistical heterogeneity across the studies [35]. $I^2 > 30\%$ was considered as at least moderate heterogeneity. In view of substantial heterogeneity being detected, we presented the pooled estimates based on the random-effects model.

Potential publication bias was assessed by Egger's test [36]. Because the sample sizes of reference groups and comparative groups were balanced in all the studies, we used Harbord's modification to Egger's test to reduce the false-positive rate [37]. The results were also confirmed by Begg's test [38] and Peters's test [39].

Potential nonlinear associations were assessed using restricted cubic splines; we used four knots at fixed percentiles 5%, 35%, 65% and 95% of the distribution [40]. The study-specific estimates were pooled by using the REML method in a random-effects meta-analysis [41].

We also conducted a sensitivity analysis to investigate the influence of a single study on the overall risk estimate by dropping one study in each turn. We performed all analyses in Stata (version 14.1; Stata Corp., College Station, TX, USA). A p value < 0.05 was considered statistically significant, except where otherwise specified.

3. Results

3.1. Eligible Studies and Characteristics

Our literature search identified 25 studies from 17 cohorts that met the eligibility criteria (Figure 1). These studies were published between 1997 and 2014 and comprised 637,922 individuals and 26,828 T2D cases after excluding duplicated cohorts (Table 1). There were 16 studies conducted in the U.S. (including Hawaii), two in Europe (Italy and Germany), and seven in Asia (five in Japan and two in China). Studies treated dietary calcium [42–44], red/processed meat [45,46], whole grain [47], fiber [14,15,48], vitamin D [43,44], carbohydrates [14], coffee [49] or glycemic load [15,48,50] as main exposures, but also reported dietary magnesium intakes which were included in our meta-analysis. The main endpoints of two studies were impaired insulin metabolism [7] and insulin resistance [22], but both studies also reported the incidence of T2D. Participants were predominately middle-aged at baseline, with a mean age of 51.2 years and a mean BMI of 25.0 kg/m^2 across the studies. The length of the follow-up period ranged from four to 20 years.

Dietary intake of magnesium was evaluated by food frequency questionnaires (FFQs) in all the studies and 13 studies indicated that the questionnaires were validated. The median magnesium intake of the different dose groups ranged from 115 mg/day in U.S. black women [18] (much lower than the US Recommended Dietary Allowance of 400 mg/day for men and 310 magnesium for women >30 years [51]) to 478 mg/day in a U.S. population [22]. T2D was ascertained by self-report and 21 studies indicated that the self-reported diagnoses were validated.

For the 16 studies with the magnesium as the main exposure, although the degree of covariate and confounder adjustment varied in the multivariate models, most studies adjusted for age, body mass index (BMI), total energy intake, smoking, physical activity, family history of diabetes and hypertension; fewer studies adjusted for intake of calcium or other nutrition supplement and education attainment. For the nine studies with other nutrients as main exposure, only crude RRs were extracted.

Table 1. Characteristics of 25 cohort studies providing risk estimates for dietary magnesium intake and T2D incidence.

First Author, Year, Study, Country	No. of Case (Cohort Size)	Years of Follow-Up	Dietary Assessment Method	Case Ascertainment	Sex, Mean Age at Baseline (Years)	Magnesium Intake (Magnesium/Day) for Highest vs. the Lowest Quantile [RR (95% CI)]	Confounders Adjusted for
Hruby, 2014, FHSO, U.S. [7]	179 (2582)	7	Validated FFQ	Validated self-report	M and F, 53.9	395 vs. 236 (0.49 (0.27, 0.88))	Age, sex, energy intake, family history of diabetes, BMI, physical activity, smoking, alcohol, hypertension, dietary fiber
Oba, 2013, JPHCPS, Japan [50]	Men: 690 (27,769)	5	Validated FFQ	Validated self-report	M: 56.5	349 vs. 232 (0.85 (0.69, 1.06))	Crude *
	Women: 500 (36,864)				F: 56.9	356 vs. 211 (0.69 (0.54, 0.88))	
Hata, 2013, Hisayama, Japan [52]	417 (1999)	15.6	FFQ	Self-report	M and F, 57.0	215 vs. 133 (0.63 (0.44, 0.90))	Age, sex, family history of diabetes, BMI. HDL cholesterol, triglycerides, hypertension, smoking, alcohol, physical activity, total energy intake, carbohydrate, crude fiber, saturated fatty acid, polyunsaturated fatty acid and vitamin C
Weng, 2012, CVDFACTS, Taiwan [53]	141 (1604)	4.6	Validated FFQ	Self-report	M and F, 50.0	406 vs. 212 (0.38 (0.21, 0.70))	Age, sex, caloric intake, residential area, family history of diabetes, BMI, education, smoking, alcohol, physical activity, hypertension, hypercholesterolemia, hypertriglyceridemia, low HDL-cholesterol
Hopping, 2010, MEC, Hawaii [21]	Men: 4555 (36,255)	14	FFQ	Validated self-report	M: 57.4	185 vs. 129 (0.77 (0.70, 0.85))	Ethnicity, BMI, physical activity, education, calories
	Women: 4032 (39,255)				F: 57.2	200 vs. 139 (0.84 (0.76, 0.93))	
Kirii, 2010, JACC, Japan [23]	Men: 237 (6480)	5	Validated FFQ	Validated self-report	M: 53.3	323 vs. 156 (0.64 (0.44, 0.91))	Age, BMI, family history of diabetes, smoking, alcohol, physical activity, green tea, coffee, total energy intake
	Women: 222 (11,112)				F: 53.1	298 vs. 159 (0.68 (0.33, 0.75))	
Nanri, 2010, JPHCPS, Japan [24]	Men: 634 (25,872)	5	FFQ	Validated self-report	M: 56.5	348 vs. 213 (0.86 (0.63, 1.16))	Age, study area, BMI, smoking, alcohol, family history of diabetes, physical activity, hypertension, coffee, calcium intake, total energy intake
	Women: 480 (33,919)				F: 57.3	333 vs. 213 (0.92 (0.66, 1.28))	
Kim, 2010, CARDIA, U.S. [22]	330 (4497)	20	Validated FFQ	Validated self-report	M and F, 24.9	478 vs. 362 (0.53 (0.32, 0.86))	Age, sex, ethnicity, study center, education, smoking, alcohol, physical activity, family history of diabetes, BMI, blood pressure, total energy intake, saturated fat, crude fiber
Kirri, 2009, JPHCPS, Japan [43]	Men: 634 (25,877)	5	FFQ	Validated self-report	M: 56.5	331 vs. 245 (0.89 (0.72, 1.10))	Crude
	Women: 480 (33,919)				F: 57.3	314 vs. 248 (0.76 (0.59, 0.98))	
Villegas, 2009, SWHS, China [20]	2270 (64,190)	7	Validated FFQ	Self-report	F: 51.0	318 vs. 214 (0.86 (0.75, 0.97))	Age, energy intake, WHR, smoking, alcohol, physical activity, income, education level, occupation, hypertension
Schulze, 2007, EPIC, Germany [19]	844 (27,550)	7	Validated FFQ	Validated self-report	M and F, 49.6	359 vs. 298 (0.75 (0.60, 0.94))	Crude
Liu, 2006, WHS, U.S. [42]	651 (14,874)	10	Validated FFQ	Validated self-report	F: 54.5	340 vs. 307 (0.88 (0.76, 1.04))	Crude
Pereira, 2006, IWHS, U.S. [49]	1415 (28,812)	11	FFQ	Validated self-report	F: 61.3	334 vs. 281 (0.60 (0.47, 0.76))	Crude

Table 1. *Cont.*

First Author, Year, Study, Country	No. of Case (Cohort Size)	Years of Follow-Up	Dietary Assessment Method	Case Ascertainment	Sex, Mean Age at Baseline (Years)	Magnesium Intake (Magnesium/Day) for Highest vs. the Lowest Quantile [RR (95% CI)]	Confounders Adjusted for
van Dam, 2006, BWHS, U.S. [18]	1964 (41,186)	8	Validated FFQ	Validated self-report	F: 38.7	244 vs. 115 (0.65 (0.54, 0.78))	Age, energy intake, BMI, smoking, alcohol, physical activity, family diabetes history, education level, calcium, coffee, sugar, soft drink, processed meat, red meat
Pittas, 2006, NHS, U.S. [44]	4843 (83,779)	20	FFQ	Validated self-report	F: 46.1	313 vs. 281 (0.79 (0.64, 0.96))	Crude
Song, 2004, WHS, U.S. [45]	708 (14,924)	8.8	Validated FFQ	Validated self-report	F: 53.9	377 vs. 305 (0.47 (0.41, 0.55))	Crude
Song 2004, WHS, U.S. [17]	918 (38,025)	6	Validated FFQ	Validated self-report	F: 53.9	399 vs. 252 (0.88 (0.71, 1.1))	Age, smoking, BMI, exercise, alcohol, family history of diabetes and total calories
Lopez-Ridaura, 2004, NHS, U.S. [16]	4085 (85,060)	18	FFQ	Validated self-report	F: 46.1	373 vs. 222 ([0.73 (0.65, 0.82))	Age, energy, family history of diabetes, BMI, physical activity, smoking, alcohol, hypertension, hypercholesterolemia, other dietary variables
Lopez-Ridaura, 2004, HPFS, U.S. [16]	1333 (42,872)	12	FFQ	Validated self-report	M: 53.3	457 vs. 270 (0.72 (0.58, 0.89))	Age, energy, family history of diabetes, BMI, physical activity, smoking, alcohol, hypertension, hypercholesterolemia, other dietary variables
Hodge, 2004, MCCS, Italy [15]	365 (31,641)	4	FFQ	Validated self-report	M and F, 54.5	Per 500 magnesium increment (0.73 (0.51, 1.04))	Age, sex, country of birth, physical activity, family history of diabetes, alcohol, education, weight change, energy intake, BMI and WHR
Schulze, 2003, NHS II, U.S. [46]	741 (92,146)	8	Validated FFQ	Validated self-report	F: 36.0	341 vs. 281 [0.26 (0.20, 0.36))	Crude
Liu, 2000, NHS, U.S. [47]	1879 (75,521)	10	Validated FFQ	Validated self-report	F: 56.5	342 vs. 248 (1.04 (0.90, 1.19))	Crude
Meyer, 2000, IWHS, U.S. [14]	1141 (35,988)	6	FFQ	Validated self-report	F: 61.5	362 vs. 220 (0.67 (0.55, 0.82))	Age, total energy intake, BMI, WTH ratio, education, smoking, alcohol intake, physical activity
Kao, 1999, ARIC, U.S. [13]	White people: 739 (9506)	6	FFQ	Validated self-report	M and F, 54.2	418 vs. 308 (1.25 (0.88, 0.1.78))	Age, sex education, family history of diabetes, BMI, WHR, physical activity, alcohol, diuretic use, dietary calcium, potassium, fasting insulin and glucose
	Black people: 367 (2622)				M and F, 53.0	374 vs. 264 (1.05 (0.58, 1.93))	
Salmeron, 1997, HPFS, U.S. [48]	523 (42,759)	6	FFQ	Validated self-report	M: 53.3	461 vs. 262 (0.72 (0.54, 0.96))	Age, BMI, alcohol, smoking, physical activity, family history of diabetes
Salmeron, 1997, NHS, U.S. [54]	915 (65,173)	6	FFQ	Validated self-report	F: 46.1	338 vs. 222 (0.62 (0.50, 0.78))	Age, BMI, alcohol, smoking, physical activity, family history of diabetes

* Simple risk ratio without any adjustment.

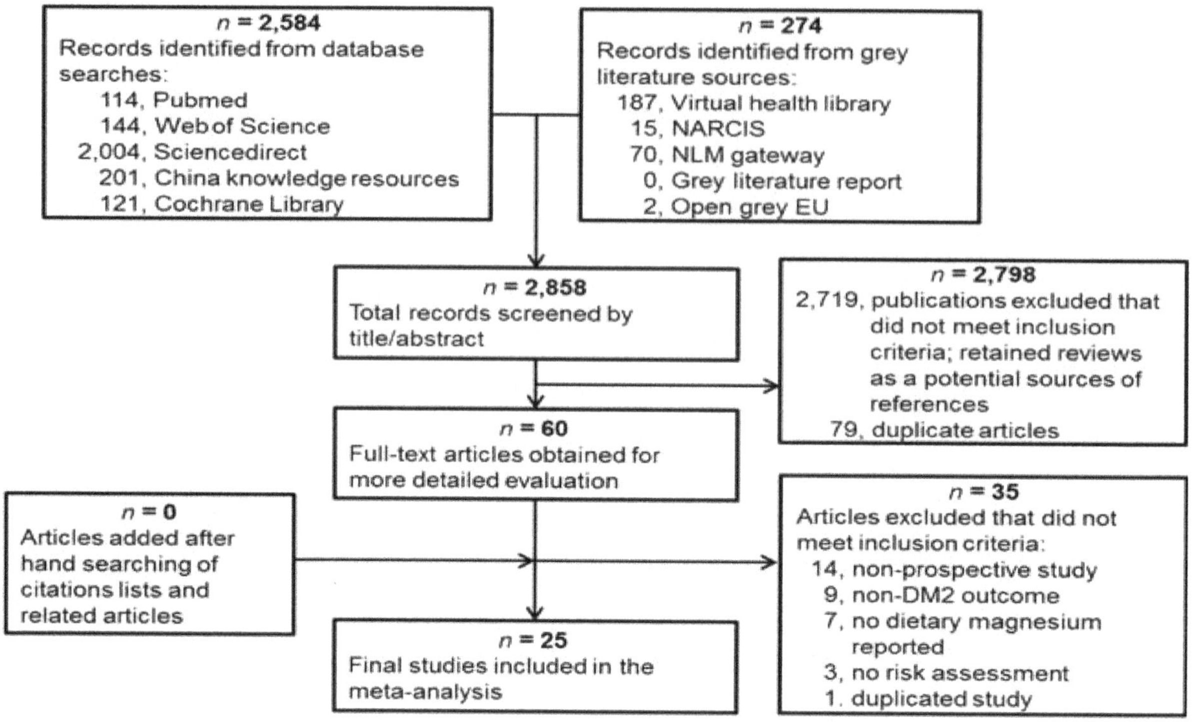

Figure 1. Screening and selection of articles on dietary magnesium intake and risk of type 2 diabetes mellitus.

3.2. *Dietary Magnesium Intake and Type 2 Diabetes Mellitus (T2D) Incidence*

We divided the increment of dietary magnesium intake into four categories, i.e., <50 mg/day, 50–99 mg/day, 100–149 mg/day and ≥150 mg/day, by subtracting the reference doses from the compared doses. Heterogeneity was found by Higgins's test, with $I^2 = 73.3\%$ ($p < 0.001$) for all compared doses, and 67.2% ($p < 0.001$), 75.0% ($p < 0.001$), 52.3% ($p = 0.005$) and 54.5% ($p = 0.031$) for four increment categories, respectively. However, the approximately symmetric funnel plot of all but four doses suggests a moderate homogeneity among the studies (Figure 2). Although there is evidence of publication bias among all compared doses for Egger's test ($p = 0.002$), Begg's, Harbord's and Peters's tests show no evidence of publication bias ($p = 0.170$, 0.401 and 0.105, respectively).

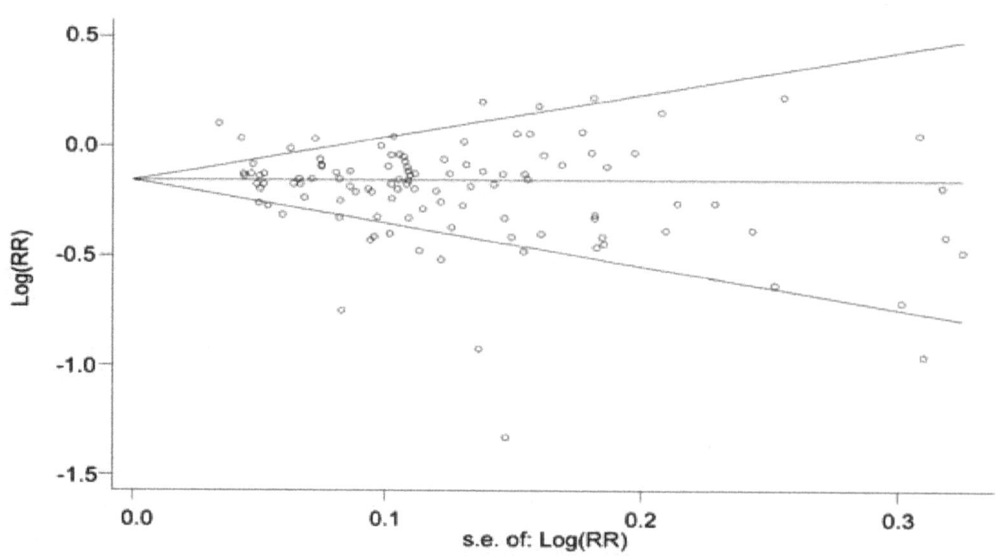

Figure 2. Funnel plot with pseudo 95% confidence limits.

The overall combined RR for T2D incidence is 0.83 (95% CI: 0.80, 0.86; $p < 0.001$) for all compared doses. The results of subgroup analysis are presented in Table 2. A statistically significant negative association between dietary magnesium and risk of T2D incidence was observed across sexes and the pooled RRs are 0.81 (95% CI: 0.77, 0.86) for women, 0.84 (95% CI: 0.80, 0.88) for men, and 0.85 (95% CI: 0.78, 0.94) for the studies that only reported sex-combined risk estimates. The association was statistically significant in all the study areas and the largest magnitude association was found among U.S. studies (pooled RR = 0.82 in U.S. vs. 0.86 in Europe and 0.85 in Asia), compared with the unadjusted associations (pooled RR = 0.81; 95% CI: 0.74, 0.88), with lower magnitude after adjustment (pooled RR = 0.83; 95% CI: 0.81, 0.86). Two studies investigated the association specially in black people and showed a statistically significant association (pooled RR = 0.82; 95% CI: 0.71, 0.94), however, it seems this is mainly observed among black women [18] rather than black men [13].

Table 2. Pooled RRs * for T2D incidence of increased dietary magnesium intake by sex, area and adjustment.

Subgroup	No. of Studies (Dose Quantiles)	RR (95% CI)	I^2 (%)	Heterogeneity-p
Sex				
Women	17 (58)	0.814 (0.774, 0.856)	82.4	<0.001
Men	7 (25)	0.838 (0.803, 0.876)	25.7	0.120
Both	7 (26)	0.854 (0.775, 0.941)	46.7	0.005
Area				
U.S.	16 (67)	0.817 (0.780, 0.857)	81.7	<0.001
Europe	2 (5)	0.858 (0.774, 0.951)	0	0.498
Asia	7 (37)	0.846 (0.811, 0.883)	10.2	0.294
Adjustment				
Adjusted †	16 (76)	0.830 (0.806, 0.855)	39.6	<0.001
Crude ‡	9 (33)	0.808 (0.741, 0.881)	87.8	<0.001
Black people	2 (7)	0.815 (0.711, 0.935)	59.3	0.022

* Random-effects model was used; † Adjusted for age, BMI, energy intake, smoking, alcohol, physical activity, calcium, sugar, soft drink, red meat family and/or other dietary intakes, and/or family history, sociodemographic factors; ‡ Simple risk ratio without any adjustment.

The dose-category-specific pooled RRs for T2D incidence from the included studies are shown in Figure 3a–d, which are 0.88 (95% CI: 0.85, 0.92), 0.81 (95% CI: 0.76, 0.86), 0.77 (95% CI: 0.70, 0.83) and 0.72 (95% CI: 0.61, 0.84) for increment <50 mg/day, 50–99 mg/day, 100–149 mg/day and ≥150 mg/day, respectively. In general, the RR decreases 4% to 7% per 50 mg/day increment (equivalent to 8% to 14% per 100 mg/day increment) in dietary magnesium intake.

3.3. Linear Dose-Response Relationship

After adjusting for age and BMI in random-effects meta-regression models, a statistically significant linear dose-response relationship between incremental dietary magnesium intake and T2D incidence was found across all the studies (see Table 3 and Figure 4). The RRs (95% CI) for the association of a 100 mg/day increment in dietary magnesium intake with T2D incidence are 0.92 (95% CI: 0.85, 0.99) and 0.88 (0.80, 0.97) for including and excluding one extreme dose, respectively. The statistically significant linear dose-response relationship was also found for men (RR = 0.87; 95% CI: 0.77, 0.98) but not for women (RR = 0.88; 95% CI = 0.76, 1.02). Regarding study areas, significantly linear dose-response relationship was only found in Asia (RR = 0.87; 95% CI: 0.77, 0.98). No significant linear dose-response relationship was found in black people (RR = 0.75; 95% CI = 0.23, 2.41).

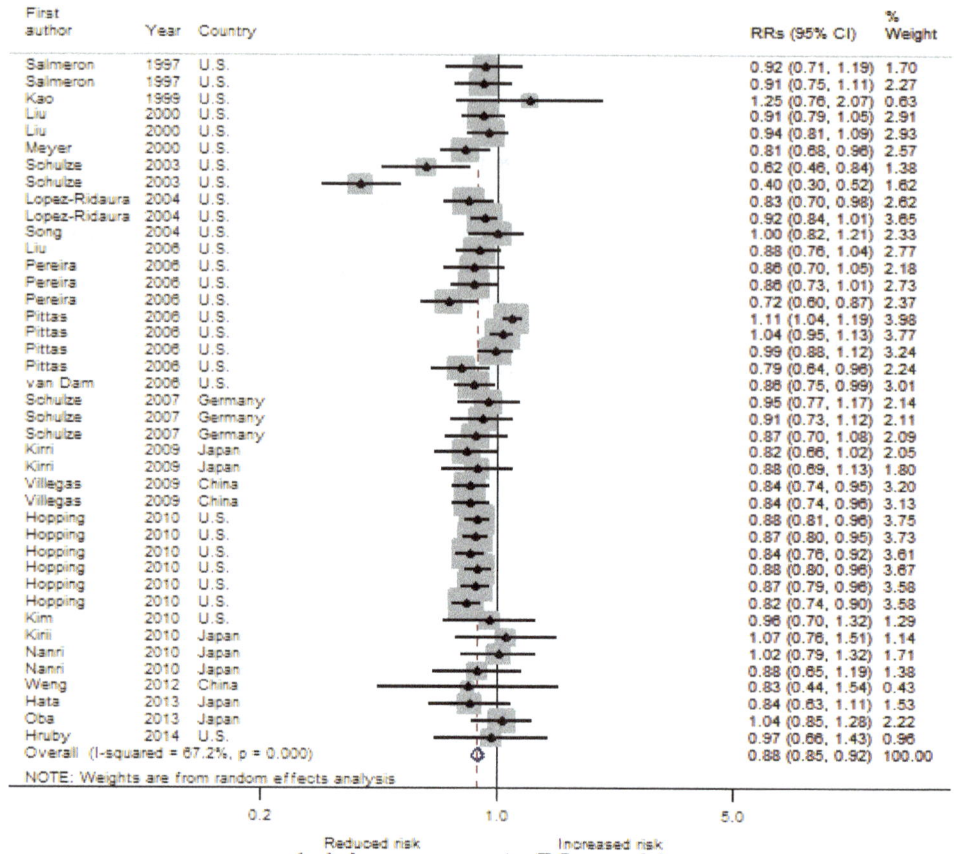

(a) Increment<50 mg/d

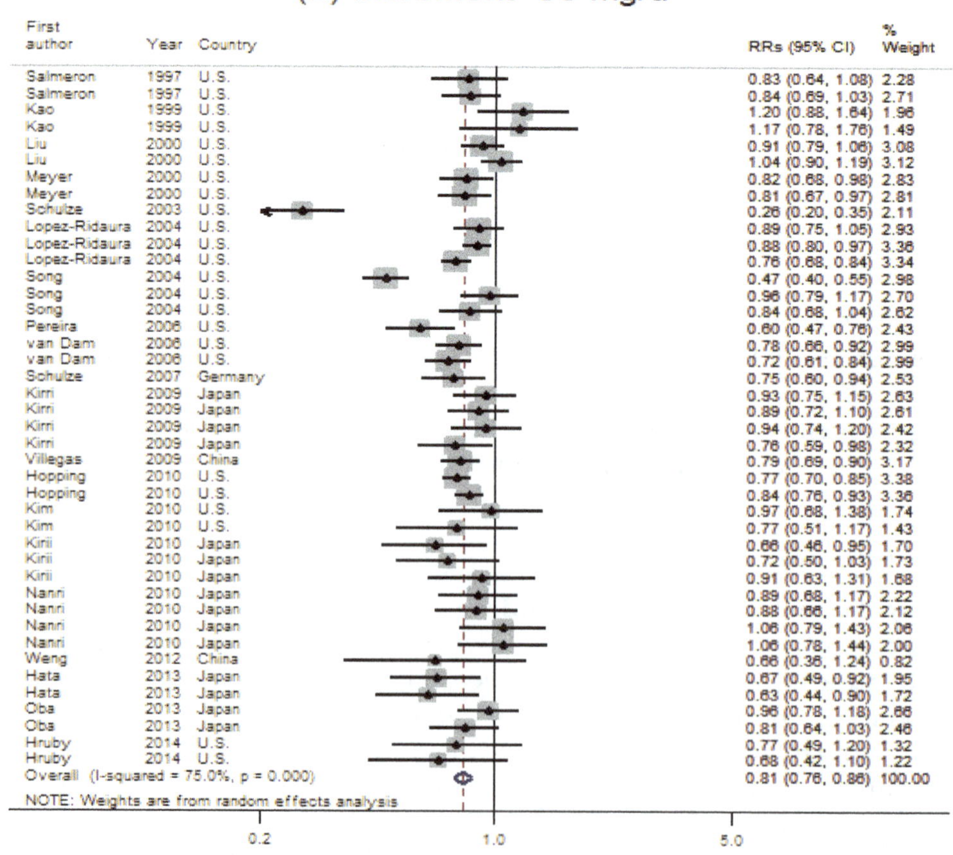

(b) Increment >=50 and <100 mg/d

Figure 3. *Cont.*

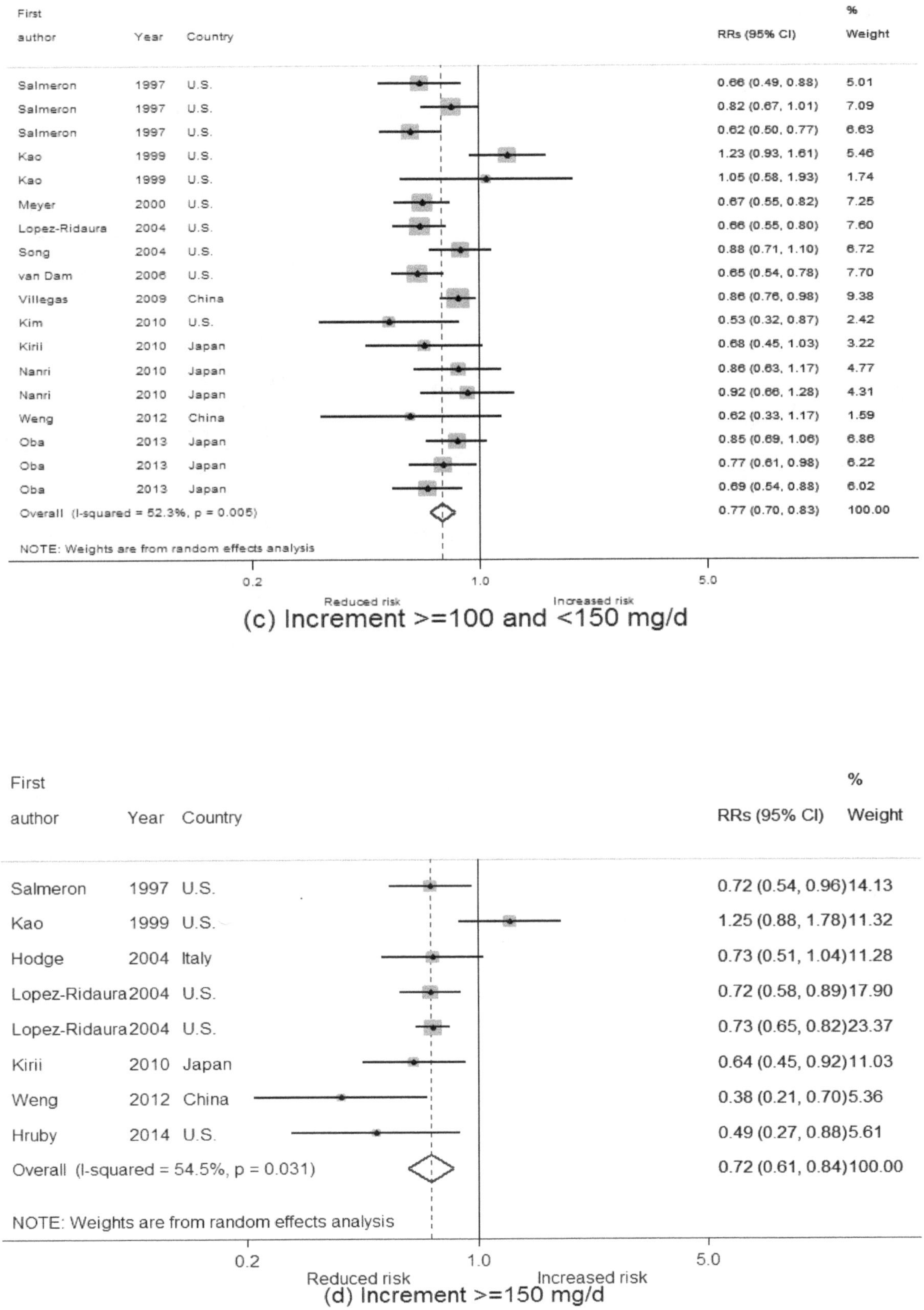

Figure 3. Relative risks (RRs) for risk of T2D incidence for different dietary magnesium increment categories: (**a**) <50 mg/day; (**b**) 50–99 mg/day; (**c**) 100–159 mg/day; (**d**) $\geq$150 mg/day.

Table 3. Estimated RRs for T2D incidence per 100 mg/day increment in dietary magnesium intake, adjusted for age and BMI.

	No. of Studies (Doses)	I^2 (%)	RR (95% CI)	*p*-Value
All studies	25 (105)	69.72	0.916 (0.852, 0.985)	0.018
All studies *	24 (104)	69.13	0.882 (0.803, 0.969)	0.010
Sex				
Women	17 (56)	78.87	0.879 (0.756, 1.023)	0.094
Men	7 (23)	0	0.865 (0.767, 0.975)	0.020
Both	7 (26)	26.51	0.935 (0.853, 1.026)	0.148
Both *	6 (25)	29.00	0.857 (0.695, 1.057)	0.141
Area				
U.S.	16 (63)	79.09	0.910 (0.796, 1.042)	0.169
Europe	2 (5)	0	1.071 (0.264, 4.351)	0.644
Europe *	1 (4)	-	-	-
Asia	7 (37)	0	0.867 (0.768, 0.978)	0.022
Adjustment				
Adjusted	16 (72)	25.73	0.911 (0.864, 0.961)	0.001
Adjusted *	15 (71)	24.09	0.885 (0.830, 0.944)	<0.001
Crude	9 (33)	85.14	0.653 (0.462, 0.924)	0.018
Black people	2 (7)	0	0.747 (0.232, 2.409)	0.486

* One extreme dose was excluded.

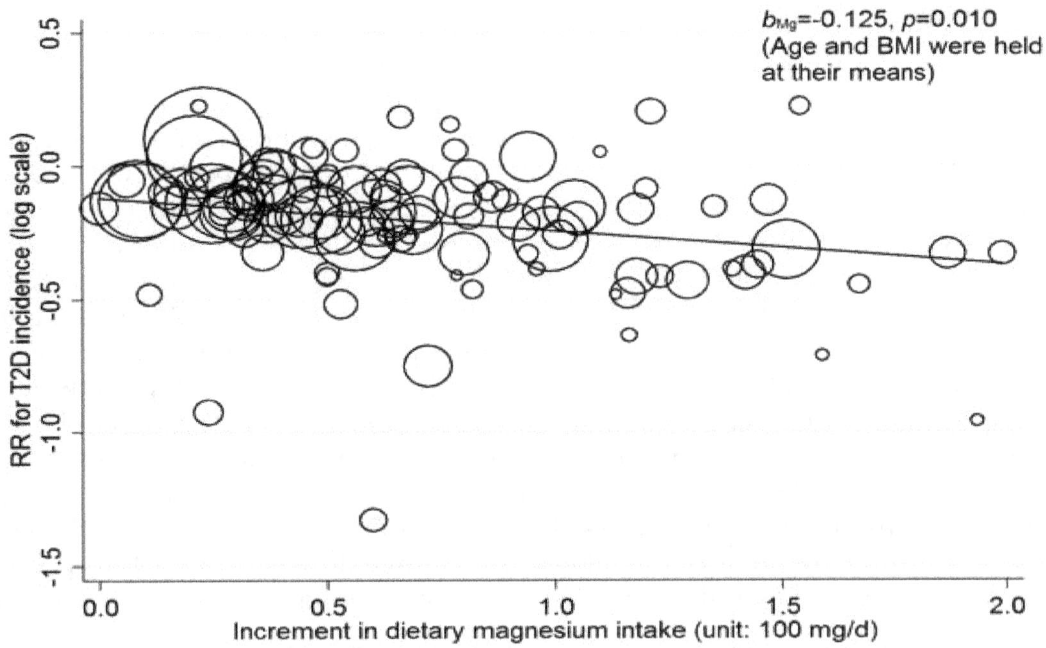

Figure 4. Dose-response relationship between risk of T2D incidence and incremental dietary magnesium intake (excluding one extreme dose). The size of the bubble reflects the study-specific analytical weight, i.e., the inverse of the variance.

In general, the risk of T2D incidence decreases by 8% (across all studies) to 13% (in the Asian population) per 100 mg/day increment in dietary magnesium intake, which is consistent with the result from dose-category-specific analysis.

3.4. Nonlinear Dose-Response Relationship

We found no evidence of nonlinear associations between dietary magnesium intake and T2D incidence across all the studies with (p = 0.665) or without (p = 0.980) one extreme dose (Figure 5), adjusting for age and BMI. For subgroup analysis, no evidence of nonlinear association was found for women (p = 0.637), men (p = 0.790), sex-combined (p = 0.987), black people (p = 0.787), U.S. population (p = 0.686), Asian population (p = 0.519), adjusted RRs (p = 0.663) and crude RRs (p = 0.250), which suggested that pooling the dose-response estimates from linear trend estimation for dietary magnesium intake and T2D incidence was appropriate. Because of insufficient dose observations, no nonlinear association was evaluated for European studies.

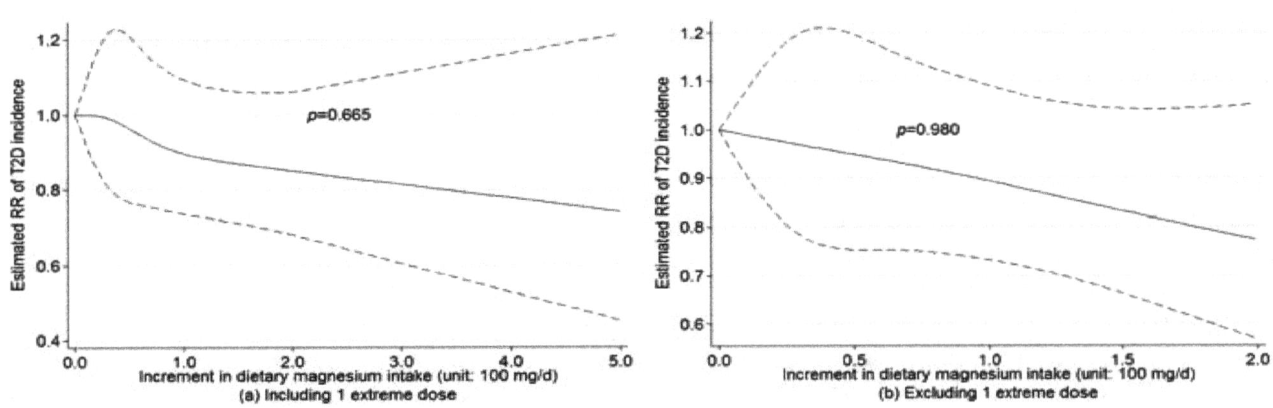

Figure 5. Examination of nonlinear association between increment in dietary magnesium intake and risk of T2D incidence by random-effects model with the use of restricted cubic splines.

3.5. Sensitivity Analysis

Regarding the combined risk of T2D incidence for all studies, the sensitivity analysis omitting one study at a time yielded statistically significant RRs within a very narrow range from 0.82 (95% CI: 0.79, 0.84) to 0.84 (95% CI: 0.81, 0.87). The subgroup analyses also showed robust results for women (RR range: 0.80, 0.84), men (RR range: 0.83, 0.85), sex-combined (RR range: 0.79, 0.88), U.S. population (RR range: 0.80, 0.84), Asian population (RR range: 0.83, 0.85), adjusted RRs (RR range: 0.82, 0.84) and crude RRs (RR range: 0.78, 0.86). However, because of a limited number of studies in Europe and black people, the sensitivity analysis generated relatively wide ranges for these two subgroups. The RR ranges were from 0.73 (95% CI: 0.51, 1.04) to 0.87 (95% CI: 0.78, 0.97) and from 0.76 (95% CI: 0.67, 0.85) to 1.17 (95% CI: 0.88, 1.54) for European studies and black people, respectively.

The sensitivity analyses for linear and nonlinear dose-response relationships between incremental dietary magnesium intake and the risk of T2D incidence show similar results. The RRs of linear dose-response relationship across all the studies are statistically significant and range from 0.88 (95% CI: 0.80, 0.97) to 0.93 (95% CI: 0.87, 1.00) when omitting one study at a time. The p-values for a nonlinear dose-response relationship across all studies range from 0.52 to 0.96 when omitting one study at a time. The results for subgroup analysis also change little except for European studies and black people (data not show). Overall, the results from sensitivity analyses indicate the robustness of our findings.

4. Discussion

This meta-analysis of 25 prospective studies showed a statistically significant negative association between dietary magnesium intake and T2D incidence. Compared with the lowest dietary magnesium consumption groups in the populations, the risk of T2D could be reduced by 19% in women and 16% in men (Table 2). The largest reduction of risk was observed for the U.S. population (18%). A statistically significant linear dose-response relationship was found between incremental dietary magnesium intake and T2D incidence across all the studies, in male and Asian populations, adjusting for age and BMI. The risk of T2D was associated with a reduction of 8%–13% per 100 g/day increment in dietary magnesium intake. After adjusting for age and BMI, we did not find a statistically significant nonlinear dose-response relationship of incremental dietary magnesium intake with T2D risk. The present systematic review, which includes a total of 637,922 participants and 26,828 T2D cases, provides the most robust evidence to date of the linear dose-response relationship between incremental dietary magnesium intake across its physiological range and risk of T2D.

4.1. Dose-Response Association of Dietary Magnesium Intake with T2D Incidence

A putative protective effect of magnesium intake against T2D incidence has been reported previously [13,14]. The negative association between magnesium intake and T2D incidence is biologically plausible and may be partially explained by its influence on glucose metabolism, insulin sensitivity and insulin action [5,6]. However, there is no conclusive evidence for the beneficial dose of dietary magnesium. For example, a meta-analysis indicated that 300 mg/day of magnesium intake was the essential dose for preventing T2D [27]. A cross-sectional study concluded that more than 300 mg/day of magnesium intake might not improve insulin sensitivity and have no influence [55]. Evidence from a prospective study showed that increased intake of magnesium might provide more benefit to participants with magnesium deficiency, as magnesium deficiency and hypomagnesaemia have been associated with the development of insulin resistance [18]. Meta-analyses of magnesium supplementation have also revealed conflicting results. A review including 12 randomized controlled trials (RCTs) assessing the efficacy of magnesium supplementation on insulin sensitivity and glucose levels included studies yielding inconsistent results [56]. However, concerning the effect of dietary magnesium intake on T2D incidence, the previous meta-analyses appeared to reach a consensus [19,25,27]. A meta-analysis of eight cohort studies showed a significant negative association (RR = 0.77; 95% CI: 0.72, 0.84). Another meta-analysis of 13 prospective cohort studies detected a significant negative association between magnesium intake and risk of T2D (RR = 0.78; 95% CI:

0.73, 0.84). A more recent meta-analysis with a total of 539,735 participants and 25,252 incident diabetes cases also indicated that magnesium intake was associated with a significant lower risk of T2D (RR = 0.77; 95% CI: 0.71, 0.82). However, there is less conclusive evidence of dose-response relationship between dietary magnesium intake and risk of T2D incidence [26]. By combining results of seven cohort studies, Larsson et al. observed a statistically significant lower risk of T2D for 100 mg/day increase in magnesium intake (RR = 0.85; 95% CI: 0.79, 0.92). Dong et al. also found a linear dose-response relationship for every 100 mg/day increment in magnesium intake (RR = 0.86; 95% CI: 0.82, 0.89) [25]. In contrast, a nonlinear relationship ($p = 0.003$) between magnesium intake and type 2 diabetes was reported by Xu et al. [27].

Our meta-analysis with a larger number of people with T2D did support existence of a statistically significant linear dose-response relationship between increased dose of dietary magnesium intake and T2D incidence among all the participants, especially in males and in Asian populations. In addition, we found no evidence of nonlinear associations between dietary magnesium intake and T2D incidence across all the studies ($p = 0.665$). The magnitude of the effect for 100 mg/day increment in magnesium intake in this meta-analysis (8%–13% reduction in risk of T2D) is comparable to those from other meta-analyses (8%–21% reduction in risk of T2D).

The discrepant findings between women and men might be due to the influence of other factors than magnesium intake. For example, the influence of magnesium on T2D incidence in women may be potentially attenuated by changed endogenous sex hormones in postmenopausal women [57,58]; which could accelerate T2D development and counteract the potentially protective influence of magnesium. The discrepancy between the Asian population and non-Asian population needs further research. However, because of the limited number of the included studies in Europe, the discrepancy may have been accidental and a chance finding cannot be ruled out.

It should be noted that our sensitivity analysis revealed robust associations for linear and nonlinear dose-response analyses among all the participants.

4.2. *Implication for Practice*

Magnesium is mainly consumed through diet, and low magnesium consumption is common worldwide. It has been estimated that magnesium intake in a normal Western diet is often inadequate for the body's needs; in the United States, 67% of women and 64% of men consume inadequate amounts of magnesium [59]. For people aged more than 30, the recommended dietary allowance (RDA) of magnesium for men and women is 350 mg/day and 420 mg/day, respectively [51]. On the basis of the studies we have reviewed, current evidence from population-based prospective cohort studies support the recommendation for increasing dietary magnesium intake.

4.3. *Strengths and Limitations*

The population-based evidence on whether increased magnesium intake may reduce T2D incidence is still sparse. To our knowledge, this study is the largest meta-analysis that investigated the dose-response relationship between dietary magnesium intake and T2D risk. It has several strengths. First, our data providing a systematic review of prospective studies represent the best available evidence of how dietary magnesium intake may influence risk of T2D incidence. Because of the lagged and cumulative effects of exposure on outcome of chronic diseases, the dose-response relationship without reversed causality would be revealed only by prospective studies rather than cross-sectional or retrospective studies. In addition, the prospective studies also minimized recall and selection bias. Second, by combining all available doses in included studies across a wide range of exposure, we increased the validity of the dose-response estimates. Our studies included 141 dietary magnesium doses and 108 risk estimates, which enabled us to estimate both linear and nonlinear dose-response relationship with a high statistical power. Third, age and BMI were adjusted for in our meta-regression model and stratified analyses were used for sex, study areas and adjustment, which reduced the potential confounding from demographic and other factors. Furthermore, the random-effects model considered the heterogeneity among studies, which resulted in a relatively conservative conclusion rather than an exaggerated one.

However, some limitations warrant consideration. First, although the majority of the studies adjusted for known risk factors for T2D incidence, such as age, BMI, smoking status, education, physical activity level and alcohol consumption, we could only retrieve age and BMI for all the studies and adjust only for them in our final model. The possible bias from residual confounders remained. Subgroup analyses that distinguish the studies with and without adjustment for these confounders would be informative. For example, we conducted the subgroup analysis for the studies adjusting for intake of cereal fiber; however, the overall RRs changed little, which were 0.892 (95% CI: 0.834, 0.954) and 0.916 (95% CI: 0.852, 0.985) for adjusted and unadjusted studies, respectively. Second, the magnesium intake in these studies were only assessed by FFQ, which do not capture the magnesium intake from drinking water and nutritional supplementation, and thereby might underestimate total magnesium intake and result in potential misclassification. However, the misclassification would most likely lead to an underestimated association. Third, influence of other nutrients or dietary components such as coffee [49], red meat [45], calcium [43] and fiber [14,19] that are correlated with dietary magnesium could not be excluded; other nutrients may have been responsible for the observed association partly or completely. Finally, publication bias may be a problem in our pooling analysis. Although we tried as much as possible to search for potential unpublished studies, no valid studies were identified from the available grey literature resources. However, the evidence (Harbord's $p = 0.401$) did not indicate notable publication bias in our meta-analysis.

5. Conclusions

In conclusion, results from this meta-analysis indicate that dietary magnesium intake is associated with a reduced risk of type 2 diabetes (T2D). The greatest magnitude in risk reduction was found in the US population. A statistically significant linear dose-response relationship was identified across all the studies, and the largest magnitude association was found in the Asian population. A 100 mg/day increment in dietary magnesium intake was associated with an 8%–13% reduction in risk of T2D. No nonlinear dose-response relationship was found between incremental dietary magnesium intake and T2D incidence. Regarding the dose-response relationship between dietary magnesium intake and T2D in populations in Africa and Europe, more evidence is needed.

Acknowledgments: X.F. is supported by the Karolinska Institutet doctoral research grant (KID-funds). Y.C. is supported by the Junior Faculty Research Grants (C62412022) of the Institute of Environmental Medicine, Karolinska Institutet, Sweden.

Author Contributions: Y.C. and J.A. designed the research; X.F. and J.H. provided study oversight and took primary responsibility for the final content of the manuscript; X.F., C.L. and M.L. undertook literature search, screening and data extraction; X.F. and H.H. performed statistical analysis; X.F. drafted the manuscript; Z.F. and S.M. revised the article critically; and all authors contributed to the manuscript writing, made critical revision, read and approved the final manuscript.

Abbreviations

CI	Confidence interval
FFQ	Food frequency questionnaires
HR	Hazard ratio
OR	Odds ratio
RCT	Randomized controlled trial
REML	Restricted maximum likelihood
RR	Relative risk
T2D	Type 2 diabetes
US	United States

References

1. Shaw, J.E.; Sicree, R.A.; Zimmet, P.Z. Global estimates of the prevalence of diabetes for 2010 and 2030. *Diabetes Res. Clin. Pract.* **2010**, *87*, 4–14. [CrossRef] [PubMed]
2. Shi, Y.; Hu, F.B. The global implications of diabetes and cancer. *Lancet* **2014**, *383*, 1947–1948. [CrossRef]
3. Colditz, G.A.; Manson, J.E.; Stampfer, M.J.; Rosner, B.; Willett, W.C.; Speizer, F.E. Diet and risk of clinical diabetes in women. *Am. J. Clin. Nutr.* **1992**, *55*, 1018–1023. [PubMed]
4. Knowler, W.C.; Barrett-Connor, E.; Fowler, S.E.; Hamman, R.F.; Lachin, J.M.; Walker, E.A.; Nathan, D.M. Reduction in the incidence of type 2 diabetes with lifestyle intervention or metformin. *N. Engl. J. Med.* **2002**, *346*, 393–403. [PubMed]
5. Barbagallo, M.; Dominguez, L.J. Magnesium metabolism in type 2 diabetes mellitus, metabolic syndrome and insulin resistance. *Arch. Biochem. Biophys.* **2007**, *458*, 40–47. [CrossRef] [PubMed]
6. Balon, T.W.; Jasman, A.; Scott, S.; Meehan, W.P.; Rude, R.K.; Nadler, J.L. Dietary magnesium prevents fructose-induced insulin insensitivity in rats. *Hypertension* **1994**, *23*, 1036–1039. [CrossRef] [PubMed]
7. Hruby, A.; Meigs, J.B.; O'Donnell, C.J.; Jacques, P.F.; McKeown, N.M. Higher magnesium intake reduces risk of impaired glucose and insulin metabolism and progression from prediabetes to diabetes in middle-aged Americans. *Diabetes Care* **2014**, *37*, 419–427. [CrossRef] [PubMed]
8. Bo, S.; Pisu, E. Role of dietary magnesium in cardiovascular disease prevention, insulin sensitivity and diabetes. *Curr. Opin. Lipidol.* **2008**, *19*, 50–56. [CrossRef] [PubMed]
9. Barbagallo, M.; Dominguez, L.J.; Galioto, A.; Ferlisi, A.; Cani, C.; Malfa, L.; Pineo, A.; Busardo, A.; Paolisso, G. Role of magnesium in insulin action, diabetes and cardio-metabolic syndrome X. *Mol. Asp. Med.* **2003**, *24*, 39–52. [CrossRef]
10. Ramadass, S.; Basu, S.; Srinivasan, A.R. Serum magnesium levels as an indicator of status of diabetes mellitus type 2. *Diabetes Metab. Syndr.* **2015**, *9*, 42–45. [CrossRef] [PubMed]
11. Ma, J.; Folsom, A.R.; Melnick, S.L.; Eckfeldt, J.H.; Sharrett, A.R.; Nabulsi, A.A.; Hutchinson, R.G.; Metcalf, P.A. Associations of serum and dietary magnesium with cardiovascular disease, hypertension, diabetes, insulin, and carotid arterial wall thickness: The aric study. Atherosclerosis risk in communities study. *J. Clin. Epidemiol.* **1995**, *48*, 927–940. [CrossRef]
12. Del Gobbo, L.C.; Song, Y.; Poirier, P.; Dewailly, E.; Elin, R.J.; Egeland, G.M. Low serum magnesium concentrations are associated with a high prevalence of premature ventricular complexes in obese adults with type 2 diabetes. *Cardiovasc. Diabetol.* **2012**, *11*, 23. [CrossRef] [PubMed]
13. Kao, W.H.; Folsom, A.R.; Nieto, F.J.; Mo, J.P.; Watson, R.L.; Brancati, F.L. Serum and dietary magnesium and the risk for type 2 diabetes mellitus: The atherosclerosis risk in communities study. *Arch. Intern. Med.* **1999**, *159*, 2151–2159. [CrossRef] [PubMed]
14. Meyer, K.A.; Kushi, L.H.; Jacobs, D.R., Jr.; Slavin, J.; Sellers, T.A.; Folsom, A.R. Carbohydrates, dietary fiber, and incident type 2 diabetes in older women. *Am. J. Clin. Nutr.* **2000**, *71*, 921–930. [PubMed]
15. Hodge, A.M.; English, D.R.; O'Dea, K.; Giles, G.G. Glycemic index and dietary fiber and the risk of type 2 diabetes. *Diabetes Care* **2004**, *27*, 2701–2706. [CrossRef] [PubMed]
16. Lopez-Ridaura, R.; Willett, W.C.; Rimm, E.B.; Liu, S.; Stampfer, M.J.; Manson, J.E.; Hu, F.B. Magnesium intake and risk of type 2 diabetes in men and women. *Diabetes Care* **2004**, *27*, 134–140. [CrossRef] [PubMed]
17. Song, Y.; Manson, J.E.; Buring, J.E.; Liu, S. Dietary magnesium intake in relation to plasma insulin levels and risk of type 2 diabetes in women. *Diabetes Care* **2004**, *27*, 59–65. [CrossRef] [PubMed]
18. Van Dam, R.M.; Hu, F.B.; Rosenberg, L.; Krishnan, S.; Palmer, J.R. Dietary calcium and magnesium, major food sources, and risk of type 2 diabetes in U.S. black women. *Diabetes Care* **2006**, *29*, 2238–2243. [CrossRef] [PubMed]
19. Schulze, M.B.; Schulz, M.; Heidemann, C.; Schienkiewitz, A.; Hoffmann, K.; Boeing, H. Fiber and magnesium intake and incidence of type 2 diabetes: A prospective study and meta-analysis. *Arch. Intern. Med.* **2007**, *167*, 956–965. [CrossRef] [PubMed]
20. Villegas, R.; Gao, Y.T.; Dai, Q.; Yang, G.; Cai, H.; Li, H.; Zheng, W.; Shu, X.O. Dietary calcium and magnesium intakes and the risk of type 2 diabetes: The Shanghai women's health study. *Am. J. Clin. Nutr.* **2009**, *89*, 1059–1067. [CrossRef] [PubMed]

21. Hopping, B.N.; Erber, E.; Grandinetti, A.; Verheus, M.; Kolonel, L.N.; Maskarinec, G. Dietary fiber, magnesium, and glycemic load alter risk of type 2 diabetes in a multiethnic cohort in Hawaii. *J. Nutr.* **2010**, *140*, 68–74. [CrossRef] [PubMed]
22. Kim, D.J.; Xun, P.; Liu, K.; Loria, C.; Yokota, K.; Jacobs, D.R., Jr.; He, K. Magnesium intake in relation to systemic inflammation, insulin resistance, and the incidence of diabetes. *Diabetes Care* **2010**, *33*, 2604–2610. [CrossRef] [PubMed]
23. Kirii, K.; Iso, H.; Date, C.; Fukui, M.; Tamakoshi, A. Magnesium intake and risk of self-reported type 2 diabetes among Japanese. *J. Am. Coll. Nutr.* **2010**, *29*, 99–106. [CrossRef] [PubMed]
24. Nanri, A.; Mizoue, T.; Noda, M.; Takahashi, Y.; Kirii, K.; Inoue, M.; Tsugane, S.; Japan Public Health Center-based Prospective Study Group. Magnesium intake and type ii diabetes in japanese men and women: The Japan public health center-based prospective study. *Eur. J. Clin. Nutr.* **2010**, *64*, 1244–1247. [CrossRef] [PubMed]
25. Dong, J.Y.; Xun, P.; He, K.; Qin, L.Q. Magnesium intake and risk of type 2 diabetes: Meta-analysis of prospective cohort studies. *Diabetes Care* **2011**, *34*, 2116–2122. [CrossRef] [PubMed]
26. Larsson, S.C.; Wolk, A. Magnesium intake and risk of type 2 diabetes: A meta-analysis. *J. Intern. Med.* **2007**, *262*, 208–214. [CrossRef] [PubMed]
27. Xu, T.; Chen, G.C.; Zhai, L.; Ke, K.F. Nonlinear reduction in risk for type 2 diabetes by magnesium intake: An updated meta-analysis of prospective cohort studies. *Biomed. Environ. Sci.* **2015**, *28*, 527–534. [PubMed]
28. Liberati, A.; Altman, D.G.; Tetzlaff, J.; Mulrow, C.; Gotzsche, P.C.; Ioannidis, J.P.A.; Clarke, M.; Devereaux, P.J.; Kleijnen, J.; Moher, D. The PRISMA statement for reporting systematic reviews and meta-analyses of studies that evaluate health care interventions: Explanation and elaboration. *PLoS Med.* **2009**, *6*, e1000100. [CrossRef] [PubMed]
29. Stroup, D.F.; Berlin, J.A.; Morton, S.C.; Olkin, I.; Williamson, G.D.; Rennie, D.; Moher, D.; Becker, B.J.; Sipe, T.A.; Thacker, S.B. Meta-analysis of observational studies in epidemiology: A proposal for reporting. Meta-analysis of observational studies in epidemiology (MOOSE) group. *JAMA* **2000**, *283*, 2008–2012. [CrossRef] [PubMed]
30. Gargon, E.; Williamson, P.R.; Clarke, M. Collating the knowledge base for core outcome set development: Developing and appraising the search strategy for a systematic review. *BMC Med. Res. Methodol.* **2015**, *15*, 26. [CrossRef] [PubMed]
31. Sanderson, S.; Tatt, I.D.; Higgins, J.P. Tools for assessing quality and susceptibility to bias in observational studies in epidemiology: A systematic review and annotated bibliography. *Int. J. Epidemiol.* **2007**, *36*, 666–676. [CrossRef] [PubMed]
32. Carletta, J. Assessing agreement on classification tasks: The kappa statistic. *Comput. Linguist.* **1996**, *22*, 249–254.
33. Rothman, K.J.; Greenland, S.; Lash, T.L. *Modern Epidemiology*; Lippincott Williams & Wilkins: Philadelphia, PA, USA, 2008.
34. Harbord, R.M.; Higgins, J.P.T. Meta-regression in Stata. *Stata J.* **2008**, *8*, 493–519.
35. Higgins, J.P.; Thompson, S.G. Quantifying heterogeneity in a meta-analysis. *Stat. Med.* **2002**, *21*, 1539–1558. [CrossRef] [PubMed]
36. Egger, M.; Davey, S.G.; Schneider, M.; Minder, C. Bias in meta-analysis detected by a simple, graphical test. *BMJ* **1997**, *315*, 629–634. [CrossRef] [PubMed]
37. Harbord, R.M.; Egger, M.; Sterne, J.A. A modified test for small-study effects in meta-analyses of controlled trials with binary endpoints. *Stat. Med.* **2006**, *25*, 3443–3457. [CrossRef] [PubMed]
38. Begg, C.B.; Mazumdar, M. Operating characteristics of a rank correlation test for publication bias. *Biometrics* **1994**, *50*, 1088–1101. [CrossRef] [PubMed]
39. Peters, J.L.; Sutton, A.J.; Jones, D.R.; Abrams, K.R.; Rushton, L. Comparison of two methods to detect publication bias in meta-analysis. *JAMA* **2006**, *295*, 676–680. [CrossRef] [PubMed]
40. Harrell, F.E., Jr.; Lee, K.L.; Pollock, B.G. Regression models in clinical studies: Determining relationships between predictors and response. *J. Natl. Cancer Inst.* **1988**, *80*, 1198–1202. [CrossRef] [PubMed]
41. Jackson, D.; White, I.R.; Thompson, S.G. Extending dersimonian and laird's methodology to perform multivariate random effects meta-analyses. *Stat. Med.* **2010**, *29*, 1282–1297. [CrossRef] [PubMed]
42. Liu, S.; Choi, H.K.; Ford, E.; Song, Y.; Klevak, A.; Buring, J.E.; Manson, J.E. A prospective study of dairy intake and the risk of type 2 diabetes in women. *Diabetes Care* **2006**, *29*, 1579–1584. [CrossRef] [PubMed]

43. Kirii, K.; Mizoue, T.; Iso, H.; Takahashi, Y.; Kato, M.; Inoue, M.; Noda, M.; Tsugane, S. Calcium, vitamin D and dairy intake in relation to type 2 diabetes risk in a Japanese cohort. *Diabetologia* **2009**, *52*, 2542–2550. [CrossRef] [PubMed]
44. Pittas, A.G.; Dawson-Hughes, B.; Li, T.; Van Dam, R.M.; Willett, W.C.; Manson, J.E.; Hu, F.B. Vitamin D and calcium intake in relation to type 2 diabetes in women. *Diabetes Care* **2006**, *29*, 650–656. [CrossRef] [PubMed]
45. Song, Y.; Manson, J.E.; Buring, J.E.; Liu, S. A prospective study of red meat consumption and type 2 diabetes in middle-aged and elderly women: The women's health study. *Diabetes Care* **2004**, *27*, 2108–2115. [CrossRef] [PubMed]
46. Schulze, M.B.; Manson, J.E.; Willett, W.C.; Hu, F.B. Processed meat intake and incidence of type 2 diabetes in younger and middle-aged women. *Diabetologia* **2003**, *46*, 1465–1473. [CrossRef] [PubMed]
47. Liu, S.; Manson, J.E.; Stampfer, M.J.; Hu, F.B.; Giovannucci, E.; Colditz, G.A.; Hennekens, C.H.; Willett, W.C. A prospective study of whole-grain intake and risk of type 2 diabetes mellitus in US women. *Am. J. Public Health* **2000**, *90*, 1409–1415. [PubMed]
48. Salmeron, J.; Ascherio, A.; Rimm, E.B.; Colditz, G.A.; Spiegelman, D.; Jenkins, D.J.; Stampfer, M.J.; Wing, A.L.; Willett, W.C. Dietary fiber, glycemic load, and risk of NIDDM in men. *Diabetes Care* **1997**, *20*, 545–550. [CrossRef] [PubMed]
49. Pereira, M.A.; Parker, E.D.; Folsom, A.R. Coffee consumption and risk of type 2 diabetes mellitus: An 11-year prospective study of 28,812 postmenopausal women. *Arch. Intern. Med.* **2006**, *166*, 1311–1316. [CrossRef] [PubMed]
50. Oba, S.; Nanri, A.; Kurotani, K.; Goto, A.; Kato, M.; Mizoue, T.; Noda, M.; Inoue, M.; Tsugane, S. Dietary glycemic index, glycemic load and incidence of type 2 diabetes in japanese men and women: The Japan public health center-based prospective study. *Nutr. J.* **2013**, *12*, 165. [CrossRef] [PubMed]
51. He, K.; Song, Y.; Belin, R.J.; Chen, Y. Magnesium intake and the metabolic syndrome: Epidemiologic evidence to date. *J. Cardiometab. Syndr.* **2006**, *1*, 351–355. [CrossRef] [PubMed]
52. Hata, A.; Doi, Y.; Ninomiya, T.; Mukai, N.; Hirakawa, Y.; Hata, J.; Ozawa, M.; Uchida, K.; Shirota, T.; Kitazono, T.; et al. Magnesium intake decreases type 2 diabetes risk through the improvement of insulin resistance and inflammation: The Hisayama study. *Diabet. Med.* **2013**, *30*, 1487–1494. [CrossRef] [PubMed]
53. Weng, L.C.; Lee, N.J.; Yeh, W.T.; Ho, L.T.; Pan, W.H. Lower intake of magnesium and dietary fiber increases the incidence of type 2 diabetes in Taiwanese. *J. Formos. Med. Assoc.* **2012**, *111*, 651–659. [CrossRef] [PubMed]
54. Salmeron, J.; Manson, J.E.; Stampfer, M.J.; Colditz, G.A.; Wing, A.L.; Willett, W.C. Dietary fiber, glycemic load, and risk of non-insulin-dependent diabetes mellitus in women. *JAMA* **1997**, *277*, 472–477. [CrossRef] [PubMed]
55. Ma, B.; Lawson, A.B.; Liese, A.D.; Bell, R.A.; Mayer-Davis, E.J. Dairy, magnesium, and calcium intake in relation to insulin sensitivity: Approaches to modeling a dose-dependent association. *Am. J. Epidemiol.* **2006**, *164*, 449–458. [CrossRef] [PubMed]
56. Rodriguez-Moran, M.; Simental, M.L.; Zambrano, G.G.; Guerrero-Romero, F. The role of magnesium in type 2 diabetes: A brief based-clinical review. *Magnes. Res.* **2011**, *24*, 156–162. [PubMed]
57. Meisinger, C.; Thorand, B.; Schneider, A.; Stieber, J.; Doring, A.; Lowel, H. Sex differences in risk factors for incident type 2 diabetes mellitus: The MONICA Augsburg cohort study. *Arch. Intern. Med.* **2002**, *162*, 82–89. [CrossRef] [PubMed]
58. Kalyani, R.R.; Franco, M.; Dobs, A.S.; Ouyang, P.; Vaidya, D.; Bertoni, A.; Gapstur, S.M.; Golden, S.H. The association of endogenous sex hormones, adiposity, and insulin resistance with incident diabetes in postmenopausal women. *J. Clin. Endocrinol. Metab.* **2009**, *94*, 4127–4135. [CrossRef] [PubMed]
59. Moshfegh, A.; Goldman, J.; Cleveland, L. *What We Eat in America, NHANES 2001–2002: Usual Nutrient Intakes from Food Compared to Dietary References Intake*; Agricultural Research Service, U.S. Department of Agriculture: Washington, DC, USA, 2005; pp. 1–56.

5

Intakes of Zinc, Potassium, Calcium and Magnesium of Individuals with Type 2 Diabetes Mellitus and the Relationship with Glycemic Control

Paula Nascimento Brandão-Lima [1], Gabrielli Barbosa de Carvalho [2], Ramara Kadija Fonseca Santos [2], Beatriz da Cruz Santos [3], Natalia Lohayne Dias-Vasconcelos [3], Vivianne de Sousa Rocha [4], Kiriaque Barra Ferreira Barbosa [1,2,3] and Liliane Viana Pires [2,3,*]

1. Health Sciences Postgraduate Program, Department of Medicine, Federal University of Sergipe, Rua Cláudio Batista, S/N, Cidade Nova, Aracaju, 49060-108 Sergipe, Brazil; paulanblima@gmail.com (P.N.B.-L.); kiribarra@yahoo.com.br (K.B.F.B.)
2. Nutrition Sciences Postgraduate Program, Department of Nutrition, Federal University of Sergipe, Avenida Marechal Rondon, S/N, Jardim Rosa Elze, São Cristovão, 49100-000 Sergipe, Brazil; gabicarvalho_31@hotmail.com (G.B.d.C.); rkadijanutri@gmail.com (R.K.F.S.)
3. Undergraduate Nutrition Program, Department of Nutrition, Federal University of Sergipe, Avenida Marechal Rondon, S/N, Jardim Rosa Elze, São Cristovão, 49100-000 Sergipe, Brazil; cruz14_bia@outlook.com (B.d.C.S.); diaslohayne@gmail.com (N.L.D.-V.)
4. Department of Nutrition, Federal University of Sergipe, Avenida Governador Marcelo Déda, 13, Centro, Lagarto, 49400-000 Sergipe, Brazil; viviannesrocha@gmail.com

* Correspondence: lvianapires@gmail.com or lvpires@usp.br

Abstract: The role of the concomitant intake of zinc, potassium, calcium, and magnesium in the glycemic control of individuals with type 2 diabetes mellitus (T2DM) has not been extensively discussed. We evaluated the relationship between the dietary intake of these micronutrients and glycemic markers in 95 individuals with T2DM (mean age 48.6 $\pm$ 8.4 years). Hierarchical grouping analysis was used to divide the individuals into two clusters according to their micronutrient intake, and differences between clusters were statistically assessed. Effects of individual and combination intake of micronutrients on glycated hemoglobin percentage (%HbA1c) were assessed using multiple linear regression and binary logistic regression analysis. We observed a high likelihood of inadequate intake of the four micronutrients. The group with lower micronutrient intake (cluster 1) displayed higher %HbA1c (p = 0.006) and triglyceride (p = 0.010) levels. High %HbA1c showed an association with cluster 1 (odds ratio (OR) = 3.041, 95% confidence interval (CI) = 1.131; 8.175) and time of T2DM diagnosis (OR = 1.155, 95% CI = 1.043; 1.278). Potassium ($\beta = -0.001$, $p = 0.017$) and magnesium ($\beta = -0.007$, $p = 0.015$) intakes were inversely associated with %HbA1c. Reduced concomitant intake of the four micronutrients studied proved to be associated with risk of increased %HbA1c in individuals with T2DM, which was particularly predicted by magnesium and potassium intakes.

Keywords: micronutrients; trace elements; food; glycated hemoglobin A; hyperglycemia

---

1. Introduction

Type 2 diabetes mellitus (T2DM) is characterized by failures in blood glucose homeostasis and is considered a global public health problem [1]. Chronic hyperglycemia leads to increased oxidative stress and production of proinflammatory cytokines, disrupting insulin signaling pathways, lipid metabolism, protein synthesis, and cell differentiation, and may alter body concentrations of micronutrients [2–5]. The maintenance of the glycemic control in individuals with T2DM involves strategies for lifestyle changes, drug therapy, and adoption of healthy eating habits [1,2]. A balanced diet with adequate nutrient content can reduce the glycated hemoglobin percentage (%HbA1c) in subjects with T2DM by 0.3–2% [6]. Over the last few years, studies have verified the participation of minerals in the synthesis, secretion, and action of insulin. Among them, the minerals zinc, potassium, calcium, and magnesium are considered essential for the homeostasis of glucose metabolism [5,7,8].

Zinc plays a key role in the insulin biosynthesis as part of the hexameric structure of this hormone, and in the sensitivity to insulin in target tissues through stimulation of insulin receptors [9,10]. Calcium and potassium regulate voltage-dependent channels in pancreatic β-cells, which are essential for insulin exocytosis [11,12]. Magnesium is important for β-cell functioning and acts as a cofactor of many enzymes involved in the glucose metabolism, like tyrosine kinase enzymes, which phosphorylate insulin receptors and trigger the signaling cascade [4,12,13].

Thus, an inadequate intake of these micronutrients may impair the insulin synthesis, secretion, and signaling pathways [4,11,14]. It is possible to observe in the literature studies that associate the low intake and serum concentration of these minerals with risk of T2DM development [2,13,15–18]. Nevertheless, studies that evaluate the relationship between the dietary intake of these minerals in glycemic control in subjects with established disease are not widely found. In addition, no studies have assessed the relationship of the concomitant intake of these four micronutrients with the glycemic control, insulin biosynthesis, and insulin sensitivity of individuals with T2DM. In this scenario, the present study aimed to evaluate the relationship of the dietary intake of zinc, potassium, calcium, and magnesium with glycemic markers in individuals with T2DM in order to expand the understanding of these relationships in glycemic control.

2. Materials and Methods

2.1. Study Design and Participants

In this cross-sectional study, to be eligible for enrollment, individuals had to be 19–59 years old and have diagnosis of T2DM. Thus, 102 individuals with T2DM who visited the Family Health Units in the state of Sergipe, Brazil, were evaluated. Exclusion criteria adopted were the use of vitamin–mineral supplements, pregnancy, status as a current smoker, and the presence of the following diseases: rheumatoid arthritis, cancer, chronic renal failure, thyroid dysfunction, and acute infections or inflammatory processes such as influenza and urinary tract infection. The study followed the guidelines of the Declaration of Helsinki and all participants provided written informed consent. The study was approved by the Ethical Committee of the Federal University of Sergipe (Approval number 1.370.831).

Venous blood samples were obtained, after an overnight fast for at least 10 hours, in ethylenediamine tetra-acetic acid (EDTA) tubes for estimation of concentration of glycated hemoglobin (HbA1c) in whole blood, and in gel tubes for the determination of fasting glucose, lipid profile, insulin, and C-peptide in serum. Measurements of anthropometric parameters, body fat percentage, and blood pressure were performed. All the measurements were realized by trained technicians, and the individuals were instructed to avoid physical activity or effort one day before the tests. In combination, dietary intake assessments of macro and micronutrients was performed. Information about socioeconomic conditions, medical history, and lifestyle were obtained using a questionnaire.

2.2. Anthropometric Parameters, Bioelectric Impedance and Blood Pressure Measurements

Weight and height measurements were performed to calculate the body mass index (BMI). The BMI was calculated by dividing the body weight value (in kilograms) by the square value of the body height (in meters). The participants were classified as malnourished (BMI < 18.5 kg/m^2), normal weight (BMI 18.5–24.9 kg/m^2) or overweight/obese (BMI $\geq$ 25 kg/m^2), assessed according to the cut-off values proposed by the World Health Organization [19]. Waist circumference was measured with a non-extendable tape positioned at the midpoint between the last floating rib and the top of the iliac crest. The cut-off point used for waist circumference was ≥80 cm for women and ≥94 cm for men [20].

Measurement of body fat percentage was performed using the BIA 310 Bioimpedance Analyzer (Biodynamics Corporation, Shoreline, WA, USA), following the manufacturer's instructions. Blood pressure was measured using aneroid sphygmomanometers and a stethoscope according to the recommendations of the Brazilian Society of Cardiology [21] at rest in a sitting position.

2.3. Biochemical Analyses

Serum concentrations of glucose, triglycerides, total cholesterol, and high-density lipoprotein cholesterol (HDL-c) were measured by an enzymatic colorimetric method using commercial kits (Labtest®, Lagoa Santa/MG, Brazil). The HbA1c was measured by immunoturbidimetric inhibition. All biochemical tests were performed using an automatic biochemical analyzer CMD 800i (Wiener Lab Group®, Rosario, Argentina). Serum insulin and C-peptide concentrations were measured by chemiluminescence using commercial kits (Abbott®, Abbott Park, IL, USA) and the automatic immunoassay analyzer Architect i1000SR (Abbott®, Abbott Park, IL, USA). The homeostasis model assessment (HOMA) was used to assess insulin sensitivity, based on C-peptide and glucose levels. Calculations were made using the HOMA calculator (University of Oxford, United Kingdom).

2.4. Food Intake

The 24-h dietary recalls over three days (including two weekdays and one weekend day) were obtained by Multiple-Pass method [22], and analyzed using the NutWin software (Department of Informatics, Paulista School of Medicine/UNIFESP, São Paulo/SP, Brazil), which includes the updated versions of the Brazilian Table of Food Composition (TACO), the Table of Nutritional Composition of Food Consumed in Brazil, the United States Department of Agriculture (USDA) Food Composition Databases, and food labels. The adequacy of usual dietary intake of nutrients by each group was evaluated according to the estimated average requirement (EAR) and adequate intake (AI) for potassium values proposed by the dietary reference intakes [23,24]. The probability of inadequate food intake by group was evaluated by z-score, which was calculated from the difference between the EAR corresponding to each nutrient and the mean ingestion of the group divided by the standard deviation of the intake. Potassium intake values were compared with AI values [24].

2.5. Statistical Analyses

The Kolmogorov–Smirnov test was used to evaluate data homogeneity. Non-homogeneous data were subjected to logarithmic transformation. The identification of individuals with inaccurate report of energy intake was performed using the methodology proposed by Mccrory et al. [25], based on the ratio between the reported energy intake and the total energy expenditure predicted, calculated by the equation of Vinken et al. [26] and considering the cut-off value of ± one standard deviation. The usual dietary intake was calculated using the Multiple Sources Method (MSM) (https://msm.dife.de/) [27]. Micronutrient intake values were adjusted for total energy intake according to residual method proposed by Willett et al. [28].

To verify associations between response variables, and to characterize individuals according to dietary intake of zinc, magnesium, calcium, and potassium, a hierarchical cluster analysis was used. From this analysis, the mean values corresponding to the energy-adjusted dietary intake of the four minerals were auto-scaled, and the similarities between the individuals calculated according to the Euclidean squared distance, while the Ward's method was used for the formation of clusters. Differences between the two clusters formed was assessed using the Student's *t*-test (for normal data distribution) or the Mann–Whitney test (for non-normal data distribution).

Regression models were used to assess the effect of the micronutrient intake on the glycemic control. Independent variables with $p \leq 0.20$ in the bivariate analyses were included in the models using the enter method. $p \leq 0.20$ was adopted according to the criterion of Wang et al. [29], established for the testing of a greater number of predictor variables in the model. Thus, a binary logistic regression model was applied using %HbA1c values above 7.0 [30] and cluster 1 (lower micronutrient intake) as risk variables. In addition, multiple regression models were applied to assess the effect of each micronutrient intake on %HbA1c separately. Multicollinearity was assessed by variance inflation factors (VIF) and no correlation was identified between the independent variables (VIF <10). Both regression models used sex, age, and time of T2DM diagnosis as adjustment variables.

The results were expressed as means and standard deviations, and as absolute and relative frequencies. A significance level of 5% was adopted for all tests. All statistical analyses were performed using SPSS for Windows Version 17.0 (SPSS Inc., Chicago, IL, USA).

3. Results

After exclusion of participants with missing dietary information, 95 individuals with T2DM were finally evaluated; 69.5% of them were female and mean age was 48.6 ± 8.4 years. Most individuals were overweight or obese (81.0%), and mean BMI and body fat percentage values were 30.22 ± 6.78 kg/m^2 and 34.98 ± 7.94%, respectively. Waist circumference measurement showed 85.3% of the participants at increased risk of obesity-associated metabolic diseases (Table 1).

Deficient glycemic control was observed, as indicated by values of fasting glucose and %HbA1c above the cut-off point for disease control (fasting glucose < 154 mg/dL; %HbA1c < 7.0) [30]. Regarding lipid profile, 73.7% of the participants presented low HDL-c levels, and 37.9%, 10.5%, and 3.1% presented hypertriglyceridemia, mixed hyperlipidemia, and hypercholesterolemia, respectively.

Table 1. Clinical, biochemical and nutrient intake variables of individuals with type 2 diabetes mellitus (T2DM).

Variables	T2DM (*n* = 95)
Age, years	48.6 ± 8.4
Sex	
Men, *n* (%)	29 (30.5)
Women, *n* (%)	66 (69.5)
Time of T2DM diagnosis [1], years	7.3 ± 6.2
Insulin therapy [2], *n* (%)	21 (22.1)
Oral antidiabetic agents [2], *n* (%)	70 (73.7)
Lipid-lowering agents [2], *n* (%)	24 (25.3)
Antihypertensive agents [2], *n* (%)	46 (48.4)
Weight, kg	78.9 ± 19.3
BMI, kg/m^2	30.2 ± 6.8
Fat mass [2], %	35.0 ± 7.9
Waist circumference, cm	99.8 ± 14.3
Men, *n* (%)	
<94 cm	8 (27.6)
≥94 cm	21 (72.4)
Women, *n* (%)	
<80 cm	6 (9.1)
≥80 cm	60 (90.9)
SBP [3], mmHg	129.2 ± 17.0
DBP [3], mmHg	83.5 ± 15.3
Fasting glucose, mg/dL	180.1 ± 84.1
%Hb1Ac	8.1 ± 2.1
Insulin, µU/mL	13.8 ± 13.5
C-peptide, ng/mL	2.7 ± 0.8
HOMA2-%B	77.0 ± 56.2
HOMA2-%S	42.8 ± 20.9
HOMA2-IR	3.3 ± 2.9
Total cholesterol, mg/dL	193.4 ± 47.3
HDL-c, mg/dL	41.1 ± 10.4
LDL-c, mg/dL	117.4 ± 39.8
Triglycerides, mg/dL	174.3 ± 117.1

Table 1. *Cont.*

Variables	T2DM (n = 95)
Energy intake, kcal/day	1469.4 ± 478.5
Protein intake, g/day	80.0 ± 20.2
Carbohydrate intake, g/day	210.1 ± 73.6
Lipid intake, g/day	37.1 ± 15.6
Zinc intake, mg/day	5.2 ± 1.5
Potassium intake, mg/day	1848.5 ± 543.4
Calcium intake, mg/day	469.0 ± 195.3
Magnesium intake mg/day	218.4 ± 68.1

Results presented in mean ± standard deviation and absolute frequency; [1] n = 91; [2] n = 93; [3] n = 89. %HbA1c: glycated hemoglobin percentage; BMI: body mass index; DBP: diastolic blood pressure; HDL-c: high-density lipoprotein cholesterol; HOMA: Homeostasis Assessment Model; LDL-c: low-density lipoprotein cholesterol; T2DM: type 2 diabetes mellitus; SBP: systolic blood pressure. Micronutrients adjusted for total energy intake using the residual method [28].

Energy intake was found to be underreported by 84.2% of the individuals. A prevalence of inadequacy in energy-adjusted zinc intake of 99.9% in males and 82.6% in females was observed. The prevalence of inadequate energy-adjusted magnesium intake for males and females was 96.4% and 74.9%, respectively. The energy-adjusted calcium intake showed a prevalence of inadequacy of 95.5%. All the individuals evaluated had energy-adjusted potassium intake below the AI values (Figure 1).

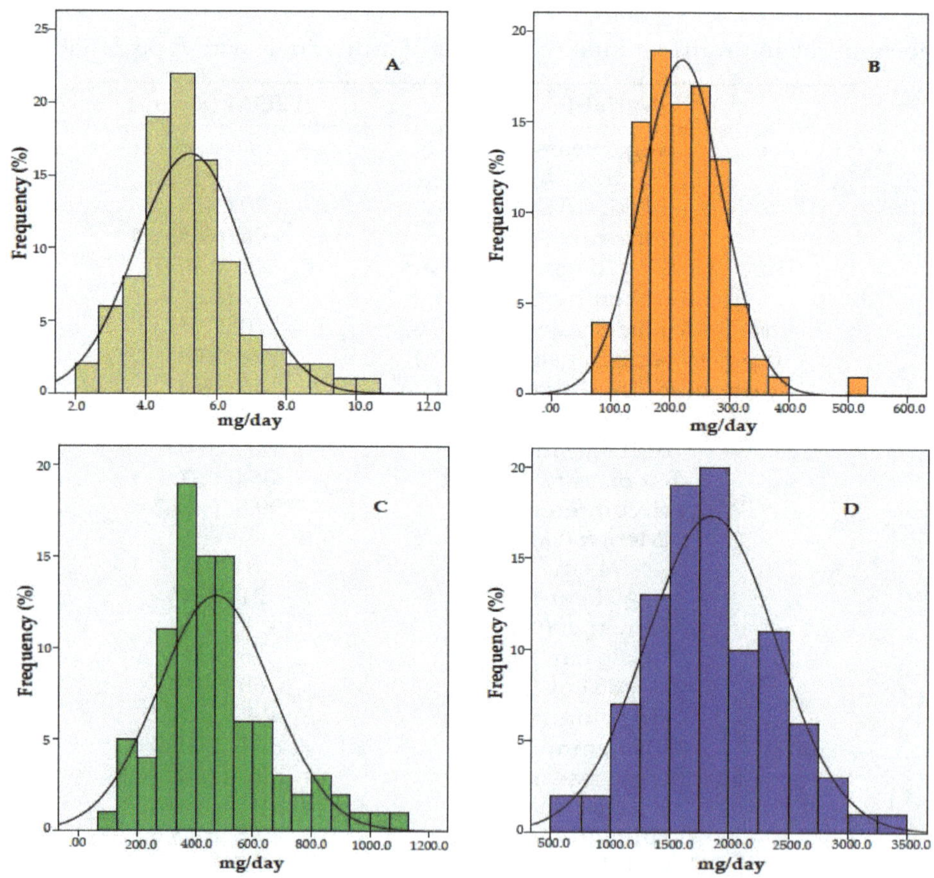

Figure 1. Histogram of energy-adjusted intake of zinc (**A**), magnesium (**B**), calcium (**C**), and potassium (**D**), and prevalence of inadequate intake in individuals with type 2 diabetes mellitus (T2DM) (n = 95). (**A**) Group intake (mean ± SD): 5.23 ± 1.53 mg/day; Z-score: 3.06 (men) and 0.94 (women). (**B**) Group intake (mean ± SD): 218.36 ± 68.13 mg/day; Z-score: 1.80 (men) and 0.67 (women). (**C**) Group intake (mean ± SD): 468.95 ± 195.3 mg/day; Z-score: 1.96 (group). (**D**) Group intake (mean ± SD): 1848.45 ± 543.43 mg/day. SD: Standard deviation.

When energy-adjusted micronutrient (zinc, potassium, calcium, and magnesium) intake was compared between clusters, the group with lower micronutrient intake (cluster 1) showed significantly higher %HbA1c ($p = 0.006$) and serum triglyceride concentration ($p = 0.01$) in comparison with the group with higher intake (cluster 2). No statistical differences were seen with regard to the other variables studied (Table 2).

Table 2. Clinical, biochemical and nutrient intake variables of individuals with type 2 diabetes mellitus (T2DM).

Variables	*Cluster* 1 ($n = 65$)	*Cluster* 2 ($n = 30$)	*p*-value
Age, years	48.6 ± 8.6	48.9 ± 7.9	0.866 ¥
Time of T2DM diagnosis, years	7.2 ± 6.4	7.4 ± 6.0	0.909
BMI, kg/m^2	30.4 ± 6.9	29.9 ± 6.7	0.762 ¥
Waist circumference, cm	100.8 ± 13.7	97.7 ± 15.5	0.332
Fat mass, %	34.6 ± 8.0	35.8 ± 7.8	0.483
Total cholesterol, mg/dL	198.8 ± 49.7	181.5 ± 40.0	0.097
HDL-c, mg/dL	41.9 ± 10.5	39.2 ± 10.3	0.247
LDL-c, mg/dL	117.9 ± 42.2	116.4 ± 34.5	0.867
Triglycerides, mg/dL	194.9 ± 131.1	129.6 ± 58.5	0.010
%Hb1Ac	8.3 ± 2.1	7.2 ± 1.7	0.006
C-peptide, ng/mL	2.7 ± 0.9	2.7 ± 0.7	0.963
Fasting glucose, mg/dL	190.3 ± 88.2	158.1 ± 70.7	0.082 ¥
Insulin, μU/mL	13.2 ± 11.7	15.1 ± 16.8	0.525
HOMA2-%B	73.7 ± 59.4	84.0 ± 48.8	0.407 ¥
Energy intake, kcal/day	1452.3 ± 471.4	1506.3 ± 499.7	0.611
Lipid intake, g/day	37.4 ± 15.1	36.5 ± 16.8	0.796
Protein intake, g/day	80.2 ± 19.7	79.4 ± 21.4	0.856
Carbohydrate intake, g/day	203.6 ± 74.1	224.2 ± 71.7	0.207
Zinc intake, mg/day	4.8 ± 1.4	6.1 ± 1.5	<0.001
Potassium intake, mg/day	1556.5 ± 344.3	2480.9 ± 301.4	<0.001
Calcium intake, mg/day	400.6 ± 136.4	616.9 ± 222.4	<0.001
Magnesium intake mg/day	191.5 ± 54.2	276.6 ± 58.5	<0.001

Results presented in mean ± standard deviation. *p*-value <0.05 was considered statistically significant. Student's *t*-test for independent samples and ¥ Mann–Whitney test. %HbA1c: glycated hemoglobin percentage; BMI: body mass index; HDL-c: high-density lipoprotein cholesterol; HOMA: Homeostasis Assessment Model; LDL-c: low-density lipoprotein cholesterol; T2DM: type 2 diabetes mellitus. Micronutrients adjusted for total energy intake using the residual method [28].

Considering the significant difference in %HbA1c between clusters, a binary logistic regression model was applied in order to investigate the risk factors for increased %HbA1c (Table 3). We found that alterations in the %HbA1c were dependent of the time (in years) taken to diagnose T2DM ($p = 0.005$) and lower micronutrient intake (cluster 1) ($p = 0.028$).

Table 3. Binary logistic regression model of glycated hemoglobin percentage (%HbA1c) and clusters formed from energy-adjusted mineral intake by individuals with type 2 diabetes mellitus (T2DM).

Dependent Variable	Covariables	OR (95% CI)	*p*-value
%Hb1Ac §	Age (years) £	0.987 (0.931; 1.046)	0.661
	Sex §	1.598 (0.580; 4.405)	0.365
	Time of T2DM diagnosis (years) £	1.155 (1.043; 1.278)	0.005
	Cluster 1 §	3.041 (1.131; 8.175)	0.028

p-value <0.05 was considered significant. *p*-value of model: 0.003 and r^2: 0.221. Hosmer and Lemeshow test: 0.591. § Variables included in the model in the dichotomous format. £ Variables included in the model in continuous format. Model adjusted by sex, age, and time of T2DM diagnosis. %HbA1c: glycated hemoglobin percentage; CI: confidence interval; OR: odds ratio; T2DM: type 2 diabetes mellitus. Risk classification used %HbA1c >7% [30] and cluster 1 with lower combined intake of zinc, potassium, calcium, and magnesium.

Multiple regression analyses showed that, for every 1 g of potassium and 100 mg of magnesium ingested, there was 1% and 0.7% reduction in %HbA1c, respectively. These results were influenced by sex and time taken to diagnose T2DM (Table 4).

Table 4. Multiple linear regression models of glycated hemoglobin percentage (%HbA1c; dependent variable) and energy-adjusted mineral intake by individuals with type 2 diabetes mellitus (T2DM).

	Independent Variables	β (95%CI)	*p*-value	r^2 Adjusted
Model 1 [1]	Age (years)	−0.032 (−0.082; 0.019)	0.216	0.143
	Sex §	1.069 (0.209; 1.930)	0.015	
	Time of T2DM diagnosis (years)	0.117 (0.051; 0.183)	0.001	
	Zinc intake (mg/day)	−0.017 (−0.283; 0.250)	0.902	
Model 2 [2]	Age (years)	−0.028 (−0.077; 0.021)	0.259	0.198
	Sex §	0.925 (0.086; 1.765)	0.031	
	Time of T2DM diagnosis (years)	1.118 (0.054; 0.182)	<0.001	
	Potassium intake (mg/day)	−0.001 (−0.002; 0.000)	0.017	
Model 3 [2]	Age (years)	−0.029 (−0.079; 0.021)	0.253	0.151
	Sex §	1.025 (0.163; 1.887)	0.020	
	Time of T2DM diagnosis (years)	0.119 (0.053; 0.184)	0.001	
	Calcium intake (mg/day)	−0.001 (−0.003; 0.001)	0.377	
Model 4 [2]	Age (years)	−0.031 (0.080; 0.017)	0.206	0.201
	Sex §	1.009 (0.177; 1.840)	0.018	
	Time of T2DM diagnosis (years)	0.117 (0.053; 0.181)	<0.001	
	Magnesium intake (mg/day)	−0.007 (−0.012; −0.001)	0.015	

[1] *p*-value of model: 0.002. [2] *p*-value of model: <0.001. β non-standardized. Variables included in the models in the continuous format and in the § dichotomous format. All models adjusted by sex, age and time of T2DM diagnosis. %HbA1c: glycated hemoglobin percentage; CI: confidence interval; T2DM: type 2 diabetes mellitus.

4. Discussion

After assessing the effect of the energy-adjusted dietary intake of zinc, potassium, calcium, and magnesium on the glycemic control of individuals with T2DM, we found a three-fold increased risk of high %HbA1c when dietary intake was reduced. In addition, potassium and magnesium intakes were predictive of %HbA1c decrease. It is noteworthy that most evaluated individuals were likely to have inadequate ingestion of these micronutrients.

The association between low micronutrient intake and deficient glycemic control is well known and poor intake of these micronutrients is widely documented in T2DM [2,3,12,31]. However, most studies looked at the intake of each micronutrient individually, and studies evaluating the concomitant intake thereof are scarce.

Epidemiological studies have shown a significant association between low daily zinc intake and risk of T2DM [10,18,32], and the risk can be reduced by 20% upon daily intake of more than 13 mg of zinc [33]. Kanoni et al. [34] found a significant correlation between zinc intake and fasting glucose values, where the daily intake of every 1 mg of zinc was able to reduce the glucose concentration by 0.02 mg/dL. The same study was included in a recent systematic review, which reported that the serum zinc concentration has been negatively correlated with %HbA1c and fasting glucose values in T2DM [16].

The role of zinc in the functioning and maintenance of pancreatic β-cell mass, insulin biosynthesis, and maturation of secretory granules is well documented [9,10]. In addition, zinc inhibits tyrosine phosphatases by stimulating auto phosphorylation of insulin receptors [14,16]. Moreover, it is essential in the redox mechanisms as a component of the superoxide dismutase enzyme, thus being helpful against the oxidative stress generated by hyperglycemia [10,14].

The role of magnesium in the glycemic control has been shown in experimental studies on rats with induced T2DM. Magnesium supplementation improved insulin secretion and sensitivity, lipid profile, and inflammatory status [35,36]. Morakinyo et al. [36] also showed that rats supplemented with magnesium improved GLUT4 translocation and, consequently, the metabolic control.

Previous evidence also points to an inverse association between magnesium intake and T2DM risk [13,37]. Hypomagnesemia and low magnesium intake are very prevalent in individuals diagnosed with T2DM, especially in those with poor glycemic control [12,31,38]. In addition, reduced plasma concentration of magnesium may lead to changes in the glycemic control, since the body distribution of this micronutrient has an impact on insulin secretion and action [12].

However, studies addressing the effect of magnesium supplementation on glycemic control are controversial. Some studies have shown positive effects of magnesium supplementation on blood glucose and %HbA1c lowering, and on the increased insulin sensitivity [8,39–41]. However, other studies did not observe such effects, which may be explained by the presence of normomagnesemia, time of supplementation, and reduced number of individuals assessed [42–47]. Two meta-analyses studies showed reduction of 0.56 mmol/L (95% confidence interval (CI) = −1.10; −0.01) [48] and 0.37 mmol/L (95% CI = −0.74; −0.00) [4], respectively, in the fasting glucose levels upon magnesium supplementation.

Magnesium is an important cofactor of enzymes involved in the glucose metabolism, in which it binds to an ATP molecule, yielding the Mg–ATP complex that acts in phosphate transfer reactions [4,12,37]. Thus, magnesium participates in the autophosphorylation of the β-subunit of insulin receptors, proliferation and maintenance of pancreatic β-cells, activity of tyrosine kinases, and stimulation of proteins and substrates of the insulin signaling cascade [12,13].

Enhanced intakes of calcium and potassium are also associated with reduced risk of T2DM [5,15], due to the combined action of these minerals in the process of insulin release [7]. Within the pancreatic β-cells, the intracellular ATP/ADP ratio that follows the glucose metabolism leads to the closure of ATP-sensitive potassium channels, and subsequent depolarization of the plasma membrane. Calcium channels are then opened, allowing the calcium influx to the cells and subsequent activation of exocytosis of the insulin granules [7,11].

The fundamental role of calcium in body weight control and, consequently, in the maintenance of insulin sensitivity in the adipose tissue, is observed in animal models. Dietary calcium induces suppression of calcitriol, thus reducing lipogenesis and increasing lipolysis. In addition, it increases the uncoupling protein-2 (UCP2) expression in the adipose tissue. UCP2 is responsible for the transport and oxidation of mitochondrial fatty acids, which reduces lipid storage and adiposity [49].

Few studies have assessed the effect of calcium intake on the glycemic control. In an eight-week study, calcium supplementation (1500 mg per day) improved the insulin sensitivity in individuals with T2DM [50]. However, insulin sensitivity was not changed after non-diabetic obese individuals underwent 24 weeks of supplementation with 1000 mg of calcium per day [49].

Furthermore, magnesium intake is likely to be a confounding factor as it is highly correlated with calcium metabolism as observed in studies addressing the association between intake of both minerals and the risk of T2DM [51,52]. A relationship between calcium and vitamin D intakes was also observed as the interaction of these nutrients leads to reduced fasting insulin and %HbA1c levels in individuals with T2DM [53].

The relation between potassium intake and variables of glycemic control in individuals with T2DM is not widely addressed in the literature. Both low potassium intake and reduced potassium concentration in serum were shown to be significantly associated with reduced insulin sensitivity and with a compensatory increase in insulin secretion [5], as well as with risk of T2DM [17,54].

Considering that the adoption of healthy dietary and body weight control patterns is fundamental for the T2DM management [1,6], a high rate of underreported energy intake is observed among individuals with T2DM in this study, and this can be the main reason for the high prevalence of overweight and obesity here documented. Underreporting is a commonly observed practice among obese individuals and can affect the estimation of nutrient intake, consequently impairing nutritional and disease assessments [55,56]. In addition, the analysis of food intake that relies on 24-hour recalls may have limitations, since this method is susceptible to inaccurate reports about both the food consumed and the size of its portions [25]. However, these limitations were mitigated after calculation of intra and interindividual variability, in combination with the adjustment for energy intake of nutrients.

Furthermore, food evaluation involves data of tables of food composition, and such tables can be different depending on where the food is produced. Therefore, similar to the present study, the use of region or country-specific food composition tables may help to correct this confounding factor.

5. Conclusions

Overall, studies evaluating the effect of the concomitant intake of micronutrients on variables of glycemic metabolism in individuals with T2DM are scarce, especially when it comes to zinc, potassium, calcium, and magnesium. This highlights the importance of our results for a better evaluation of usual food intake in this population, which is a simple and low-cost procedure, as %HbA1c is routinely measured in individuals with T2DM and it is the gold standard for glycemic control evaluation.

Therefore, inadequate concomitant intake of zinc, potassium, calcium, and magnesium is related to poor glycemic control in individuals with T2DM, and the intakes of magnesium and potassium are predictors of %HbA1c reduction. Further studies on dietary intake of individuals with T2DM and their relation with glucose metabolism are needed.

Author Contributions: P.N.B.-L. and L.V.P. designed the study; All authors performed the analysis and contributed to the writing of the manuscript. All authors approved the final version of the manuscript.

Acknowledgments: The authors would like to thank the research volunteers, Alan Santos Oliveira for the support in data collection, the National Council for Scientific and Technological Development (CNPq) for the financial support, the Foundation for Research and Technological Innovation Support of the State of Sergipe (Fapitec/SE), and the Coordination of Improvement of Higher Education Personnel (CAPES).

References

1. International Diabetes Federation. *IDF Diabetes Atlas*, 8th ed.; IDF: Brussels, Belgium, 2017.
2. Shah, M.; Vasandani, C.; Adams-Huet, B.; Garg, A. Comparison of nutrient intakes in South Asians with type 2 diabetes mellitus and controls living in the United States. *Diabetes Res. Clin. Pract.* **2018**, *138*, 47–56. [CrossRef] [PubMed]
3. Perez, A.; Rojas, P.; Carrasco, F.; Basfi-fer, K.; Perez-Bravo, F.; Codoceo, J.; Inostroza, J.; Galgani, J.E.; Gilmore, L.A.; Ruz, M. Association between zinc nutritional status and glycemic control in individuals with well-controlled type-2 diabetes. *J. Trace Elem. Med. Biol.* **2018**, *50*, 560–565. [CrossRef] [PubMed]
4. Veronese, N.; Watutantrige-Fernando, S.; Luchini, C.; Solmi, M.; Sartore, G.; Sergi, G.; Manzato, E.; Barbagallo, M.; Maggi, S.; Stubbs, B. Effect of magnesium supplementation on glucose metabolism in people with or at risk of diabetes: A systematic review and meta-analysis of double-blind randomized controlled trials. *Eur. J. Clin. Nutr.* **2016**, *70*, 1354–1359. [CrossRef] [PubMed]
5. Chatterjee, R.; Biggs, M.L.; de Boer, I.H.; Brancati, F.L.; Svetkey, L.P.; Barzilay, J.; Djoussé, L.; Ix, J.H.; Kizer, J.R.; Siscovick, D.S.; et al. Potassium and Glucose Measures in Older Adults: The Cardiovascular Health Study. *J. Gerontol. A Biol. Sci. Med. Sci.* **2015**, *70*, 255–261. [CrossRef] [PubMed]
6. American Diabetes Association. Lifestyle Management: Standards of Medical Care in Diabetes-2018. *Diabetes Care* **2018**, *41*, S38–S50. [CrossRef] [PubMed]
7. Fu, Z.; Gilbert, E.R.; Liu, D. Regulation of insulin synthesis and secretion and pancreatic Beta-cell dysfunction in diabetes. *Curr. Diabetes Rev.* **2013**, *9*, 25–53. [CrossRef]
8. Solati, M.; Ouspid, E.; Hosseini, S.; Soltani, N.; Keshavarz, M.; Dehghani, M. Oral magnesium supplementation in type II diabetic patients. *Med. J. Islam. Repub. Iran* **2014**, *28*, 67.
9. Wijesekara, N.; Chimienti, F.; Wheeler, M.B. Zinc, a regulator of islet function and glucose homeostasis. *Diabetes Obes. Metab.* **2009**, *11*, 202–214. [CrossRef]
10. Sun, Q.; Van Dam, R.M.; Willett, W.C.; Hu, F.B. Prospective Study of Zinc Intake and Risk of Type 2 Diabetes in Women. *Diabetes Care* **2009**, *32*, 629–634. [CrossRef]

11. Bonfanti, D.H.; Alcazar, L.P.; Arakaki, P.A.; Martins, L.T.; Agustini, B.C.; de Moraes Rego, F.G.; Frigeri, H.R. ATP-dependent potassium channels and type 2 diabetes mellitus. *Clin. Biochem.* **2015**, *48*, 476–482. [CrossRef]
12. Sales, C.H.; Pedrosa, L.F.; Lima, J.G.; Lemos, T.M.; Colli, C. Influence of magnesium status and magnesium intake on the blood glucose control in patients with type 2 diabetes. *Clin. Nutr.* **2011**, *30*, 359–364. [CrossRef] [PubMed]
13. Hruby, A.; Meigs, J.B.; O'Donnell, C.J.; Jacques, P.F.; McKeown, N.M. Higher magnesium intake reduces risk of impaired glucose and insulin metabolism and progression from prediabetes to diabetes in middle-aged americans. *Diabetes Care* **2014**, *37*, 419–427. [CrossRef] [PubMed]
14. Chabosseau, P.; Rutter, G.A. Zinc and Diabetes. *Arch. Biochem. Biophys.* **2016**, *611*, 79–85. [CrossRef] [PubMed]
15. Villegas, R.; Gao, Y.T.; Dai, Q.; Yang, G.; Cai, H.; Li, H.; Zheng, W.; Shu, X.O. Dietary calcium and magnesium intakes and the risk of type 2 diabetes: The Shanghai Women's Health Study. *Am. J. Clin. Nutr.* **2009**, *89*, 1059–1067. [CrossRef] [PubMed]
16. de Carvalho, G.B.; Brandão-Lima, P.N.; Maia, C.S.; Barbosa, K.B.F.; Pires, L.V. Zinc's role in the glycemic control of patients with type 2 diabetes: A systematic review. *BioMetals* **2017**, *30*, 151–162. [CrossRef] [PubMed]
17. Chatterjee, R.; Colangelo, L.A.; Yeh, H.C.; Anderson, C.A.; Daviglus, M.L.; Liu, K.; Brancati, F.L. Potassium intake and risk of incident type 2 diabetes mellitus: The Coronary Artery Risk Development in Young Adults (CARDIA) Study. *Diabetologia* **2012**, *55*, 1295–1303. [CrossRef] [PubMed]
18. Drake, I.; Hindy, G.; Ericson, U.; Orho-Melander, M. A prospective study of dietary and supplemental zinc intake and risk of type 2 diabetes depending on genetic variation in SLC30A8. *Genes Nutr.* **2017**, *12*, 30. [CrossRef] [PubMed]
19. World Health Organization. *Obesity: Preventing and Managing the Global Epidemic*; WHO Technical Report Series 894; WHO: Geneva, Switzerland, 2000; ISBN 92 4 120894 5.
20. World Health Organization. *Waist Circumference and Waist-Hip Ratio: Report of a WHO Expert Consultation*; World Health Organization: Geneva, Switzerland, 2011; ISBN 978 92 4 150149 1.
21. Brazilian Society of Cardiology. *7ª Diretriz Brasileira de Hipertensão Arterial*; Arq Bras Cardiol: Rio de janeiro, Brazil, 2016; ISSN 0066-782X.
22. Guenther, P.M.; DeMaio, T.J.; Ingwersen, L.A.; Berlin, M. The multiple-pass approach for the 24 hour recall in the Continuing Survey of food intakes by individuals (CSFII) 1994–1996. In Proceedings of the 2nd International Conference on Dietary Assessment Methods, Boston, MA, USA, 22–24 January 1995.
23. Institute of Medicine. *Dietary Reference Intakes for Calcium and Vitamin D*; National Academy of Sciences: Washington, DC, USA, 2011; ISBN 978-0-309-16394-1.
24. Institute of Medicine. *Dietary Reference Intakes: The Essential Guide to Nutrient Requirements*; National Academy of Sciences: Washington, DC, USA, 2006; ISBN 978-0-309-10091-5.
25. Mccrory, M.A.; Hajduk, C.L.; Roberts, S.B. Procedures for screening out inaccurate reports of dietary energy intake. *Public Health Nutr.* **2002**, *5*, 873–882. [CrossRef] [PubMed]
26. Vinken, A.G.; Bathalon, G.P.; Sawaya, A.L.; Dallal, G.E.; Tucker, K.L.; Roberts, S.B. Equations for predicting the energy requirements of healthy adults aged 18–81 y. *Am. J. Clin. Nutr.* **1999**, *69*, 920–926. [CrossRef]
27. German Institute of Human Nutrition Potsdam-Rehbrücke (DIfE). *The Multiple Source Method (MSM)*; DIfE: Nuthetal, Germany, 2012; Available online: https://msm.dife.de (accessed on 25 April 2018).
28. Willett, W.C.; Howe, G.R.; Kushi, L.H. Adjustment for total energy intake in epidemiologic studies. *Am. J. Clin. Nutr.* **1997**, *65*, 1220S–1231S. [CrossRef] [PubMed]
29. Wang, Q.; Koval, J.J.; Mills, C.A.; Lee, K.-I.D. Determination of the Selection Statistics and Best Significance Level in Backward Stepwise Logistic Regression. *Commun. Stat. Simul. C* **2007**, *37*, 62–72. [CrossRef]
30. American Diabetes Association. Glycemic Targets: Standards of Medical Care in Diabetes-2018. *Diabetes Care* **2018**, *41*, S55–S64. [CrossRef]
31. Sampaio, F.A.; Feitosa, M.M.; Sales, C.H.; Silva, D.M.C.; Cruz, K.J.C.; Oliveira, F.E.; Colli, C.; Marreiro, D.N. Influence of magnesium on biochemical parameters of iron and oxidative stress in patients with type 2 diabetes. *Nutr. Hosp.* **2014**, *30*, 570–576. [CrossRef]

32. Eshak, E.S.; Iso, H.; Maruyama, K.; Muraki, I.; Tamakoshi, A. Associations between dietary intakes of iron, copper and zinc with risk of type 2 diabetes mellitus: A large population-based prospective cohort study. *Clin. Nutr.* **2018**, *37*, 667–674. [CrossRef] [PubMed]
33. Vashum, K.P.; McEvoy, M.; Shi, Z.; Milton, A.H.; Islam, M.R.; Sibbritt, D.; Patterson, A.; Byles, J.; Loxton, D.; Attia, J. Is dietary zinc protective for type 2 diabetes? Results from the Australian longitudinal study on women's health. *BMC Endocr. Disord.* **2013**, *13*, 40. [CrossRef] [PubMed]
34. Kanoni, S.; Nettleton, J.A.; Hivert, M.F.; Ye, Z.; van Rooij, F.J.; Shungin, D.; Sonestedt, E.; Ngwa, J.S.; Wojczynski, M.K.; Lemaitre, R.N.; et al. Total Zinc Intake May Modify the Glucose-Raising Effect of a Zinc Transporter (SLC30A8) Variant: A 14-Cohort Meta-analysis. *Diabetes* **2011**, *60*, 2407–2416. [CrossRef] [PubMed]
35. Ige, A.O.; Ajayi, O.A.; Adewoye, E.O. Anti-inflammatory and insulin secretory activity in experimental type-2 diabetic rats treated orally with magnesium. *J. Basic Clin. Physiol. Pharmacol.* **2018**, *29*, 507–514. [CrossRef] [PubMed]
36. Morakinyo, A.O.; Samuel, T.A.; Adekunbi, D.A. Magnesium upregulates insulin receptor and glucose transporter-4 in streptozotocin-nicotinamide-induced type-2 diabetic rats. *Endocr. Regul.* **2018**, *52*, 6–16. [CrossRef]
37. Dong, J.Y.; Xun, P.; He, K.; Qin, L.Q. Magnesium Intake and Risk of Type 2 Diabetes: Meta-analysis of prospective cohort studies. *Diabetes Care* **2011**, *34*, 2116–2122. [CrossRef]
38. Barbagallo, M.; Dominguez, L.J. Magnesium and type 2 diabetes. *World J. Diabetes* **2015**, *6*, 1152–1157. [CrossRef]
39. Rodríguez-Morán, M.; Guerrero-Romero, F. Oral magnesium supplementation improves insulin sensitivity and metabolic control in type 2 diabetic subjects: A randomized double-blind controlled trial. *Diabetes Care* **2003**, *26*, 1147–1152. [CrossRef]
40. Paolisso, G.; Sgambato, S.; Pizza, G.; Passariello, N.; Varricchio, M.; D'Onofrio, F. Improved insulin response and action by chronic magnesium administration in aged NIDDM subjects. *Diabetes Care* **1989**, *12*, 265–269. [CrossRef]
41. Paolisso, G.; Scheen, A.; Cozzolino, D.; Di Maro, G.; Varricchio, M.; D'Onofrio, F.; Lefebvre, P.J. Changes in glucose turnover parameters and improvement of glucose oxidation after 4-week magnesium administration in elderly noninsulin-dependent (type II) diabetic patients. *J. Clin. Endocrinol. Metab.* **1994**, *78*, 1510–1514. [CrossRef] [PubMed]
42. Navarrete-Cortes, A.; Ble-Castillo, J.L.; Guerrero-Romero, F.; Cordova-Uscanga, R.; Juárez-Rojop, I.E.; Aguilar-Mariscal, H.; Tovilla-Zarate, C.A.; Lopez-Guevara Mdel, R. No effect of magnesium supplementation on metabolic control and insulin sensitivity in type 2 diabetic patients with normomagnesemia. *Magnes. Res.* **2014**, *27*, 48–56. [CrossRef] [PubMed]
43. Lima, M.L.; Cruz, T.; Pousada, J.C.; Rodrigues, L.E.; Barbosa, K.; Cangucu, V. The Effect of Magnesium Supplementation in Increasing Doses on the Control of Type 2 Diabetes. *Diabetes Care* **1998**, *21*, 682–686. [CrossRef]
44. de Valk, H.W.; Verkaaik, R.; van Rijn, H.J.; Geerdink, R.; Struyvenberg, A. Oral magnesium supplementation in insulin-requiring Type 2 diabetic patients. *Diabet. Med.* **1998**, *15*, 503–507. [CrossRef]
45. Gullestad, L.; Jacobsen, T.; Dolva, L. Effect of Magnesium Treatment on Glycemic Control and Metabolic Parameters in NIDDM Patients. *Diabetes Care* **1994**, *17*, 460–461. [CrossRef] [PubMed]
46. Purvis, J.R.; Cummings, D.M.; Landsman, P.; Carroll, R.; Barakat, H.; Bray, J.; Whitley, C.; Horner, R.D. Effect of oral magnesium supplementation on selected cardiovascular risk factors in non-insulin-dependent diabetics. *Arch. Fam. Med.* **1994**, *3*, 503–508. [CrossRef] [PubMed]
47. Eibl, N.L.; Kopp, H.P.; Nowak, H.R.; Schnack, C.J.; Hopmeier, P.G.; Schernthaner, G. Hypomagnesemia in Type II Diabetes: Effect of a 3-month replacement therapy. *Diabetes Care* **1995**, *18*, 188–192. [CrossRef]
48. Song, Y.; He, K.; Levitan, E.B.; Manson, J.E.; Liu, S. Effects of oral magnesium supplementation on glycaemic control in Type 2 diabetes: A meta-analysis of randomized double-blind controlled trials. *Diabet. Med.* **2006**, *23*, 1050–1056. [CrossRef]
49. Shalileh, M.; Shidfar, F.; Haghani, H.; Eghtesadi, S.; Heydari, I. The influence of calcium supplement on body composition, weight loss and insulin resistance in obese adults receiving low calorie diet. *J. Res. Med. Sci.* **2010**, *15*, 191–201.

50. Pikilidou, M.I.; Lasaridis, A.N.; Sarafidis, P.A.; Befani, C.D.; Koliakos, G.G.; Tziolas, I.M.; Kazakos, K.A.; Yovos, J.G.; Nilsson, P.M. Insulin sensitivity increase after calcium supplementation and change in intraplatelet calcium and sodium-hydrogen exchange in hypertensive patients with Type 2 diabetes. *Diabet. Med.* **2009**, *26*, 211–219. [CrossRef] [PubMed]
51. Dong, J.Y.; Qin, L.Q. Dietary calcium intake and risk of type 2 diabetes: Possible confounding by magnesium. *Eur. J. Clin. Nutr.* **2012**, *66*, 408–410. [CrossRef] [PubMed]
52. Van Dam, R.M.; Hu, F.B.; Rosenberg, L.; Krishnan, S.; Palmer, J.R. Dietary Calcium and Magnesium, Major Food Sources, and Risk of Type 2 Diabetes in U.S. Black Women. *Diabetes Care* **2006**, *29*, 2238–2243. [CrossRef] [PubMed]
53. Santos, R.K.F.; Brandão-Lima, P.N.; Tete, R.M.D.D.; Freire, A.R.S.; Pires, L.V. Vitamin D ratio and glycaemic control in individuals with type 2 diabetes mellitus: A systematic review. *Diabetes Metab. Res. Rev.* **2018**, *34*, 1–11. [CrossRef] [PubMed]
54. Chatterjee, R.; Yeh, H.C.; Shafi, T.; Selvin, E.; Anderson, C.; Pankow, J.S.; Miller, E.; Brancati, F. Serum and dietary potassium and risk of incident type 2 diabetes mellitus: The Atherosclerosis Risk in Communities (ARIC) study. *Arch. Intern. Med.* **2010**, *170*, 1745–1751. [CrossRef] [PubMed]
55. Becker, W.; Welten, D. Under-reporting in dietary surveys—Implications for development of food-based dietary guidelines. *Public Health Nutr.* **2001**, *4*, 683–687. [CrossRef] [PubMed]
56. Mirmiran, P.; Esmaillzadeh, A.; Azizi, F. Under-reporting of energy intake affects estimates of nutrient intakes. *Asia Pac. J. Clin. Nutr.* **2006**, *15*, 459–464. [PubMed]

6

The Association between Vitamin D Deficiency and Diabetic Retinopathy in Type 2 Diabetes

Bang-An Luo [1], Fan Gao [2] and Lu-Lu Qin [2,3,*]

1 Department of Mental Health, Brain Hospital of Hunan Province, Changsha 410007, Hunan, China; luo276@126.com
2 Department of Social Medicine and Health Management, Xiangya School of Public Health, Central South University, Changsha 410078, Hunan, China; gfydsl@163.com
3 Department of Prevention Medicine, Medical School, Hunan University of Chinese Medicine, Changsha 410208, Hunan, China
* Correspondence: powerestlulu@163.com

Abstract: Emerging evidence from in vivo and in vitro studies have shown that vitamin D may play an important role in the development of diabetic retinopathy (DR), but individually published studies showed inconclusive results. The aim of this study was to quantitatively summarize the association between vitamin D and the risk of diabetic retinopathy. We conducted a systematic literature search of Pubmed, Medline, and EMBASE updated in September 2016 with the following keywords: "vitamin D" or "cholecalciferol" or "25-hydroxyvitamin D" or "25(OH)D" in combination with "diabetic retinopathy" or "DR". Fifteen observational studies involving 17,664 subjects were included. In this meta-analysis, type 2 diabetes patients with vitamin D deficiency (serum 25(OH)D levels <20 ng/mL) experienced a significantly increased risk of DR (odds ratio (OR) = 2.03, 95% confidence intervals (CI): 1.07, 3.86), and an obvious decrease of 1.7 ng/mL (95% CI: −2.72, −0.66) in serum vitamin D was demonstrated in the patients with diabetic retinopathy. Sensitivity analysis showed that exclusion of any single study did not materially alter the overall combined effect. In conclusion, the evidence from this meta-analysis indicates an association between vitamin D deficiency and an increased risk of diabetic retinopathy in type 2 diabetes patients.

Keywords: vitamin D; diabetic retinopathy; type 2 diabetes; meta-analysis

---

1. Introduction

Diabetes mellitus (DM) is a large public health problem which affects more than 300 million individuals in the world, with significant morbidity and mortality worldwide [1]. In addition to the deleterious effects of the disease itself, its long-term complications can conspicuously decrease the quality of life of diabetes patients. Diabetes patients with uncontrolled or poorly-controlled blood glucose are at high risk of microvascular complications. Diabetic retinopathy (DR) is among the most common diabetic complications, and is the leading cause of blindness among working-aged individuals worldwide [2]. The prevalence of DR varies from 20% to 80% in different studies. Recent estimates suggest that the number of people with diabetic retinopathy will increase to 191 million by 2030 [3]. Diabetic retinopathy has a complex process. Many risk factors for DR have been established, such as poor glycemic control, long duration of diabetes, smoking, inflammation, obesity, and hypertension. Stratton et al. have given evidence that poor glycemic control and long duration of diabetes are independent risk factors of DR [4]. Praidou et al. found that increased physical activity is associated with less severe levels of DR, independent of the effects of HbA1c and body mass index (BMI) [5]. However, detailed pathophysiological mechanisms and other DR risk factors are not fully clarified.

Vitamin D is a multi-functional fat-solute metabolite required for humans' growth and development. Vitamin D deficiency (VDD) is seen across all ages, races, and geographic regions. Due to the wide functionality of vitamin D and because vitamin D deficiency is epidemic, vitamin D's non-classical functions are gaining more attention for the close association between vitamin D deficiency and cancers, infectious diseases, autoimmune diseases, diabetes, and diabetic complications [6–8]. The prevalence of vitamin D deficiency is high in type 2 diabetes mellitus (T2DM) patients [9–11]. Vitamin D receptors are expressed extensively in the retina [12], and an animal study showed that calcitriol was a potent inhibitor of retinal neovascularization in an oxygen-induced ischemic retinopathy mouse model [13]. This evidence indicated that vitamin D may play a role in the pathogensis of diabetic retinopathy.

While there are accumulating studies on the effect of vitamin D on diabetic retinopathy, the association between vitamin D and diabetic retinopathy are conflicting. According to some studies, vitamin D deficiency is associated with an increasing risk of diabetic retinopathy. Patrick et al. found an association between serum 25-hydroxyvitamin D concentration and diabetic retinopathy in a cohort of 1790 type 2 diabetes patients [14]. Inukai et al. reported that serum 25-hydroxyvitamin D (25(OH)D) levels were decreased in type 2 patients with retinopathy when compared with type 2 patients who had no microangiopathy [15]. However, others suggested that no significant differences in vitamin D status were found between type 2 diabetes with or without diabetic retinopathy. Alam et al. found no association between serum 25(OH)D levels and the presence and the severity of diabetic retinopathy [16].

Currently, there is insufficient evidence showing whether serum vitamin D deficiency is related to diabetic retinopathy, and the determination of this relationship has rarely been conducted. To address these issues, we carried out this meta-analysis by pooling the results from observation studies to examine the potential association between vitamin D and diabetic retinopathy.

2. Methods

2.1. Data Sources

Relevant articles were identified by a systematic literature search of Pubmed, Medline, and EMBASE through September 2016, using the following keywords: "vitamin D" or "cholecalciferol" or "25-hydroxyvitamin D" or "25(OH)D" in combination with "diabetic retinopathy" or "retinopathy" or "DR". Additionally, we manually searched all eligible original articles, reviews, and other relevant articles. This meta-analysis was performed following the guidelines for observation study protocols (Meta-analysis Of Observational Studies in Epidemiology (MOOSE) guidelines) [17].

2.2. Study Selection

Original articles evaluating the relationship between serum vitamin D status and diabetic retinopathy were reviewed and selected if they met the following inclusion criteria: (a) the study population was type 2 diabetes patients; (b) DR was the outcome, and the control group consisted of type 2 diabetes patients without DR; (c) the study presented sample sizes and odds ratios (OR) with 95% confidence intervals (CI) or information that could be used to infer these results; (d) vitamin D deficiency was defined as a 25(OH)D level below 20 ng/mL, and vitamin D insufficiency was defined as 25(OH)D levels of 21–29 ng/mL; (e) the study was published in English; and (f) the study met the predefined methodological quality assessment criteria for observational studies (Supplementary Data Box 1). Animal experiments, chemistry, or cell-line studies and editorials, commentaries, review articles, and case reports were excluded. Other exclusion criteria consisted of studies with a score of 0 for any item or a total score <7 out of 10 maximal points [18].

Two independent reviewers (Bang-An Luo and Fan Gao) reviewed all the literature searches and acquired full-length articles for all citations meeting the predefined selection criteria. Final inclusion or exclusion decisions were made after reading the full text. We resolved any disagreements through consensus or arbitration by a third reviewer (Lu-Lu Qin).

The following information was extracted from each article: the last name of first author, publication year, location of study, study design, sample size, 25(OH)D assay methods, 25(OH)D concentration, and the prevalence of vitamin D deficiency. In the case of relevant missing data, contacts were made to the main authors for more information.

2.3. Statistical Analysis

We performed this meta-analysis with RevMan Software (Version 5.2, Cochrane Collaboration, London, UK). The odds ratio (OR) and weight mean difference (WMD) were used as measures of associations between vitamin D status and risk for DR. If the OR and 95% CI were not available for the meta-analysis, these data were extracted from the selected articles to construct 2 × 2 tables of serum low vitamin D status versus the presence or absence of diabetic retinopathy.

We used forest plots to visually assess pooled estimates and corresponding 95% CIs for each study. The heterogeneity among the results of the included studies was evaluated with I^2 statistical tests. The percentage of $I^2 < 25$, near 50, and >75 indicated low, moderate, and high heterogeneity, respectively. A fixed-effects model or a random-effects model was used to combine the study results according to the heterogeneity. Once the effects were found to be heterogeneous ($I^2 > 50\%$), a random effects model was used. Otherwise, a fixed effect model was used.

Potential publication bias was assessed using the funnel plots. A sensitivity analysis was conducted to test the robustness of results, as well as to investigate the effect of a single article on the overall risk estimated by removing one article in each turn. Additionally, a subgroup analysis was performed to explore the possible explanations for heterogeneity. All the p-values were for a two-tailed and $p < 0.05$ was considered as statistically significant.

3. Results

3.1. Search Results

Of the 238 articles identified from our initial search, a total of 15 studies were finally identified as eligible for inclusion in this meta-analysis through a strict screening process (Figure 1). The quality assessment showed that the quality scores of these studies ranged from 8.5 to 10 according to the MOOSE guidelines, which indicates that all of the selected studies were of high quality (Supplementary Table S1).

3.2. Characteristics of the Included Studies

The characteristics of these articles in this meta-analysis are summarized in Table 1. These studies were published from 2000 to 2016. Among these studies, nine were conducted in Asia, two each in North America and Europe, one in Africa, and one each in three countries (Australia, New Zealand, and Finland). Seven studies had cross-sectional design, five were case–control, two were prospective cohort, and one had a retrospective cohort design. Four different assay techniques were used to measure the serum 25(OH)D levels, and four different ways were used to diagnose DR. Eight of the included studies explored the association between vitamin D deficiency and diabetic retinopathy, four explored the association between vitamin D insufficiency and diabetic retinopathy, and ten explored the mean difference in vitamin D status among diabetic retinopathy and non-diabetic retinopathy.

The diversity of participant characteristics was considerable in these studies. Out of 17,664 participants, 3455 (19.6%) were diagnosed with diabetic retinopathy, consisting of different ages and races. In addition, the age of type 2 diabetes participants were older than 18 years and the mean BMI—if provided by articles—varied from 13.9 to 42.0 kg/m^2. The vitamin D status of diabetic retinopathy ranged from 9.2 to 32.6 ng/mL.

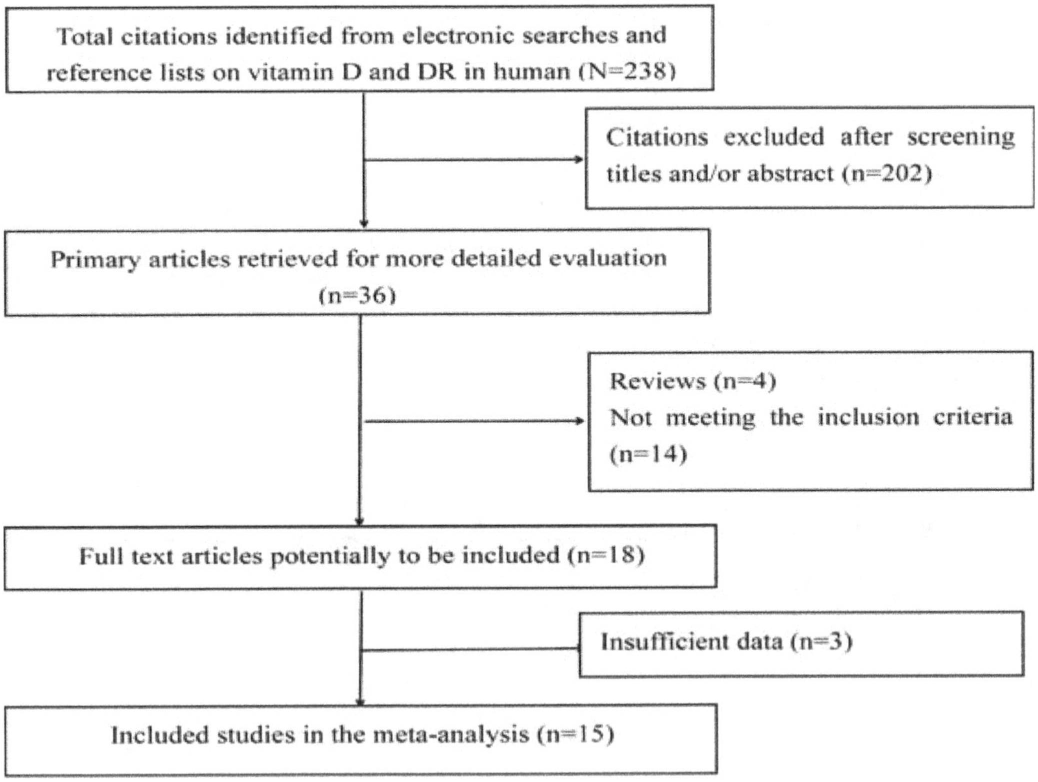

Figure 1. Flow chart of literature search and study selection.

3.3. *Main Analysis*

The relationship between serum vitamin D deficiency (VDD) and the risk of diabetic retinopathy is shown in Figure 2 and Supplementary Table S2. Eight studies involving 13,435 participants were included. As the results of this meta-analysis show, type 2 diabetes with vitamin D deficiency (serum 25(OH)D levels <20 ng/mL) had an increased risk of developing diabetic retinopathy (OR = 2.03, 95% CI: 1.07, 3.86) in the random-effects model.

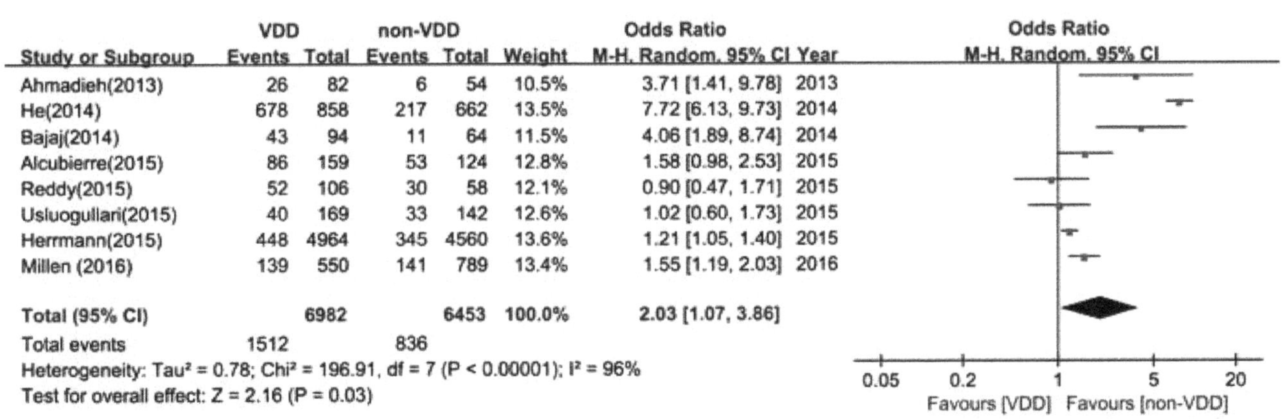

Figure 2. The meta-analysis of the association between vitamin D deficiency (VDD) and diabetic retinopathy (DR).

Based on four studies, the pooled OR for vitamin D insufficiency (VDI, serum 25(OH)D levels <30 ng/mL) was calculated as (OR = 0.89, 95% CI: 0.20, 4.02) (Supplementary Table S2 and Supplementary Figure S1). Only the result of vitamin D deficiency showed that low serum vitamin D status increased the risk of diabetic retinopathy.

The comparison of the mean difference between the DR group and the control group (non-DR group) is shown in Figure 3. From the results of the random-effects model, the pooled effect was −1.7 ng/mL (95% CI: −2.75, −0.66) and significant heterogeneity was observed ($I^2 = 80\%$, $p < 0.001$). It showed that serum 25(OH)D levels were significantly lower in diabetic retinopathy patients than the control in type 2 diabetes. This result demonstrated that vitamin D deficiency is significantly related with an increased risk of DR.

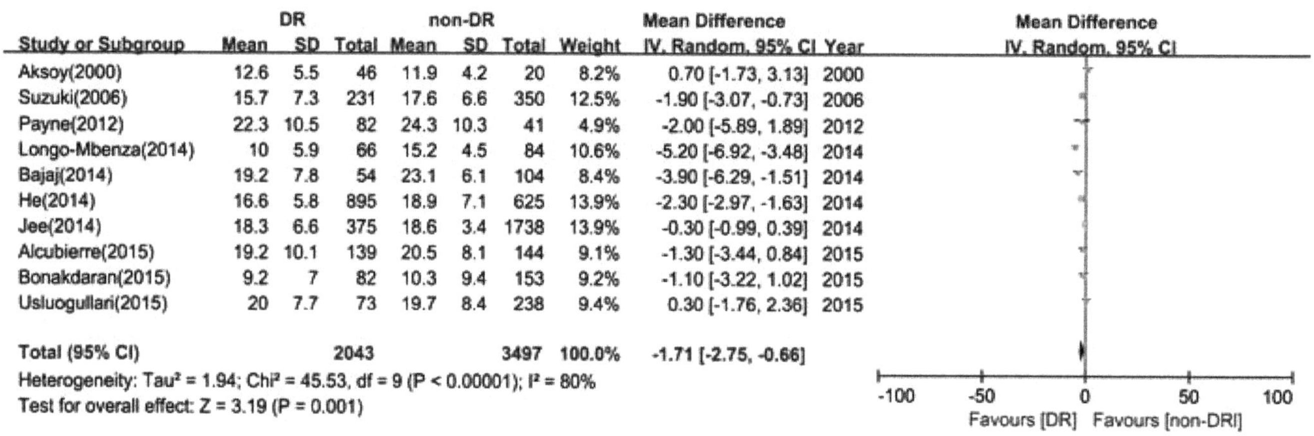

Figure 3. Meta-analysis of the association between 25-hydroxyvitamin D (25(OH)D) levels and DR.

Table 1. Characteristics of observational studies included in this meta-analysis.

Author and Year	Country	Study Design	Sample Size (*n*)	VD Assay Method	DR Diagnosis	VDD Prevalence (%)		Mean 25(OH)D ng/mL (SD)		Significant	Adjustment
						DR	NDR	DR	NDR		
Aksoy (2000) [19]	Turkey	Cross-sectional	66	RIA	Ophthalmologists	NA	NA	12.6 ± 5.5	11.9 ± 4.2	Yes	No
Suzuki (2006) [20]	Japan	Case–control	581	RIA	Ophthalmologists	NA	NA	15.7 ± 7.3	17.6 ± 6.6	Yes	Age, BMI, duration, HbA1c, treatment
Payne (2012) [21]	US	Cross-sectional	123	CL	Ophthalmologists	NA	NA	22.3 ± 10.5	24.3 ± 10.3	Yes	Multivitamin use
Ahmadieh (2013) [22]	Lebanon	Cross-sectional	136	RIA	Ophthalmologists	78.8	53.8	NA	NA	Yes	BMI, duration, smoking
Bajaj (2014) [23]	Indian	Case–control	158	NA	Ophthalmologists	79.6	49.0	NA	NA	Yes	No
He (2014) [24]	China	Cross-sectional	1520	CL	The International Clinical DR Severity Scale	75.7	63.6	16.6 ± 5.8	18.9 ± 7.1	Yes	Age, sex, duration
Jee (2014) [25]	Korea	Cross-sectional	2113	RIA	The Early Treatment Diabetic Retinopathy Study severity scale	NA	NA	18.3 ± 6.6	18.7 ± 3.4	Yes	Sex
Longo-Mbenza (2014) [26]	Congo	Case–control	150	HPLC	The modified Airlie House classification system	NA	NA	10 ± 5.9	15.2 ± 4.5	Yes	No
Alcubierre (2015) [27]	Spain	Case–control	283	CL	Ophthalmologists	61.9	50.7	19.2 ± 10.1	20.5 ± 8.1	Yes	Race, season, physical activity
Bonakdaran (2015) [10]	Iran	Cross-sectional	235	RIA	Ophthalmologists	NA	NA	9.2 ± 7.0	10.3 ± 9.4	No	Age, sex, duration, BMI, HbA1c,BMI, sex, HbA1c
Herrmann (2015) [28]	Australia, New Zealand, and Finland	Prospective	9524	CL	Ophthalmologists	56.5	51.7	NA	NA	Yes	Age, sex, et al. *
Reddy (2015) [29]	Indian	Case–control	164	HPLC	The modified Airlie House classification system	27.0	23.0	NA	NA	No	Duration
Usluogullari (2015) [30]	Turkey	Retrospective	557	HPLC	Ophthalmologists	45.2	54.2	20.0 ± 7.7	19.7 ± 8.4	No	Age, BMI, sex, HbA1c
Zoppini (2015) [31]	Italy	Cross-sectional	715	CL	Ophthalmologists	NA	NA	NA	NA	Yes	Age
Millen (2016) [32]	US	Prospective	1339	LC-MS	The modified Airlie House classification system	49.6	38.8	NA	NA	Yes	Race, duration, HbA1c, hypertension

DR: diabetic retinopathy; VD: vitamin D; VDD: vitamin D deficiency; NDR: no diabetic retinopathy; NA: not available. CL: chemiluminescence; HPLC: high performance liquid chromatography; RIA: radioimmunoassay; LC-MS: high-sensitivity mass spectrometry; SD: standard deviation; et al. *: diabetes duration, HbA 1c, systolic blood pressure, BMI, lipids (triglycerides and high-density lipoprotein (HDL) and low-density lipoprotein (LDL) cholesterol), smoking, baseline use of oral hypoglycemic agents, and baseline use of insulin.

3.4. Sensitivity and Subgroup Analysis

To explore the impact of various exclusion criteria on the overall risk estimate, we conducted sensitivity and subgroup analyses to examine the potential sources of heterogeneity in this meta-analysis. In the result of the pooled ORs, the study conducted in China [24] was responsible for most of the heterogeneity in this meta-analysis. After excluding this study, the heterogeneity was down to 67% and the pooled OR was 1.50 (95% CI: 1.41, 1.98). Besides, there were no obvious changes in the pooled ORs as a result of the exclusion of any other single study. In the comparison of the mean difference between the DR group and the control group, moderate heterogeneity ($I^2 = 70\%$, $p < 0.001$) was observed among the remaining studies after the exclusion Jee's study [25]. Jee's study was responsible for most of the heterogeneity. Further exclusion of any single study did not alter the overall combined relative risk, with a range from −2.2 ng/mL (−3.28, −1.17) to −1.6 ng/mL (−2.43, −0.69), and each outcome had statistical significance.

In the subgroup with study design, there were moderate heterogeneities in cross-sectional and prospective cohort studies for the pooled OR ($I^2 = 52\%$, $p = 0.15$ for cross-sectional studies; $I^2 = 61\%$, $p = 0.11$ for prospective cohort studies) (Supplementary Materials Figure S2). We found that there were obvious heterogeneities in the cross-sectional and the case–control studies for the pooled WMD ($I^2 = 79\%$, $p = 0.0007$ for cross-sectional studies; $I^2 = 76\%$, $p = 0.006$ for case–control studies) (Supplementary Materials Figure S3). In the subgroup with VD assay methods, there were high heterogeneities in the chemiluminescence (CL) vitamin D assay method for the pooled OR ($I^2 = 99\%$, $p < 0.0001$), and the study conducted in China [24] was responsible for the heterogeneities. After excluding this study, the heterogeneity in the CL subgroup was down to 8% and the pooled OR was 1.25 (95% CI: 1.06, 1.48) (Supplementary Materials Figure S4). In the subgroup with DR diagnosis, there were modern heterogeneities in the ophthalmologists group (OR = 1.71, 95% CI: 1.11, 2.62, $I^2 = 74\%$, $p = 0.0004$) (Supplementary Materials Figure S5). Subgroup analyses of BMI, season, duration of diabetes, race, and age were not conducted due to insufficient data in some studies.

3.5. Publication Bias

No obvious publication bias was observed in the funnel plots of this meta-analysis (Supplementary Materials Figure S6).

4. Discussion

Vitamin D's non-classical functions have attracted much public health attention for its closer association with some diseases. This is the first meta-analysis of the relationship between serum vitamin D status and DR in type 2 diabetes. In this meta-analysis, the results of 15 observational studies provided strong evidence that serum 25(OH)D levels were associated with an increased risk of DR in type 2 diabetes patients. Both the results of the pooled OR for vitamin D deficiency (serum 25(OH)D levels <20 ng/mL) and the pooled effect of WMD showed that the serum 25(OH)D levels in type 2 diabetes had a relationship with DR, while the pooled OR for vitamin D insufficiency (serum 25(OH)D levels <30 ng/mL) did not. Considering the results of vitamin D deficiency and that serum 25(OH)D levels were more reliable and accurate than the result of vitamin D insufficiency (only four studies), we concluded that low 25(OH)D levels were associated with an increased risk of DR.

The quality of the studies included in this meta-analysis was high. From the funnel plots, we concluded that there was no obvious publication bias in this meta-analysis. We further conducted sensitivity and subgroup analyses to explore potential sources of heterogeneity. From the forest plots, we observed high heterogeneity among the pooled OR and WMD as the association of DR (Figures 2 and 3), which was not surprising given the different characteristics of participants and adjustments for confounding factors. Regarding the results of sensitivity analyses, two studies probably contributed to the heterogeneity [24,25]. After excluding the two studies, there was moderate heterogeneity, and there may be other factors contributing to the heterogeneity in this study. Firstly, there was no consensus on the levels of vitamin D denoting deficiency and insufficiency, and the diagnosis standards of DR might not be uniform among different ophthalmologists in these studies. Secondly, there were four methods for measuring vitamin D, such as HPLC (high performance liquid chromatography) and RIA (radioimmunoassay). Thirdly, the time of collecting blood sample were different. Fourthly, the heterogeneity might be a result of differences in the study populations—there were several races included in this meta-analysis. Fifthly, the duration of diabetes, the age of patients, the diet, the treatment of diabetes, and the sunlight exposure are confounding factors in this meta-analysis. Hence, more studies are needed to give full proof.

There is an epidemic of vitamin D deficiency around the world [6]. From this meta-analysis, the prevalence of vitamin D deficiency was high among type 2 diabetes patients, although it may vary from different latitude, ethnicity, body mass index, season, and supplementation of vitamin D. VDD was consistent with previous studies [9–11]. For patients with diabetes, the association with vitamin D deficiency and risk of developing diabetes has been acknowledged. Vitamin D deficiency is associated with an increased risk for diabetes [9,22,29].

In patients with diabetic retinopathy, the level of serum 25(OH)D was lower than patients without diabetic retinopathy. The characteristic feature of diabetic retinopathy is the appearance of vascular lesions of increasing severity, ending up in the growth of new vessels (neovascularization). Vitamin D has anti-inflammation properties and inhibits vascular smooth muscle cell growth and effects on the expression of transforming growth factor β1 [13,33–35]. Vitamin D is an important regulator of hundreds of genes regulating key biological processes from cell division to apoptosis [36]. It is well known that poor glycemic control is a risk factor for the development and progression of DR, and vitamin D deficiency has been shown to impair insulin synthesis and secretion in animal models of diabetes [37]. On the other hand, an optimal concentration of vitamin D is strongly proven to be necessary for efficient insulin secretion and function [38–40], and vitamin D receptors (VDR) are ubiquitously expressed in every human tissue, including retina. Active vitamin D mediates its biological function by binding to vitamin D receptors. Vitamin D receptors have been found to be associated with insulin secretion and sensitivity, and have been identified in pancreatic beta cells [41]. Additionally, some genes associated with the development of diabetic retinopathy have been found, such as *Bsm1*, *rs2228570*, and *TT*. So, vitamin D status is related with the development and progression of diabetic retinopathy among type 2 diabetes patients.

Increasing studies have given more evidence of this. Annwelier et al. found that the serum 25(OH)D levels were associated with optic chiasm volume [42], and in a vitro experiment, vitamin D was found to inhibit neovascularization in retinal tissue in a model of ischemic retinopathy [13]. What is more, proof of the VDR polymorphisms related with diabetic retinopathy was found. Hong et al. showed that patients with the B allele (BB or Bb) of Bsm1 polymorphism in VDR were associated with lower risk of diabetic retinopathy compared to patients without the B allele (bb) in Korean type 2 diabetic patients [41]. Bucan et al. showed that the bb genotype in VDR has a higher risk of developing diabetic retinopathy [43]. Zhong et al. found that rs2228570 was associated with increased risk of diabetic retinopathy in Han Chinese type 2 diabetes patients [44]. Benjamin et al. reported that the anticipation of retinopathy onset is significantly associated with the exaggeration of oxidative stress biomarkers or decrease of antioxidants in African type 2 diabetics, and supplementation with vitamin D should be recommended as complement therapies of T2DM [26]. Therefore, low serum 25(OH)D levels are association with an increased risk of diabetic retinopathy, but more studies are required to identify the mechanism of the relationship between vitamin D and diabetic retinopathy fully.

It is well known that one of the two major sources of vitamin D is cutaneous synthesis by solar ultraviolet B radiation and the other is dietary intake. The cutaneous synthesis of vitamin D is affected by many factors, such as season, latitude, time of day, skin pigmentation, the amount of skin exposed, and whether makeup with sunscreen is used, so serum 25-hydroxyvitamin D levels vary between areas and persons. Hence, dietary vitamin D supplementation and physical activity might be a feasible way for patients with diabetes to maintain sufficient 25-hydroxyvitamin D levels. Physical activity may increase blood 25-hydroxyvitamin D concentrations as a consequence of an associated increase in sunlight exposure. Praidou et al. reported that increased physical activity is associated with less severe levels of diabetic retinopathy, independent of the effects of HbA1c and BMI [5]. Lee et al. showed that 3 months of vitamin D supplementation improved neuropathic symptoms by 50% in diabetic patients whose 25-hydroxyvitamin D status was deficient at baseline [45]. However, there has yet to be a dietary vitamin D supplementation trial on diabetic retinopathy. Thus, large randomized controlled trials researching on reducing diabetic retinopathy in type 2 diabetes are needed to accurately evaluate the potential benefits of these low-cost interventions in the future.

Diabetic retinopathy may develop and progress to advanced stages without producing any immediate symptoms to the patient. Screening for DR is essential in order to establish early treatment of sight-threatening retinopathy and has been demonstrated to be successful at achieving vision loss [46]. Considering the heavy burden of DR and the association between serum 25(OH)D level and diabetic retinopathy, low 25(OH)D levels may help us to find more early stage diabetic retinopathy patients. Therefore, screening low 25(OH)D levels may be a potential simple way for screening diabetic retinopathy among type 2 diabetes in primary hospitals—especially where there is a shortage of ophthalmic equipment or ophthalmologists.

The main strength of this study is giving strong evidence of the association of serum vitamin D and diabetic retinopathy. However, there were several limitations in this study. Firstly, different diagnostic criteria of diabetic retinopathy and different measured assays could have influenced the pooled effect. Secondly, there were some confounding factors in this meta-analysis, such as age, race, diet, the treatment of diabetes, sun exposure, physical activity, and so on. Some, but not all, of the studies generated adjusted OR, so we could not pool the findings by adjusting for confounding factors. Thirdly, there was a lack of access to complete data of all related published papers, despite correspondence with the authors. Fourthly, the association between vitamin D and the severity of diabetic retinopathy was not analyzed in this meta-analysis because of a lack of enough data and information. Finally, only published articles in English were included.

5. Conclusions

In conclusion, this meta-analysis indicates an association between vitamin D deficient type 2 diabetes mellitus patients and an increased risk of diabetic retinopathy. Type 2 diabetes patients with vitamin D deficiency experienced an increased risk of diabetic retinopathy. However, further studies are required to better understand the relationship between vitamin D deficient type 2 diabetes patients and diabetic retinopathy, and well-designed randomized controlled trials are needed to determine the explicit effect of vitamin D supplementation on the prevention of diabetic retinopathy. Considering the high prevalence of vitamin D deficiency and the burden of the diabetic retinopathy, screening type 2 diabetes patients who are at risk of vitamin D deficiency should be considered.

Supplementary Materials:
Table S1. Quality scores of included studies on vitamin D status and pregnancy outcomes. Table S2. Results of meta-analysis according to 25-hydroxyvitamin D (25(OH)D) level. DR: diabetic retinopathy; NDR: no diabetic retinopathy. Figure S1. Meta-analysis of the association between vitamin D insufficiency (<30 ng/mL) and DR. Figure S2. Subgroup analysis of pooled ORs according to study design. Figure S3. Subgroup analysis of weight mean difference (WMD) according to study design. Figure S4. Subgroup analysis of pooled ORs according to vitamin D assay method. Figure S5. Subgroup analysis of pooled ORs according to different DR diagnosis. Figure S6. Result of funnel plots.

Author Contributions: All authors participated in the process of this meta-analysis.

References

1. Sherwin, R.; Jastreboff, A.M. Year in diabetes 2012: the diabetes tsunami. *J. Clin. Endocrinol. Metab.* **2012**, *97*, 4293–4301. [CrossRef] [PubMed]
2. Klein, B.E. Overview of epidemiologic studies of diabetic retinopathy. *Ophthalmic Epidemiol.* **2007**, *14*, 179–183. [CrossRef] [PubMed]

3. Zheng, Y.; He, M.; Congdon, N. The worldwide epidemic of diabetic retinopathy. *Indian J. Ophthalmol.* **2012**, *60*, 428–431. [PubMed]
4. Stratton, I.M.; Kohner, E.M.; Aldington, S.J.; Turner, R.C.; Holman, R.R.; Manley, S.E.; Matthews, D.R. UKPDS50: Risk factors for incidence and progression of retinopathy in Type II diabetes over 6 years from diagnosis. *Diabetologia* **2001**, *44*, 156–163. [CrossRef] [PubMed]
5. Praidou, A.; Harris, M.; Niakas, D.; Labiris, G. Physical activity and its correlation to diabetic retinopathy. *J. Diabetes Complicat.* **2017**, *31*, 456–461. [CrossRef] [PubMed]
6. Holick, M.F. Vitamin D deficiency. *N. Engl. J. Med.* **2007**, *357*, 266–281. [CrossRef] [PubMed]
7. Holick, M.F.; Chen, T.C. Vitamin D deficiency: A worldwide problem with health consequences. *Am. J. Clin. Nutr.* **2008**, *87*, 1080s–1086s. [CrossRef] [PubMed]
8. Mitri, J.; Muraru, M.D.; Pittas, A.G. Vitamin D and Type 2 diabetes: A systematic review. *Eur. J. Clin. Nutr.* **2011**, *65*, 1005–1015. [CrossRef] [PubMed]
9. Rhee, S.Y.; Hwang, Y.C.; Chung, H.Y.; Woo, J.T. Vitamin D and diabetes in Koreans: Analyses based on the Fourth Korea National Health and Nutrition Examination Survey (KNHANES), 2008–2009. *Diabet. Med.* **2012**, *29*, 1003–1010. [CrossRef] [PubMed]
10. Bonakdaran, S.; Shoeibi, N. Is there any correlation between vitamin D insufficiency and diabetic retinopathy? *Int. J. Ophthalmol.* **2015**, *8*, 326–331. [PubMed]
11. Isaia, G.; Giorgino, R.; Adami, S. High prevalence of hypovitaminosis D in female type diabetic population. *Diabetes Care* **2001**, *24*, 1496. [CrossRef] [PubMed]
12. Taverna, M.J.; Selam, J.L.; Slama, G. Association between a protein polymorphism in the start codon of the vitamin D receptor gene and severe diabetic retinopathy in C-peptide-negative type 1 diabetes. *J. Clin. Endocrinol. Metab.* **2005**, *90*, 4803–4808. [CrossRef] [PubMed]
13. Albert, D.M.; Scheef, E.A.; Wang, S.; Mehraein, F.; Darjatmoko, S.R.; Sorenson, C.M.; Sheibani, N. Calcitriol is a potent inhibitor of retinal neovascularization. *Investig. Ophthalmol. Vis. Sci.* **2007**, *48*, 2327–2334. [CrossRef] [PubMed]
14. Patrick, P.A.; Visintainer, P.F.; Shi, Q.; Weiss, I.A.; Brand, D.A. Vitamin D and Retinopathy in Adults with Diabetes Mellitus. *Arch. Ophthalmol.* **2012**, *130*, 756–760. [CrossRef] [PubMed]
15. Inukai, T.; Fujiwara, Y.; Tayama, K.; Aso, Y.; Takemura, Y. Alterations in serum levels of 1 alpha, 25(OH)2 D3 and osteocalcin in patients with early diabetic nephropathy. *Diabetes Res. Clin. Pract.* **1997**, *38*, 53–59. [CrossRef]
16. Alam, U.; Amjad, Y.; Chan, A.W.; Asghar, O.; Petropoulos, I.N.; Malik, R.A. Vitamin D Deficiency Is Not Associated with Diabetic Retinopathy or Maculopathy. *J. Diabetes Res.* **2016**, *2016*, 6156217. [CrossRef] [PubMed]
17. Stroup, D.F.; Berlin, J.A.; Morton, S.C.; Olkin, I.; Williamson, G.D.; Rennie, D.; Moher, D.; Becker, B.J.; Sipe, T.A.; Thacker, S.B. Meta-analysis of observational studies in epidemiology: A proposal for reporting. Meta-analysis of observational studies in epidemiology (moose) group. *JAMA* **2000**, *283*, 2008–2012. [CrossRef] [PubMed]
18. Duckitt, K.; Harrington, D. Risk factors for pre-eclampsia at antenatal booking: Systematic review of controlled studies. *BMJ (Clin. Res. Ed.)* **2005**, *330*, 565. [CrossRef] [PubMed]
19. Aksoy, H.; Akçay, F.; Kurtul, N.; Baykal, O.; Avci, B. Serum 1,25 Dihydroxy Vitamin D (1,25(OH)2D3), 25 Hydroxy Vitamin D (25(OH)D) and Parathormone Levels in Diabetic Retinopathy. *Clin. Biochem.* **2000**, *33*, 47–51. [CrossRef]
20. Suzuki, A.; Kotake, M.; Ono, Y.; Kato, T.; Oda, N.; Hayakawa, N.; Hashimoto, S.; Itoh, M. Hypovitaminosis D in type 2 diabetes mellitus: Association with microvascular complications and type of treatment. *Endocr. J.* **2006**, *53*, 503–510. [CrossRef] [PubMed]
21. Payne, J.F.; Ray, R.; Watson, D.G.; Delille, C.; Rimler, E.; Cleveland, J.; Lynn, M.J.; Tangpricha, V.; Srivastava, S.K. Vitamin D Insufficiency in Diabetic Retinopathy. *Endocr. Pract.* **2012**, *18*, 185–193. [CrossRef] [PubMed]
22. Ahmadieh, H.; Azar, S.T.; Lakkis, N.; Arabi, A. Hypovitaminosis D in Patients with Type 2 Diabetes Mellitus: A Relation to Disease Control and Complications. *ISRN Endocrinol.* **2013**, *2013*, 641098. [CrossRef] [PubMed]
23. Bajaj, S.; Singh, R.P.; Dwivedi, N.C.; Singh, K.; Gupta, A.; Mathur, M. Vitamin D levels and microvascular complications in type 2 diabetes. *Indian J. Endocrinol. Metab.* **2014**, *18*, 537–541. [CrossRef] [PubMed]

24. He, R.; Shen, J.; Liu, F.; Zeng, H.; Li, L.; Yu, H.; Lu, H.; Lu, F.; Wu, Q.; Jia, W. Vitamin D deficiency increases the risk of retinopathy in Chinese patients with Type 2 diabetes. *Diabet. Med.* **2014**, *31*, 1657–1664. [CrossRef] [PubMed]
25. Jee, D.; Han, K.; Kim, E.C. Inverse Association between High Blood 25 Hydroxyvitamin D Levels and Diabetic Retinopathy in a Representative Korean Population. *PLoS ONE* **2014**, *9*, e115199. [CrossRef] [PubMed]
26. Longo-Mbenza, B.; Mvitu Muaka, M.; Masamba, W.; Muizila Kini, L.; Longo Phemba, I.; Kibokela Ndembe, D.; Tulomba Mona, D. Retinopathy in non diabetics, diabetic retinopathy and oxidative stress: A new phenotype in Central Africa? *Int. J. Ophthalmol.* **2014**, *7*, 293–301. [PubMed]
27. Alcubierre, N.; Valls, J.; Rubinat, E.; Cao, G.; Esquerda, A.; Traveset, A.; Granado-Casas, M.; Jurjo, C.; Mauricio, D. Vitamin D Deficiency Is Associated with the Presence and Severity of Diabetic Retinopathy in Type 2 Diabetes Mellitus. *J. Diabetes Res.* **2015**, *2015*, 374178. [CrossRef] [PubMed]
28. Herrmann, M.; Sullivan, D.R.; Veillard, A.S.; McCorquodale, T.; Straub, I.R.; Scott, R.; Laakso, M.; Topliss, D.; Jenkins, A.J.; Blankenberg, S.; Burton, A.; et al. Serum 25-Hydroxyvitamin D: A Predictor of Macrovascular and Microvascular Complications in Patients With Type 2 Diabetes. *Diabetes Care* **2015**, *38*, 521–528. [CrossRef] [PubMed]
29. Reddy, G.B.; Sivaprasad, M.; Shalini, T.; Satyanarayana, A.; Seshacharyulu, M.; Balakrishna, N.; Viswanath, K.; Sahay, M. Plasma vitamin D status in patients with type 2 diabetes with and without retinopathy. *Nutrition* **2015**, *31*, 959–963. [CrossRef] [PubMed]
30. Usluogullari, C.A.; Balkan, F.; Caner, S.; Ucler, R.; Kaya, C.; Ersoy, R.; Cakir, B. The relationship between microvascular complications and vitamin D deficiency in type 2 diabetes mellitus. *BMC Endocr. Disord.* **2015**, *15*, 33. [CrossRef] [PubMed]
31. Zoppini, G.; Galletti, A.; Targher, G.; Brangani, C.; Pichiri, I.; Trombetta, M.; Negri, C.; de Santi, F.; Stoico, V.; Cacciatori, V.; et al. Lower levels of 25-hydroxyvitamin D3 are associated with a higher prevalence of microvascular complications in patients with type 2 diabetes. *BMJ Open Diabetes Res. Care* **2015**, *3*, e000058. [CrossRef] [PubMed]
32. Millen, A.E.; Sahli, M.W.; Nie, J.; LaMonte, M.J.; Lutsey, P.L.; Klein, B.E.; Mares, J.A.; Meyers, K.J.; Andrews, C.A.; Klein, R. Adequate vitamin D status is associated with the reduced odds of prevalent diabetic retinopathy in African Americans and Caucasians. *Cardiovasc. Diabetol.* **2016**, *15*, 128. [CrossRef] [PubMed]
33. Zittermann, A.; Koerfer, R. Protective and toxic effects of vitamin D on vascular calcification: Clinical implications. *Mol. Asp. Med.* **2008**, *29*, 423–432. [CrossRef] [PubMed]
34. Targher, G.; Bertolini, L.; Padovani, R.; Zenari, L.; Scala, L.; Cigolini, M.; Arcaro, G. Serum 25-hydroxyvitamin D3 concentrations and carotid artery intima–media thickness among Type 2 diabetic patients. *Clin. Endocrinol. (Oxf.)* **2006**, *65*, 593–597. [CrossRef] [PubMed]
35. Ren, Z.; Li, W.; Zhao, Q.; Ma, L.; Zhu, J. The impact of 1,25-dihydroxy vitamin D3 on the expressions of vascular endothelial growth factor and transforming growth factor-b1 in the retinas of rats with diabetes. *Diabetes Res. Clin. Pract.* **2012**, *98*, 474–480. [CrossRef] [PubMed]
36. Temmerman, J.C. Vitamin D and cardiovascular disease. *J. Am. Coll. Nutr.* **2011**, *30*, 167–170. [CrossRef] [PubMed]
37. Mathieu, C.; Gysemans, C.; Giulietti, A.; Bouillon, R. Vitamin D and diabetes. *Diabetologia* **2005**, *48*, 1247–1257. [CrossRef] [PubMed]
38. Michos, E.D. Vitamin D deficiency and the risk of incident Type 2 diabetes. *Future Cardiol.* **2009**, *5*, 15–18. [CrossRef] [PubMed]
39. Danescu, L.G.; Levy, S.; Levy, J. Vitamin D and diabetes mellitus. *Endocrine* **2009**, *35*, 11–17. [CrossRef] [PubMed]
40. Cavalier, E.; Delanaye, P.; Souberbielle, J.C.; Radermecker, R.P. Vitamin D and type 2 diabetes mellitus: where do we stand? *Diabetes Metab.* **2011**, *37*, 265–272. [CrossRef] [PubMed]
41. Hong, Y.J.; Kang, E.S.; Ji, M.J.; Choi, H.J.; Oh, T.; Koong, S.S.; Jeon, H.J. Association between Bsm1 Polymorphism in Vitamin D Receptor Gene and Diabetic Retinopathy of Type 2 Diabetes in Korean Population. *Endocrinol. Metab. (Seoul)* **2015**, *30*, 469–474. [CrossRef] [PubMed]

42. Annweiler, C.; Beauchet, O.; Bartha, R.; Graffe, A.; Milea, D.; Montero-Odasso, M. Association between serum 25-hydroxyvitamin D concentration and optic chiasm volume. *J. Am. Geriatr. Soc.* **2013**, *61*, 1026–1028. [CrossRef] [PubMed]
43. Bućan, K.; Ivanisević, M.; Zemunik, T.; Boraska, V.; Skrabić, V.; Vatavuk, Z.; Galetović, D.; Znaor, L. Retinopathy and nephropathy in type 1 diabetic patients association with polymorphysms of vitamin D-receptor, TNF, Neuro-D and IL-1 receptor 1 genes. *Coll. Antropol.* **2009**, *33*, 99–105. [PubMed]
44. Zhong, X.; Du, Y.; Lei, Y.; Liu, N.; Guo, Y.; Pan, T. Effects of vitamin D receptor gene polymorphism and clinical characteristics on risk of diabetic retinopathy in Han Chinese type 2 diabetes patients. *Gene* **2015**, *566*, 212–216. [CrossRef] [PubMed]
45. Lee, P.; Chen, R. Vitamin D as an analgesic for patients with type 2 diabetes and neuropathic pain. *Arch. Intern. Med.* **2008**, *168*, 771–772. [CrossRef] [PubMed]
46. Stitt, A.W.; Curtis, T.M.; Chen, M.; Medina, R.J.; McKay, G.J.; Jenkins, A.; Gardiner, T.A.; Lyons, T.J.; Hammes, H.P.; Simó, R.; et al. The progress in understanding and treatment of diabetic retinopathy. *Prog. Retin. Eye Res.* **2016**, *51*, 156–186. [CrossRef] [PubMed]

7

Effects of Tempeh Fermentation with *Lactobacillus plantarum* and *Rhizopus oligosporus* on Streptozotocin-Induced Type II Diabetes Mellitus in Rats

Ying-Che Huang [1], Bo-Hua Wu [2], Yung-Lin Chu [3], Wen-Chang Chang [4,†] and Ming-Chang Wu [1,2,*,†]

1 Graduate Institute of Bioresources, National Pingtung University of Science and Technology, Pingtung 91201, Taiwan; huangleo0811@gmail.com
2 Department of Food Science, National Pingtung University of Science and Technology, Pingtung 91201, Taiwan; david9097@yahoo.com.tw
3 International Master's Degree Program in Food Science, International College, National Pingtung University of Science and Technology, Pingtung 91201, Taiwan; ylchu@mail.npust.edu.tw
4 Department of Food Science, National Chiayi University, Chiayi 60004, Taiwan; d99641001@ntu.edu.tw
* Correspondence: mcwu@mail.npust.edu.tw
† These authors contributed equally to this work.

Abstract: The increased consumption of high fat-containing foods has been linked to the prevalence of obesity and abnormal metabolic syndromes. *Rhizopus oligosporus*, a fungus in the family Mucoraceae, is widely used as a starter for homemade tempeh. Although *R. oligosporus* can prevent the growth of other microorganisms, it grows well with lactic acid bacteria (LAB). *Lactobacillus plantarum* can produce β-glucosidase, which catalyzes the hydrolysis of glucoside isoflavones into aglycones (with greater bioavailability). Therefore, the development of a soybean-based functional food by the co-inoculation of *R. oligosporus* and *L. plantarum* is a promising approach to increase the bioactivity of tempeh. In this study, the ameliorative effect of *L. plantarum* in soy tempeh on abnormal carbohydrate metabolism in high-fat diet (HFD)-induced hyperglycemic rats was evaluated. The co-incubation of *L. plantarum* with *R. oligosporus* during soy tempeh fermentation reduced the homeostatic model assessment of insulin resistance, HbA1c, serum glucose, total cholesterol, triglyceride, free fatty acid, insulin, and low-density lipoprotein contents, and significantly increased the high-density lipoprotein content in HFD rats. It also increased the LAB counts, as well as the bile acid, cholesterol, triglyceride, and short-chain fatty acid contents in the feces of HFD rats. Our results suggested that the modulation of serum glucose and lipid levels by LAB occurs via alterations in the internal microbiota, leading to the inhibition of cholesterol synthesis and promotion of lipolysis. Tempeh, which was produced with both *L. plantarum* and *R. oligosporus*, might be a beneficial dietary supplement for individuals with abnormal carbohydrate metabolism.

Keywords: tempeh; lactic acid bacteria; short chain fatty acids; metabolic syndrome; high fat diet; feces

---

1. Introduction

The consumption of fast food, fried food, and high-fat foods is increasing along with changes in lifestyle. Therefore, the incidence of metabolic syndrome is increasing and is expected to become a major issue worldwide. It is characterized by high blood pressure, high blood sugar, hypertriglyceridemia, obesity, and low high-density lipoprotein (HDL) levels in the blood. In addition, metabolic syndrome is associated with an increased risk of type II diabetes and cardiovascular diseases. Therefore, the WHO predicts that the prevalence of diabetes mellitus (DM) will increase to 5.92 billion individuals by 2035, and Asia is one of the regions with the highest patient population [1]. Preliminary estimates are predicted to increase to 42.3 million for patients with diabetes mellitus in Asia in 2080 from 20.8 million populations in 2000, and economic development, high-fat foods, fried food, etc., are likely to be the primary underlying causes [1].

Lactobacillus has wide applications in probiotics and has many advantages among humans and animals. It will be beneficial to administer active microorganisms to hosts when probiotics are supplied in sufficient quantity [2]. The study also shows that probiotics play an important role in preventing and treating chronic metabolic diseases or immune-related diseases. Many studies have shown that lactic acid bacteria (LAB) are beneficial for human health, e.g., they could decrease the total cholesterol in blood and they have favorable effects in patients with type II diabetes [2]. It remarkably increased fecal and bile acid cholesterol levels after administration of *Lactobacillus plantarum*. Furthermore, it helped decrease the total blood cholesterol levels after moderate intake of *Lactobacillus plantarum* [2,3]. Recently, numerous phytochemicals have been reported in soybeans and fermented soybean products. In particular, isoflavones genistein and daidzein are beneficial for humans and isoflavones can prevent cardiovascular diseases, cancers, metabolic syndrome, or help to treat osteoporosis because it can mimic estrogen in humans [2,4]. Furthermore, certain animal studies reported that isoflavones can either decrease body weight or increase insulin levels; moreover, it plays an important role in modulating serum glucose levels in diabetic rats [2]. Numerous complex compounds are metabolized/decomposed by microorganisms to generate compounds of higher nutritional value, such as increasing aglycone during soybean fermentation [4].

Tempeh is a fermented soybean product that originated in Indonesia. Tempeh is rich in soy protein and genistein, which have beneficial effects on the regulation of high blood sugar and prevent diabetes [5]. The processing of tempeh involves the addition of *Rhizopus* spp. to cooked, peeled soybeans for fermentation at 37 °C for five days. The weather in Indonesia is wet and hot, and accordingly, tempeh can be made at room temperature [6]. Some studies have reported that tempeh, which prevents diarrhea and anemia and is richer in vitamins and minerals than unfermented soybean, contains many vitamins B_{12} and antioxidants [4]. Furthermore, genistein, daidzein, and β-sitosterol in tempeh prevent cancers, cardiovascular diseases, type II diabetes, and blood glucose regulation [7]. Tempeh also significantly decreases phytic acid and trypsin (antinutritive factors) levels during fermentation. This is one of the reasons why tempeh is popular, especially among vegetarians, in Asia, Europe, and the Americas because of its beneficial functions [4,7,8].

Many studies have shown that fermented soybean and LAB are effective for the prevention of type II diabetes [9,10]. However, the effects of the co-fermentation of *Lactobacillus plantarum* and *Rhizopus oligosporus* on type II diabetes have not been evaluated. Therefore, we prepared tempeh while using both *L. plantarum* and *R. oligosporus* (a common fungus used as a starter for tempeh) and administered it to rat models of diabetes, with HFD-induced high serum glucose and cholesterol. The objective of this study was to develop a strategy to improve the quality of life in patients with metabolic syndrome based on alternative food therapy.

2. Materials and Methods

2.1. Sample Preparation

Kaohsiung Number 9 soybeans were used for co-fermented tempeh. Soybeans were washed and soaked for 12 h and the outer membranes were removed. After drying, water (twice the weight of soybeans) and 1% lactic acid were added, followed by cooking at 100 °C for 30 min. Next, *L. plantarum* and *R. oligosporus* were inoculated at 30 °C in a fermentative environment for 48 h after samples were cooled. Normal tempeh was prepared according to the same procedure with only *R. oligosporus*. All of the samples were stored at −20 °C in a refrigerator until the central temperature reached −18 °C, and samples were then freeze-dried for 48 h. After the water was removed, samples were milled and stored at −20°C. In addition, normal diet (LabDiet 5001) was purchased from Young Li Trading Co., Ltd. (New Taipei, Taiwan) The composition of the HFD was normal diet: cholesterol: coconut oil = 73:2:25 [11].

2.2. Animals and Diets

Eight-week-old male Sprague–Dawley (SD) rats were obtained from BioLASCO Taiwan Co., Ltd. (Taipei, Taiwan). The animals were housed in a room with an alternate light/dark cycle (12 h), a temperature of 25 ± 2 °C, and a relative humidity of 55−60%. All rats were fed experimental diets ad libitum with free access to drinking water at all times. After two weeks of adaptive feeding, the rats were randomly assigned to groups of eight animals each and fed different experimental diets as follows: rats in the control group were fed a normal chow diet with 13.5% kcal fat (Laboratory Rodent Diet 5001; Lab Diet/PMI Nutrition International, Purina Mills LLC, Gray Summit, MO, USA) and rats in the negative control group and treatment groups were fed the HFD (coconut oil 25%, cholesterol 2%, feed powder 73%) modified, as described in Gandhi et al. [11]. Diabetes was induced by treatment with 30 mg/kg STZ and 45 mg/kg nicotinamide for four weeks. Rats were induced by 20 mg/kg STZ again if their serum glucose levels did not reach 150 mg/dL after one week of induction. Rats in the treatment groups (8 rats/group) were separated into the normal diet group (control group), negative control group (HFD, SH group), and positive control group fed pioglitazone (10 mg/kg body weight/day, SHP group) in the last four weeks. The other rats were orally administered cooked soybean (40 mg/kg body weight/day, SHS group), tempeh (40 mg/kg body weight/day, SHL group), or probiotic fermented tempeh (40 mg/kg body weight/day, SHTL group) in the last four weeks. The total study period was 14 weeks for all groups. Food intake and body weight were measured weekly for the duration of the experiment. The animals were maintained in accordance with the National Pingtung University of Science and Technology and Tajen University guidelines for the care and use of laboratory animals. The animal study protocols were approved by the Ethics Committee at the Tajen University (Approval No. 105-10).

2.3. Serum Samples

All blood samples were solidified at room temperature for 30 min after collection. Centrifugation at 3000× g for 20 min, the supernatant was obtained and stored at −80°C before analysis.

2.4. Fasting Serum Glucose

Before the fasting serum glucose test, all rats were fasted overnight (14–16 h). Blood from the tail artery was collected (0.1 mL/rat) and analyzed while using a blood-glucose meter.

2.5. Oral Glucose Tolerance Test (OGTT)

The OGTT assay followed a similar protocol to that of the fasting serum glucose test. All of the rats were fasted overnight (14–16 h) and weighed. Blood was then collected from the tail artery (0.1 mL/rat) and analyzed using a blood-glucose meter. All animals received 1.5 g of glucose/kg body weight. Blood was sampled from the tail vessels of conscious animals before the load (t = 0) and 30, 60, 90, and 120 min after glucose administration. The samples were allowed to clot for 30 min, centrifuged (3000× g, 20 min), and evaluated while using a blood-glucose meter.

2.6. Biochemical Measurements

Commercial kits for determining the levels of free fatty acids (FFA), HbA1c, high-density-lipoprotein-cholesterol (HDL-C), insulin, and low-density-lipoprotein-cholesterol (LDL-C) in rats were obtained from Randox Laboratories (Crumlin, Co., Antrim, UK). The biochemical assays were performed according to the protocols provided by Randox Laboratories.

2.7. Homeostasis Model Assessment-Insulin Resistance (HOMA-IR)

The homeostasis model assessment for insulin resistance (HOMA-IR) was calculated via the following equation: fasting serum insulin (mU/L) × fasting glucose (mmol/L)/22.5 [12].

2.8. Stool Assay

Total LAB in stool samples were determined while using a 1.0-g stool sample diluted 10–1000 times with double distilled endotoxin-free water. Next, 1.0 mL of the sample was added to Lactic Acid Bacteria Count Plates 6461 (3M Petrifilm, St. Paul, MN, USA). Samples were analyzed after incubation for 48 h at 37 °C. For short chain fatty acid (SCFA) detection, the protocol described by Holben [13] was used, with modifications. First, 910 μL of absolute alcohol and 90 μL of pivalic acid (5 mg/mL) were added to 0.5 g of the stool sample and vortexed for 2 min. Next, 500 μL of 0.8 M perchloric acid was added and vortexed for 5 min, followed by centrifugation for 1 min at 13,000 rpm. Then, 0.5 mL of the supernatant was mixed with 50 μL of 4 M KOH for 5 min, and 250 μL of oxalic acid solution was added at 4 °C for 60 min. Finally, the sample was centrifuged for 1 min at 13000 rpm again and the supernatant was passed through a 0.22-μm filter. All of the samples were analyzed while using Mass Selective Detector 5973Network, HP-INNOWax (Capillary column: 30 m, inner diameter: 0.25 mm, particle size: 0.25 μm, detector: Mass Selective Detector 5973Network, gas: Helium, split rate: 5:1, column flow rate: 2 mL/min, total flow rate: 15 mL/min, injector temperature = 200 °C, oven temperature = 100 °C, detector temperature = 200 °C, initial temperature = 100 °C for 1 min, heating procedure of 2 °C/min until reaching 110 °C for 2 min, then 3 °C/min until reaching 170 °C for 1 min, final heating at 10 °C/min until reaching 200 °C for 2 min). Each sample (1 μL) was used for gas chromatography injection for 32 min, and then a mass spectrometer was used to compare acetic acid, propionate, and butyrate, as described previously [13]. Cholesterol, triglycerides, and cholic acid were analyzed while using ELISA kits (BioVision Inc., Milpitas, CA, USA). All tests were performed according to the protocols provided by BioVision Inc.

2.9. Next-Generation Sequencing Analysis of Stool Samples

2.9.1. Amplicon Library Construction and Sequencing

Total bacterial DNA from 5 g of rat feces was isolated and purified using the PowerSoil® DNA Isolation Kit (Mo Bio, Qiagen, Hilden, Germany). A 16S rDNA region (V3–V5 hypervariable region) from purified total bacterial DNA was amplified via PCR to produce 400-bp DNA fragments for further purification. The specific PCR primers were as follows: forward primer overhang adaptor (5′–TCGTCGGCAGCGTCAGATGTGTATAA GAGACAG–3′) and reverse primer overhang adaptor (5′–GTCTCGTGGGCTCGGAGATGTG TATAAGAGACAG–3′). Amplicons were generated while using a high-fidelity polymerase (AccuPrime; Invitrogen, Carlsbad, CA, USA), purified using a Magnetic Bead Capture Kit (Ampure; Agencourt, Beverly, MA, USA), and quantified using a fluorometric kit (QuantIT PicoGreen; Invitrogen, Carlsbad, CA, USA). PCR conditions were 30 cycles of 30 s at 95 °C, 30 s at 55 °C, and 30 s at 72 °C, and a final extension for 5 min at 72 °C. The purified amplicons were then pooled in equimolar concentrations using a SequalPrep Plate Normalization Kit (Invitrogen, Carlsbad, CA, USA). The final concentration of the library was determined using an SYBR Green Quantitative PCR (qPCR) assay and the size distribution of the library was determined using Caliper LabChip. 16S rRNA-specific regions were then sequenced using a MiSeq sequencer (Illumina, San Diego, CA, USA).

2.9.2. Bioinformatic Analysis

Raw reads from the MiSeq sequencer for the metagenomic workflow were analyzed while using QIIME (http://qiime.org/). Reference sequences in Greengenes gg_13_8 (99_otus.fasta) were used in the analysis (Greengenes database, http://greengenes.lbl.gov/). The Ribosomal Database Project (RDP) classifier (http://rdp.cme.msu.edu/classifier/) was used to classify the 16S rDNA sequences into distinct taxonomic categories that are based on sequence alignments. The operational taxonomic units (OTUs) for Lactobacillus species were determined by BLAST searches and groups were preliminarily assigned by alignments with the NCBI genome database. All 16S rDNA sequences were mapped to the RDP database while using QIIME and divided into groups corresponding to their taxonomy at the level of order and were then assigned to OTUs. A sequence similarity exceeding 0.95 was the threshold for OTUs, according to the value for species distinction in microbiology.

2.10. Statistical Analysis

All results are reported as means ± SD and the differences between the control and tempeh-treated groups were analyzed by one-way analysis of variance (ANOVA) and Duncan's multiple range tests (IBM SPSS Statistics 19, North Castle, NY, USA) with a significance threshold of $p < 0.05$.

3. Results

3.1. Hyperglycemic Rat Model

We induced DM in rats by STZ after 10 weeks of feeding on the HFD. The fasting serum glucose level was significantly higher ($p < 0.05$) in the STZ treatment group than in normal rats provided the chow diet (Figure 1).

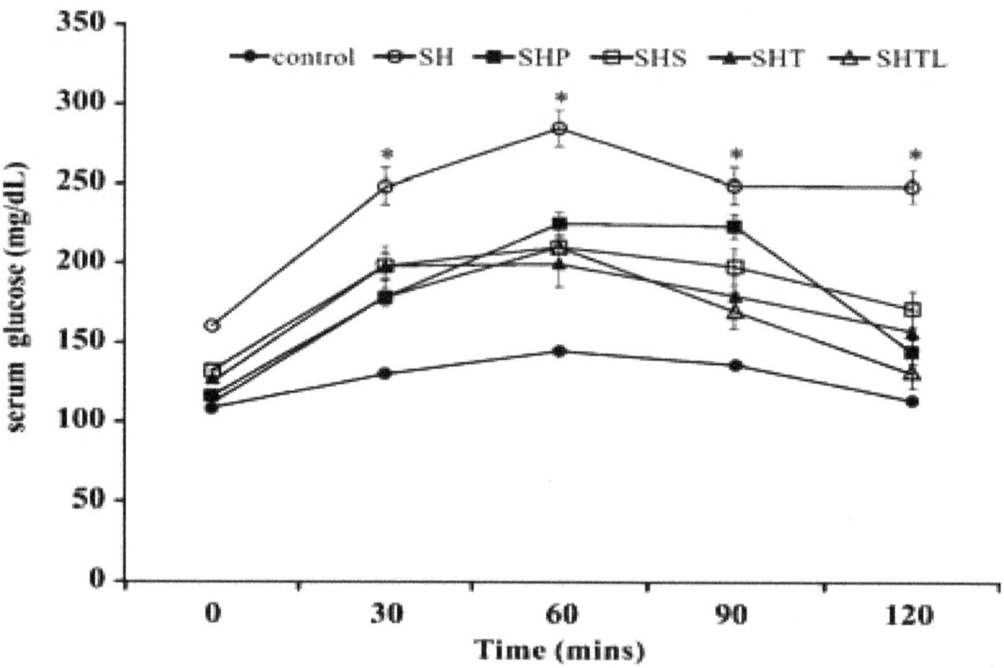

Figure 1. Oral glucose tolerance test (OGTT) for streptozotocin (STZ)-induced diabetic rats fed a high-fat diet for 14 weeks and administered *Lactobacillus plantarum* co-fermented tempeh orally during the last 4 weeks. Control: normal diet; SH: Streptozotocin (STZ 30 mg/kg, Nicotinamide 45 mg/kg) + High fat diet (Coconut oil 25%, Cholesterol 2%, Feed powder 73%); SHP: Streptozotocin (STZ 30 mg/kg, Nicotinamide 45 mg/kg) + High fat diet (Coconut oil 25%, Cholesterol 2%, Feed powder 73%) + Pioglitazone (10 mg/kg body weight); SHS: Streptozotocin (STZ 30 mg/kg, Nicotinamide 45 mg/kg) + High fat diet (Coconut oil 25%, Cholesterol 2%, Feed powder 73%) + Unfermented soybean (40 mg/kg body weight); SHT: Streptozotocin (STZ 30 mg/kg: Nicotinamide 45 mg/kg) + High fat diet (Coconut oil 25%, Cholesterol 2%, Feed powder 73%) + Tempeh (40 mg/kg body weight); SHTL: Streptozotocin (STZ 30 mg/kg, Nicotinamide 45 mg/kg) + High fat diet (Coconut oil 25%, Cholesterol 2%, Feed powder 73%) + Tempeh + *Lactobacillus plantarum* (40 mg/kg body weight). * Indicates a significant difference ($p < 0.05$) compared with the control group at the same time point. Results are expressed as mean values ± SD. ($n = 8$/group).

3.2. Oral Glucose Tolerance Test

In the treatment groups, serum glucose levels were ameliorated in DM rats after 14 weeks of HFD feeding (Figure 1). The serum glucose levels in the SH group (HFD) after the oral administration of glucose at 30, 60, 90, and 120 min were significantly higher than those of other treatment groups ($p < 0.05$). In addition, the OGTT showed that 40 mg/kg soybean (SHS group) and 40 mg/kg tempeh (SHT group) reduced the serum glucose level in STZ-induced DM rats. Moreover, the SHTL treatment group (40 mg/kg) exhibited significantly lower serum glucose levels than those in other treatment groups that are based on the OGTT ($p < 0.05$).

3.3. Effects of Various Treatments on Serum Biochemistry in DM Rats

In our serum biochemistry analysis, we observed significantly increased TG, cholesterol, LDL, FFA, serum glucose, HbA1C, and insulin levels, but reduced HDL levels in DM rats in the SH group after 14 weeks of the HFD ($p < 0.05$) (Table 1). The SH group achieved insulin resistance based on the HOMA-IR values. However, the SHS (40 mg/kg), SHT (40 mg/kg), and SHTL (40 mg/kg) treatments resulted in significant decreases in TG, cholesterol, LDL, FFA, serum glucose, HbA1C, and insulin levels, but increased HDL levels in DM rats ($p < 0.05$). In addition, the SHTL (40 mg/kg) treatment group exhibited the greatest improvements in all serum biochemical parameters, indicating that it could alleviate the symptoms of DM in rats; this group also exhibited improved insulin-resistance based on the HOMA-IR calculation.

Table 1. Selected serum biochemical parameters for STZ-induced diabetic rats fed a high-fat diet for 14 weeks and administered *Lactobacillus plantarum* co-fermented tempeh orally during the last 4 weeks.

Items/Groups	Control	SH	SHP	SHS	SHT	SHTL
Triglyceride (mg/dL)	55.11 ± 20.0^{bcd}	118.1 ± 35.8^{a}	49.30 ± 8.52^{cd}	71.50 ± 17.2^{bc}	76.40 ± 24.7^{b}	47.90 ± 9.95^{d}
Cholesterol-total (mg/dL)	53.50 ± 6.86^{c}	90.33 ± 11.1^{a}	66.50 ± 13.4^{bc}	79.67 ± 14.4^{ab}	69.67 ± 14.4^{bc}	65.50 ± 9.98^{bc}
HDL-cholesterol (mg/dL)	40.56 ± 7.78^{ab}	35.71 ± 4.59^{b}	34.20 ± 6.16^{b}	45.13 ± 10.3^{a}	40.29 ± 4.08^{ab}	40.14 ± 3.42^{ab}
Cholesterol/HDL-C	1.41 ± 0.07^{b}	2.12 ± 0.35^{a}	2.04 ± 0.36^{a}	2.02 ± 0.15^{a}	1.94 ± 0.16^{a}	2.01 ± 0.17^{a}
LDL-cholesterol (mg/dL)	7.89 ± 2.23^{c}	36.00 ± 8.68^{a}	23.63 ± 7.20^{b}	28.75 ± 9.77^{b}	24.78 ± 6.29^{b}	25.00 ± 5.24^{b}
Free-fatty acid (mmol/L)	1.43 ± 0.61^{b}	2.31 ± 0.25^{a}	1.16 ± 0.06^{b}	1.55 ± 0.23^{b}	1.36 ± 0.31^{b}	1.41 ± 0.24^{b}
Glucose AC (mg/dL)	100 ± 8.4^{c}	199 ± 42.3^{a}	125 ± 34.6^{bc}	151 ± 25.5^{b}	141 ± 24.8^{b}	109 ± 17.3^{c}
HbA1C (%)	4.02 ± 0.13^{d}	6.96 ± 1.05^{a}	5.17 ± 0.97^{bc}	5.58 ± 1.42^{b}	5.51 ± 1.25^{b}	4.42 ± 0.32^{cd}
Insulin (ng/mL)	2.48 ± 2.11^{b}	9.99 ± 5.46^{a}	1.61 ± 0.81^{b}	2.11 ± 0.67^{b}	2.61 ± 0.53^{b}	1.65 ± 0.53^{b}
HOMA-IR	0.55 ± 0.18^{c}	4.46 ± 0.95^{a}	0.54 ± 0.19^{c}	0.89 ± 0.17^{bc}	1.07 ± 0.36^{b}	0.59 ± 0.16^{c}

Control: normal diet; SH: Streptozotocin (STZ 30 mg/kg, Nicotinamide 45 mg/kg) + High fat diet (Coconut oil 25%, Cholesterol 2%, Feed powder 73%); SHP: Streptozotocin (STZ 30 mg/kg, Nicotinamide 45 mg/kg) + High fat diet (Coconut oil 25%, Cholesterol 2%, Feed powder 73%) + Pioglitazone (10 mg/kg body weight); SHS: Streptozotocin (STZ 30 mg/kg, Nicotinamide 45 mg/kg) + High fat diet (Coconut oil 25%, Cholesterol 2%, Feed powder 73%) + Unfermented soybean (40 mg/kg body weight); SHT: Streptozotocin (STZ 30 mg/kg: Nicotinamide 45 mg/kg) + High fat diet (Coconut oil 25%, Cholesterol 2%, Feed powder 73%) + Tempeh (40 mg/kg body weight); SHTL: Streptozotocin (STZ 30 mg/kg, Nicotinamide 45 mg/kg) + High fat diet (Coconut oil 25%, Cholesterol 2%, Feed powder 73%) + Tempeh + *Lactobacillus plantarum* (40 mg/kg body weight). a~d letters are significantly different from all samples tested ($p < 0.05$). Results are expressed as mean values ± SD. ($n = 8$/group).

3.4. Changes in Total Lactic Acid Bacteria in Diabetes Mellitus (DM) Rat Stools

There were no significant differences in the total LAB content in the rat stool samples before treatment among groups (Table 2). However, the total LAB content was lower in the SH group than in the Normal group. The total LAB contents were significantly higher in the SHT and SHTL groups than in the SH group in DM rats ($p < 0.05$). The total LAB content in the stool sample in the SHTL group was higher than those in other groups. However, the total LAB content in stool samples in the SHP group was significantly lower than those in all DM rats ($p < 0.05$).

Table 2. Lactic acid bacteria counts (Log CFU/g) in STZ-induced diabetic rats in different treatment groups.

Items/Groups	Control	SH	SHP	SHS	SHT	SHTL
Week 0	7.66 ± 0.04 [a]	7.65 ± 0.09 [a]	7.64 ± 0.01 [a]	7.59 ± 0.05 [a]	7.75 ± 0.08 [ab]	7.67 ± 0.05 [a]
Week 4	8.91 ± 0.07 [a]	8.09 ± 0.06 [c]	7.71 ± 0.27 [d]	8.04 ± 0.16 [c]	8.31 ± 0.04 [bc]	8.44 ± 0.05 [b]

Control: normal diet; SH: Streptozotocin (STZ 30 mg/kg, Nicotinamide 45 mg/kg) + High fat diet (Coconut oil 25%, Cholesterol 2%, Feed powder 73%); SHP: Streptozotocin (STZ 30 mg/kg, Nicotinamide 45 mg/kg) + High fat diet (Coconut oil 25%, Cholesterol 2%, Feed powder 73%) + Pioglitazone (10 mg/kg body weight); SHS: Streptozotocin (STZ 30 mg/kg, Nicotinamide 45 mg/kg) + High fat diet (Coconut oil 25%, Cholesterol 2%, Feed powder 73%) + Unfermented soybean (40 mg/kg body weight); SHT: Streptozotocin (STZ 30 mg/kg: Nicotinamide 45 mg/kg) + High fat diet (Coconut oil 25%, Cholesterol 2%, Feed powder 73%) + Tempeh (40 mg/kg body weight); SHTL: Streptozotocin (STZ 30 mg/kg, Nicotinamide 45 mg/kg) + High fat diet (Coconut oil 25%, Cholesterol 2%, Feed powder 73%) + Tempeh + *Lactobacillus plantarum* (40 mg/kg body weight). a~d letters are significantly different from all samples tested ($p < 0.05$). Results are expressed as mean values ± SD. (n = 8/group).

3.5. Changes in Short Chain Fatty Acids (SCFAs) in DM Rat Stools

For STZ-induced DM rat groups within two weeks, there were no significant differences in acetic acid, propionic acid, and butyric acid in comparison with those in the SH group in DM rats (data not shown). However, the DM rats had higher SCFA contents than the rats fed a normal diet (Table 3). After four weeks of oral administration, the SHTL group exhibited significantly increased acetic acid, propionic acid, butyric acid, and valeric acid in stool samples compared with those in the SH group in DM rats ($p < 0.05$). The increases in acetic acid, propionic acid, and butyric acid in the SHTL group were the greatest when compared with those of other treatment groups.

Table 3. Changes in short- and medium-chain fatty acid in the feces in STZ-induced diabetic rats fed a high-fat diet for 14 weeks and administered *Lactobacillus plantarum* co-fermented tempeh orally during the last four weeks.

Week	Items	Groups					
		Control	SH	SHP	SHS	SHT	SHTL
4	Acetic acid_C2	4.16 ± 0.41 [d]	5.21 ±0.11 [c]	5.30 ± 0.29 [c]	5.93 ± 0.31 [c]	6.86 ± 0.28 [b]	7.86 ±0.64 [a]
	Propanoic acid_C3	0.55 ± 0.11 [c]	0.70 ± 0.17 [bc]	0.84 ± 0.19 [abc]	1.01 ± 0.16 [ab]	0.87 ± 0.07 [ab]	1.13 ± 0.07 [a]
	Butyric acid_C4	0.51 ± 0.06 [abc]	0.27 ± 0.02 [c]	0.45 ± 0.06 [bc]	0.70 ± 0.21 [ab]	0.57 ± 0.28 [abc]	0.83 ± 0.11 [a]
	Isobutyic acid_C4t	0.00 ± 0.01 [a]	0.04 ± 0.05 [a]	0.02 ± 0.01 [a]	0.01 ± 0.02 [a]	0.04 ± 0.02 [a]	0.05 ± 0.01 [a]
	Valeric acid_C5	0.03 ± 0.01 [ab]	0.00 ± 0.00 [b]	0.01 ± 0.02 [b]	0.09 ± 0.07 [ab]	0.05 ± 0.03 [ab]	0.11 ± 0.04 [a]
	Isovaleric acid_C5t	0.02 ± 0.01 [a]	0.05 ± 0.06 [a]	0.05 ± 0.01 [a]	0.05 ± 0.01 [a]	0.06 ± 0.03 [a]	0.08 ± 0.02 [a]
	Caproic acid_C6	0.00 ± 0.00 [a]	0.00 ± 0.00 [a]	0.00 ± 0.00 [a]	0.00 ± 0.00 [a]	0.01 ± 0.01 [a]	0.01 ± 0.02 [a]

Control: normal diet; SH: Streptozotocin (STZ 30 mg/kg, Nicotinamide 45 mg/kg) + High fat diet (Coconut oil 25%, Cholesterol 2%, Feed powder 73%); SHP: Streptozotocin (STZ 30 mg/kg, Nicotinamide 45 mg/kg) + High fat diet (Coconut oil 25%, Cholesterol 2%, Feed powder 73%) + Pioglitazone (10 mg/kg body weight); SHS: Streptozotocin (STZ 30 mg/kg, Nicotinamide 45 mg/kg) + High fat diet (Coconut oil 25%, Cholesterol 2%, Feed powder 73%) + Unfermented soybean (40 mg/kg body weight); SHT: Streptozotocin (STZ 30 mg/kg: Nicotinamide 45 mg/kg) + High fat diet (Coconut oil 25%, Cholesterol 2%, Feed powder 73%) + Tempeh (40 mg/kg body weight); SHTL: Streptozotocin (STZ 30 mg/kg, Nicotinamide 45 mg/kg) + High fat diet (Coconut oil 25%, Cholesterol 2%, Feed powder 73%) + Tempeh + *Lactobacillus plantarum* (40 mg/kg body weight). a~d letters are significantly different from all samples tested ($p < 0.05$). Results are expressed as mean values ± SD. (n = 8/group).

3.6. Changes in Total Cholesterol, Bile Acid, and TG in DM Rat Stools

As shown in Table 4, there were no significant differences in stool weight, cholesterol (TC), bile acid, and TG before treatment among samples. However, the SH group had the lowest weights and excretion of TC and bile acid from the stool at 14 weeks among all the DM groups ($p < 0.05$). The SHT and SHTL groups exhibit greater bile acid contents than those of other groups in stool samples ($p < 0.05$), especially the SHTL group, which exhibited the highest bile acid excretion at 14 weeks in the DM rats ($p < 0.05$). The TG content in the SH group was significantly lower than those in the control, SHP, SHT, and SHTL groups. The excretion of TC, bile acid, and TG in the SHTL group was significantly higher than that in the SH group ($p < 0.05$).

Table 4. Changes in weight, cholesterol, bile acid, and triglyceride contents in feces in STZ-induced diabetic rats fed a high-fat diet for 14 weeks and administered *Lactobacillus plantarum* co-fermented tempeh orally during the last 4 weeks.

Week	Items	Groups					
		Control	SH	SHP	SHS	SHT	SHTL
Week 0							
	Feces weight (g)	81.7 ± 1.75	81.0 ± 5.00	81.7 ± 3.06	80.7 ± 3.73	80.3 ± 4.30	81.7 ± 4.16
	cholesterol content (mg/g)	1.56 ± 0.31	1.47 ± 0.57	1.67 ± 0.16	1.66 ± 0.34	1.60 ± 0.26	1.43 ± 0.18
	Bile acid content (μg/g)	6.35 ± 0.51	6.22 ± 0.49	6.54 ± 0.41	6.84 ± 0.59	6.48 ± 0.35	6.56 ± 0.36
	Triglyceride content (μg/g)	57.52 ± 2.85	57.14 ± 3.48	58.12 ± 4.98	58.28 ± 2.78	57.04 ± 4.62	57.28 ± 2.14
Week 4							
	Feces weight (g)	81.7 ± 3.80 ^{c}	79.7 ± 3.06 ^{c}	83.0 ± 9.8 ^{bc}	96.7 ± 4.16 ^{ab}	100.0 ± 6.00 ^{a}	104.0 ± 6.27 ^{a}
	cholesterol content (mg/g)	4.90 ± 1.32 ^{d}	27.5 ± 0.93 ^{c}	29.2 ± 2.62 ^{bc}	29.0 ± 3.13 ^{bc}	32.1 ± 2.44 ^{b}	35.6 ± 1.34 ^{a}
	Bile acid content (μg/g)	4.63 ± 0.55 ^{d}	176.4 ± 0.44 ^{b}	247.7 ± 3.73 ^{a}	115.9 ± 2.76 ^{c}	173.0 ± 6.78 ^{b}	248.2 ± 3.86 ^{a}
	Triglyceride content (μg/g)	68.97 ± 1.76 ^{a}	47.63 ± 3.45 ^{c}	57.48 ± 2.01 ^{b}	43.11 ± 0.24 ^{c}	67.16 ± 3.15 ^{a}	72.29 ± 8.87 ^{a}

Control: normal diet; SH: Streptozotocin (STZ 30 mg/kg, Nicotinamide 45 mg/kg) + High fat diet (Coconut oil 25%, Cholesterol 2%, Feed powder 73%); SHP: Streptozotocin (STZ 30 mg/kg, Nicotinamide 45 mg/kg) + High fat diet (Coconut oil 25%, Cholesterol 2%, Feed powder 73%) + Pioglitazone (10 mg/kg body weight); SHS: Streptozotocin (STZ 30 mg/kg, Nicotinamide 45 mg/kg) + High fat diet (Coconut oil 25%, Cholesterol 2%, Feed powder 73%) + Unfermented soybean (40 mg/kg body weight); SHT: Streptozotocin (STZ 30 mg/kg: Nicotinamide 45 mg/kg) + High fat diet (Coconut oil 25%, Cholesterol 2%, Feed powder 73%) + Tempeh (40 mg/kg body weight); SHTL: Streptozotocin (STZ 30 mg/kg, Nicotinamide 45 mg/kg) + High fat diet (Coconut oil 25%, Cholesterol 2%, Feed powder 73%) + Tempeh + *Lactobacillus plantarum* (40 mg/kg body weight). a~d letters are significantly different from all samples tested ($p < 0.05$). Results are expressed as mean values ± SD. ($n = 8$/group).

3.7. Microbiota Analysis of DM Rats

We evaluated the distribution of gut bacteria by next-generation sequencing. The SH, SHP, SHS, and SHT groups exhibited a change in the dominant bacteria to Bacteroides in STZ-induced DM rats, and the second most dominant bacteria changed to Prevotella (Figure 2). Interestingly, in the SHTL group, the dominant bacteria in the stool samples was Lactobacillus (36.29%) after the oral administration of tempeh co-fermented with *L. plantarum* (40 mg/kg) in DM rats. The second most dominant bacterium in the SHTL group was Bacteroides (29.58%). The Lactobacillus content in the SHTL group was greater than that in the SH group by 34.2%.

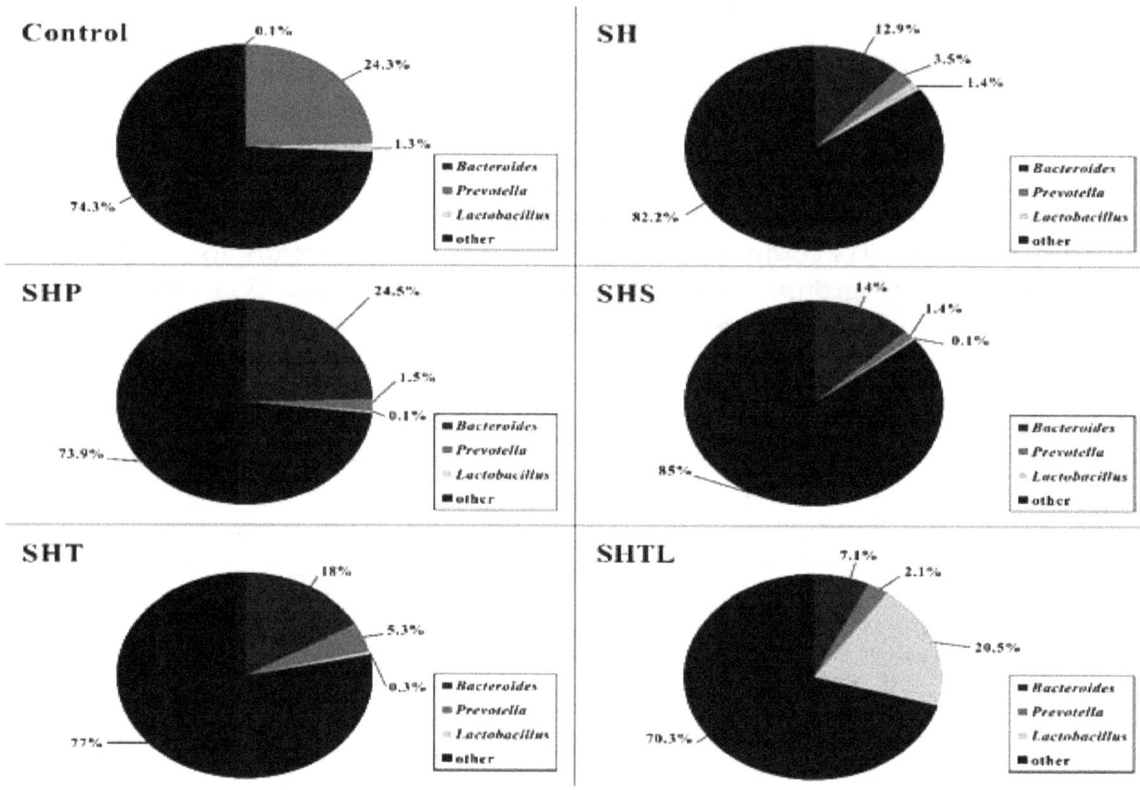

Figure 2. Changes in bacterial distribution in feces in STZ-induced diabetic rats fed a high-fat diet for 14 weeks and administered *Lactobacillus plantarum* co-fermented tempeh orally during the last 4 weeks. Control: normal diet; SH: Streptozotocin (STZ 30 mg/kg, Nicotinamide 45 mg/kg) + High fat diet (Coconut oil 25%, Cholesterol 2%, Feed powder 73%); SHP: Streptozotocin (STZ 30 mg/kg, Nicotinamide 45 mg/kg) + High fat diet (Coconut oil 25%, Cholesterol 2%, Feed powder 73%) + Pioglitazone (10 mg/kg body weight); SHS: Streptozotocin (STZ 30 mg/kg, Nicotinamide 45 mg/kg) + High fat diet (Coconut oil 25%, Cholesterol 2%, Feed powder 73%) + Unfermented soybean (40 mg/kg body weight); SHT: Streptozotocin (STZ 30 mg/kg: Nicotinamide 45 mg/kg) + High fat diet (Coconut oil 25%, Cholesterol 2%, Feed powder 73%) + Tempeh (40 mg/kg body weight); SHTL: Streptozotocin (STZ 30 mg/kg, Nicotinamide 45 mg/kg) + High fat diet (Coconut oil 25%, Cholesterol 2%, Feed powder 73%) + Tempeh + *Lactobacillus plantarum* (40 mg/kg body weight). Results are expressed as mean values ± SD. ($n = 8$/group).

4. Discussion

High serum glucose is a symptom of diabetes, and postprandial hyperglycemia is a metabolic phenomenon in type II diabetes [14,15]. Therefore, the objective of diabetes therapy is to control the fasting and postprandial serum glucose concentrations. Soybean isoflavones can be transformed from glycosides to aglycones by probiotics, and aglycone-isoflavones have better bioavailability in humans [16]. After treatment for four weeks, rats in each group were fasted for 12 h and then evaluated by OGTT (Figure 1). In our study, the SHTL group had better OGGT results in the late stage, and this was attributed to the high bioavailability of isoflavones from *L. plantarum* fermented with *Rhizopus oryzae* in tempeh in DM rats. Although the SHS and SHT groups had isoflavones, they exhibited decreased serum glucose in the OGTT. The higher serum glucose levels that were observed in the SHTL group than in other groups may reflect the higher aglycone-isoflavone content in the SHTL group. These results are consistent with previous findings [17].

The syndromes of insulin resistance are caused by abnormal responses of human tissues (such as the muscle, liver, adipocyte, and central nervous system tissues) to insulin, thereby inducing dysfunctions in glucose and lipid metabolism [18–22]. Insulin resistance normally co-exists with high blood pressure, hypertriglyceridemia, decreased HDL, increased LDL, and multiple metabolic disorder syndromes in animals. Hence, these syndromes could induce severe complications in patients with type II diabetes [23,24]. Animal and human studies consistently demonstrate that Lactobacillus can reduce the total cholesterol and LDL levels in the blood [25–27]. In addition, epidemiological and other studies have shown that isoflavonoids (genistein) in soybean could improve type II DM by regulating the metabolism of glucose and lipids [28,29]. Many studies have shown that isoflavonoids and daidzein of the soybean could reduce serum glucose levels in animals with DM [30–32]. As shown in Table 1, the SHLT co-fermentative group had better bioavailability, decreased TG and LDL levels, and increased HDL levels in the serum. Additionally, serum glucose and HbA1C levels were effectively regulated in the SHLT group. However, isoflavonoids (genistein) not only improved the metabolism of serum glucose, but also reduced the HOMA-IR value in DM rats. Our results were similar to those of Kwon (2010), who showed that fermented soybean can decrease TC and TG levels in the liver and can regulate the metabolism of serum glucose in SD rats [33].

Microbes that are beneficial to hosts are referred to as probiotics [34]. These probiotics, including LAB, need to survive in gastric acid and bile acid conditions in animals [35]. LAB can inhibit potential pathogen proliferation, decrease serum cholesterol levels, and regulate the immune system [36]. Furthermore, LAB in the stool can protect against gastric acid and bile acid damage. The consumption of soybean products also increases SCFAs, lactic acid bacteria, and the volume of stool [37]. Table 2 shows that total LAB increased significantly in soybean-fed groups. In particular, the SHLT group had the highest total LAB count in the stool. These findings are consistent with those of Panasevich [37].

Many studies have shown that increased dietary fiber intake can improve stool excretion, stimulate segmented colon movement, and improve blood sugar control [38–43]. Probiotics can produce active metabolites, such as SCFAs, in the gut. SCFAs are also a product of dietary fiber fermentation. They include acetate, propionate, and butyrate [44,45]. Some studies have shown that acetate is the most abundant SCFA in the serum and it can regulate inflammation and protect against the invasion of pathogens [46–48]. Propionate can decrease total cholesterol levels [49]. Butyrate can improve HFD-induced obesity and insulin sensitivity [50,51]. Table 3 demonstrates that the SHLT group exhibited increased acetate, propionate, and butyrate in the stool when compared with the levels in other groups. The results of Schneider (2006) supported our results for stool SCFAs [52].

Protein, isoflavones, or dietary fiber in soybeans would affect the metabolism of cholesterol [53–55]. LAB can improve the absorption of isoflavones by regulating β-galactosidase and glucosidase activity [56]. Glucosides of isoflavones are transformed to aglycone-isoflavones with better bioavailability via Lactobacillus [57]. In addition, increased consumption of aglycone-isoflavones improves fatty liver diseases [58]. Some results have demonstrated that the intake of soy products with dietary fiber can decrease serum total cholesterol and LDL-C levels, and the interaction of bile acid and microbes also regulates liver fat and the metabolism of cholesterol [59–61]. Recent studies have shown that the gut microbiota can affect intestinal-liver circulation and bile acid metabolism because it can produce new bile acid via decarboxylation, replacing the bile acid that is consumed by intestinal-liver circulation and decreasing the serum cholesterol level [62,63]. The consumption of dietary soy products can increase Lactobacillus spp. in the stool and promotes the activity of bile hydrolase [64]. Nagata (1982) also found that soy products could increase the bile acid content in rat feces and affects the metabolism of liver cholesterol, since bile acid synthesis requires cholesterol [65,66]. These results may be explained by the stimulation of bile acid secretion and the activity of 7α-hydroxylase cholesterol synthesis induced by LAB and isoflavones [67–69].

Prebiotics are a good source of probiotics and regulate cholesterol and blood sugar. They are typically derived from cereal fibers, such as β-dextran, arabinoxylan, inulin, galactose, and fructooligosaccharides [70,71]. Wang (2012) found that hemicellulose from cereals is composed of β-dextran, which can compete with cholesterol binding sites on LDL. Therefore, the consumption of dietary cereal fiber can decrease the serum levels of LDL and cholesterol [72,73]. Moreover, LAB can reduce blood cholesterol by various mechanisms, e.g., the inhibition of cholesterol synthesis enzymes, stimulation of cholesterol excretion in feces, and inhibition of cholesterol recycling, which can increase the synthesis of cholic acid [74]. Table 4 shows that the SHLT group exhibited dramatically increased levels of stool cholesterol and triglycerides. It is possible that LAB decreased cholesterol by each of these mechanisms, but it decreases blood cholesterol by increasing bile acid synthesis.

The gut microbiota is substantially influenced by the diet and it affects human health via microbial metabolism [75]. The gut microbiota in the human colon is also affected by the diet and induces metabolic diseases, like type II diabetes. In other words, dietary changes can improve physiological metabolism in humans by modifying microbial metabolic processes [76,77]. In a comparison of the gut microbiota, 53% of children in the African countryside, but not in Europe, had Prevotella. This may be explained by dietary differences since children in the African countryside consume cereal, soy, and vegetables and European children consume more protein and animal fat (and exhibit abundant Bacteroides in the gut) [78]. Prevotella and Bacteroides are major microbes in the human colon, and their distribution and metabolic activity are related to the diet. For example, Prevotella is abundant in those who eat a high fiber diet, but Bacteroides is abundant in those who eat high protein and high-fat diets [77]. Figure 2 also shows that the dominant bacteria in our HFD group were Bacteroides, but those in the normal control group were Prevotella.

Stool samples of children in the African countryside have four times higher levels of propionate and butyrate than those of samples from European children [78], and this difference might reflect the consumption of soy products, which increases Lactobacillus in stool samples [79]. Probiotics can increase SCFA production [79]. As shown in Figure 2, Lactobacillus was more abundant in the SHTL group than in other groups. Accordingly, the acetate, propionate, and butyrate contents were the highest in the stool samples of the SHTL group. These findings suggest that the SHTL group exhibits decreased serum glucose via increases in the proliferation of Lactobacillus and improvements in SCFA excretion.

5. Conclusions

The effects of *L. plantarum* co-incubated with *R. oligosporus* to produce soy tempeh on diabetes have not been evaluated. The present results demonstrate that *L. plantarum* co-incubation in soy tempeh ameliorates hyperglycemia, hyperlipidemia, and hyperinsulinemia by altering the intestinal bacterial distribution and increasing intestinal SCFA release in HFD-fed rats. These findings suggest that soy tempeh that is produced by co-incubation with *L. plantarum* has therapeutic effects and is a potential dietary supplement for preventing the progression of DM.

Author Contributions: Conceptualization, W.-C.C.; Data curation, Y.-C.H. and B.-H.W.; Funding acquisition, M.-C.W.; Methodology, B.-H.W.; Project administration, Y.-C.H. and W.-C.C.; Software, Y.-L.C.; Supervision, W.-C.C. and M.-C.W.; Validation, M.-C.W.; Writing—original draft, Y.-C.H. and W.-C.C.; Writing—review & editing, W.-C.C. and M.-C.W.

References

1. Guariguata, L.; Whiting, D.R.; Hambleton, I.; Beagley, J.; Linnenkamp, U.; Shaw, J.E. Global estimates of diabetes prevalence for 2013 and projections for 2035. *Diabetes Res. Clin. Pract.* **2014**, *103*, 137–149. [CrossRef] [PubMed]
2. Huang, Y.; Wang, X.; Wang, J.; Wu, F.; Sui, Y.; Yang, L.; Wang, Z. *Lactobacillus plantarum* strains as potential probiotic cultures with cholesterol-lowering activity. *J. Dairy Sci.* **2013**, *96*, 2746–2753. [CrossRef] [PubMed]
3. Panwar, H.; Calderwood, D.; Gillespie, A.L.; Wylie, A.R.; Graham, S.F.; Grant, I.R.; Green, B.D. Identification of lactic acid bacteria strains modulating incretin hormone secretion and gene expression in enteroendocrine cells. *J. Funct. Foods* **2016**, *23*, 348–358. [CrossRef]
4. Barus, T.; Wati, L.; Suwanto, A. Diversity of protease-producing *Bacillus* spp. from fresh Indonesian tempeh based on 16S rRNA gene sequence. *HAYATI J. Biosci.* **2017**, *24*, 35–40. [CrossRef]
5. Behloul, N.; Wu, G. Genistein: A promising therapeutic agent for obesity and diabetes treatment. *Eur. J. Pharmacol.* **2013**, *698*, 31–38. [CrossRef] [PubMed]

6. Jeleń, H.; Majcher, M.; Ginja, A.; Kuligowski, M. Determination of compounds responsible for tempeh aroma. *Food Chem.* **2013**, *141*, 459–465. [CrossRef] [PubMed]
7. Haron, H.; Ismail, A.; Shahar, S.; Azlan, A.; Peng, L.S. Apparent bioavailability of isoflavones in urinary excretions of postmenopausal Malay women consuming tempeh compared with milk. *Int. J. Food Sci. Nutr.* **2011**, *62*, 642–650. [CrossRef] [PubMed]
8. Ahmad, A.; Ramasamy, K.; Majeed, A.B.A.; Mani, V. Enhancement of β-secretase inhibition and antioxidant activities of tempeh, a fermented soybean cake through enrichment of bioactive aglycones. *Pharm. Biol.* **2015**, *53*, 758–766. [CrossRef] [PubMed]
9. Zhang, X.M.; Zhang, Y.B.; Chi, M.H. Soy protein supplementation reduces clinical indices in type 2 diabetes and metabolic syndrome. *Yonsei Med. J.* **2016**, *57*, 681–689. [CrossRef] [PubMed]
10. Feizollahzadeh, S.; Ghiasvand, R.; Rezaei, A.; Khanahmad, H.; Hariri, M. Effect of probiotic soy milk on serum levels of adiponectin, inflammatory mediators, lipid profile, and fasting blood glucose among patients with type II diabetes mellitus. *Probiotics Antimicrob. Proteins* **2017**, *9*, 41–47. [CrossRef] [PubMed]
11. Gandhi, G.R.; Stalin, A.; Balakrishna, K.; Ignacimuthu, S.; Paulraj, M.G.; Vishal, R. Insulin sensitization via partial agonism of PPARγ and glucose uptake through translocation and activation of GLUT4 in PI3K/p-Akt signaling pathway by embelin in type 2 diabetic rats. *Biochim. Biophys. Acta* **2013**, *1830*, 2243–2255. [CrossRef] [PubMed]
12. Matthews, D.R.; Hosker, J.P.; Rudenski, A.S.; Naylor, B.A.; Treacher, D.F.; Turner, R.C. Homeostasis model assessment: Insulin resistance and β-cell function from fasting plasma glucose and insulin concentrations in man. *Diabetologia* **1985**, *28*, 412–419. [CrossRef] [PubMed]
13. Holben, W.E.; Williams, P.; Saarinen, M.; Särkilahti, L.K.; Apajalahti, J.H.A. Phylogenetic analysis of intestinal microflora indicates a novel Mycoplasma phylotype in farmed and wild salmon. *Microb. Ecol.* **2002**, *44*, 175–185. [CrossRef] [PubMed]
14. Ramu, R.; Shirahatti, P.S.; Zameer, F.; Dhananjaya, B.L.; Prasad, N. Assessment of in vivo antidiabetic properties of umbelliferone and lupeol constituents of banana (*Musa* sp. var. Nanjangud Rasa Bale) flower in hyperglycaemic rodent model. *PLoS ONE* **2016**, *11*, e0151135.
15. Lebovitz, H.E. Postprandial hyperglycaemic state: Importance and consequences. *Diabetes Res. Clin. Pract.* **1998**, *40*, S27–S28. [PubMed]
16. Ali, A.A.; Velasquez, M.T.; Hansen, C.T.; Mohamed, A.I.; Bhathena, S.J. Modulation of carbohydrate metabolism and peptide hormones by soybean isoflavones and probiotics in obesity and diabetes. *J. Nutr. Biochem.* **2005**, *16*, 6993–6999. [CrossRef] [PubMed]
17. Park, S.; Kim, D.S.; Kim, J.H.; Kim, J.S.; Kim, H.J. Glyceollin-containing fermented soybeans improve glucose homeostasis in diabetic mice. *Nutrition* **2012**, *28*, 204–211. [CrossRef] [PubMed]
18. Himsworth, H.P. Diabetes mellitus: Its differentiation into insulin-sensitive and insulin-insensitive types. *Lancet* **1936**, *227*, 127–130. [CrossRef]
19. Yalow, R.S.; Berson, S.A. Plasma insulin concentrations in nondiabetic and early diabetic subjects: Determinations by a new sensitive immuno-assay technic. *Diabetes* **1960**, *9*, 254–260. [CrossRef] [PubMed]
20. Kahn, C.R.; Flier, J.S.; Bar, R.S.; Archer, J.A.; Gorden, P.; Martin, M.M. The syndromes of insulin resistance and acanthosis nigricans: Insulin-receptor disorders in man. *N. Engl. J. Med.* **1976**, *294*, 739–745. [CrossRef] [PubMed]
21. Olefsky, J.; Farquhar, J.W.; Reaven, G. Relationship between fasting plasma insulin level and resistance to insulin-mediated glucose uptake in normal and diabetic subjects. *Diabetes* **1973**, *22*, 507–513. [CrossRef] [PubMed]
22. Kolterman, O.G.; Insel, J.; Saekow, M.; Olefsky, J.M. Mechanisms of insulin resistance in human obesity: Evidence for receptor and postreceptor defects. *J. Clin. Investig.* **1980**, *65*, 1272–1284. [CrossRef] [PubMed]
23. Howard, G.O.; Leary, D.H.; Zaccaro, D.; Haffner, S.; Rewers, M.; Hamman, R. Insulin sensitivity and atherosclerosis. *Circulation* **1996**, *93*, 1809–1817. [CrossRef] [PubMed]
24. Yip, J.; Facchini, F.S.; Reaven, G.M. Resistance to insulin-mediated glucose disposal as a predictor of cardiovascular disease. *J. Clin. Endocrinol. MeTab.* **1998**, *83*, 2773–2776. [CrossRef] [PubMed]
25. Park, S.C.; Hwang, M.H.; Kim, Y.H.; Kim, J.C.; Song, J.C.; Lee, K.W. Comparison of pH and bile resistance of Lactobacillus acidophilus strains isolated from rat, pig, chicken, and human sources. *World J. Microbiol. Biotechnol.* **2006**, *22*, 35–37. [CrossRef]

26. Danielson, A.D.; Peo, E.R., Jr.; Shahani, K.M.; Lewis, A.J.; Whalen, P.J.; Amer, M.A. Anticholesteremic property of Lactobacillus acidophilus yogurt fed to mature boars. *J. Anim. Sci. Technol.* **1989**, *67*, 966–974. [CrossRef]
27. Liong, M.T.; Shah, N.P. Effects of a Lactobacillus casei synbiotic on serum lipoprotein, intestinal microflora, and organic acids in rats. *J. Dairy Sci.* **2006**, *89*, 1390–1399. [CrossRef]
28. Choi, M.S.; Jung, U.J.; Yeo, J.K.; Kim, M.J.; Lee, M.K. Genistein and daidzein prevent diabetes onset by elevating insulin level and altering hepatic gluconeogenic and lipogenic enzyme activities in non-obese diabetic (NOD) mice. *Diabetes Metab. Res. Rev.* **2008**, *24*, 74–81. [CrossRef] [PubMed]
29. Ding, M.; Pan, A.; Manson, J.E.; Willett, W.C.; Malik, V.; Rosner, B. Consumption of soy foods and isoflavones and risk of type 2 diabetes: A pooled analysis of three US cohorts. *Eur. J. Clin. Nutr.* **2016**, *70*, 1381. [CrossRef] [PubMed]
30. Mezei, O.; Banz, W.J.; Steger, R.W.; Peluso, M.R.; Winters, T.A.; Shay, N. Soy isoflavones exert antidiabetic and hypolipidemic effects through the PPAR pathways in obese Zucker rats and murine RAW 264.7 cells. *J. Nutr.* **2003**, *133*, 1238–1243. [CrossRef] [PubMed]
31. Park, S.A.; Choi, M.S.; Cho, S.Y.; Seo, J.S.; Jung, U.J.; Kim, M.J. Genistein and daidzein modulate hepatic glucose and lipid regulating enzyme activities in C57BL/KsJ-db/db mice. *Life Sci.* **2006**, *79*, 1207–1213. [CrossRef] [PubMed]
32. Lee, J.S. Effects of soy protein and genistein on blood glucose, antioxidant enzyme activities, and lipid profile in streptozotocin-induced diabetic rats. *Life Sci.* **2006**, *79*, 1578–1584. [CrossRef] [PubMed]
33. Kwon, D.Y.; Daily, J.W.; Kim, H.J.; Park, S. Antidiabetic effects of fermented soybean products on type 2 diabetes. *Nutr. Res.* **2010**, *30*, 1–13. [CrossRef] [PubMed]
34. Anandharaj, M.; Sivasankari, B.; Santhanakaruppu, R.; Manimaran, M.; Rani, R.P.; Sivakumar, S. Determining the probiotic potential of cholesterol-reducing Lactobacillus and Weissella strains isolated from gherkins (fermented cucumber) and south Indian fermented koozh. *Res. Microbiol.* **2015**, *166*, 428–439. [CrossRef] [PubMed]
35. Erkkilä, S.; Petäjä, E. Screening of commercial meat starter cultures at low pH and in the presence of bile salts for potential probiotic use. *Meat Sci.* **2000**, *55*, 297–300. [CrossRef]
36. Tsai, Y.T.; Cheng, P.C.; Fan, C.K.; Pan, T.M. Time-dependent persistence of enhanced immune response by a potential probiotic strain Lactobacillus paracasei subsp. paracasei NTU 101. *Int. J. Food Microbiol.* **2008**, *128*, 219–225. [CrossRef] [PubMed]
37. Panasevich, M.R.; Schuster, C.M.; Phillips, K.E.; Meers, G.M.; Chintapalli, S.V.; Wankhade, U. Soy compared with milk protein in a Western diet changes fecal microbiota and decreases hepatic steatosis in obese OLETF rats. *J. Nutr. Biochem.* **2017**, *46*, 125–136. [CrossRef] [PubMed]
38. Shankardass, K.; Chuchmach, S.; Chelswick, K.; Stefanovich, C.; Spurr, S.; Brooks, J. Bowel function of long-term tube-fed patients consuming formulae with and without dietary fiber. *J. Parenter. Enteral. Nutr.* **1990**, *14*, 508–512. [CrossRef] [PubMed]
39. Schneider, S.M.; Pouget, I.; Staccini, P.; Rampal, P.; Hebuterne, X. Quality of life in long-term home enteral nutrition patients. *Clin. Nutr.* **2000**, *19*, 23–28. [CrossRef] [PubMed]
40. Cabré, E. Fibre supplementation of enteral formula-diets: A look to the evidence. *Clin. Nutr.* **2004**, *1*, 63–71. [CrossRef]
41. Meier, R.; Gassull, M.A. Consensus recommendations on the effects and benefits of fibre in clinical practice. *Clin. Nutr.* **2004**, *1*, 73–80. [CrossRef]
42. Hofman, Z.; Van Drunen, J.D.E.; De Later, C.; Kuipers, H. The effect of different nutritional feeds on the postprandial glucose response in healthy volunteers and patients with type II diabetes. *Eur. J. Clin. Nutr.* **2004**, *58*, 1553. [CrossRef] [PubMed]
43. Read, N.W. Diarrhee motrice. *Clin. Gastroenterol.* **1986**, *15*, 657–686. [PubMed]
44. Russell, W.R.; Hoyles, L.; Flint, H.J.; Dumas, M.E. Colonic bacterial metabolites and human health. *Curr. Opin. Microbiol.* **2013**, *16*, 246–254. [CrossRef] [PubMed]
45. Topping, D.L.; Clifton, P.M. Short-chain fatty acids and human colonic function: Roles of resistant starch and nonstarch polysaccharides. *Physiol. Rev.* **2001**, *81*, 1031–1064. [CrossRef] [PubMed]
46. Fukuda, S.; Toh, H.; Hase, K.; Oshima, K.; Nakanishi, Y.; Yoshimura, K.; Taylor, T.D. Bifidobacteria can protect from enteropathogenic infection through production of acetate. *Nature* **2011**, *469*, 543–547. [CrossRef] [PubMed]

47. Maslowski, K.M.; Vieira, A.T.; Ng, A.; Kranich, J.; Sierro, F.; Yu, D. Regulation of inflammatory responses by gut microbiota and chemoattractant receptor GPR43. *Nature* **2009**, *461*, 1282. [CrossRef] [PubMed]
48. Hara, H.; Haga, S.; Aoyama, Y.; Kiriyama, S. Short-chain fatty acids suppress cholesterol synthesis in rat liver and intestine. *J. Nutr.* **1999**, *129*, 942–948. [CrossRef] [PubMed]
49. Hughes, S.A.; Shewry, P.R.; Gibson, G.R.; McCleary, B.V.; Rastall, R.A. In vitro fermentation of oat and barley derived β-glucans by human faecal microbiota. *FEMS Microbiol. Ecol.* **2008**, *64*, 482–493. [CrossRef] [PubMed]
50. Arora, T.; Sharma, R.; Frost, G. Propionate. Anti-obesity and satiety enhancing factor? *Appetite* **2011**, *56*, 511–515. [CrossRef] [PubMed]
51. Lin, H.V.; Frassetto, A.; Kowalik, E.J.; Nawrocki, A.R.; Lu, M.M.; Kosinski, J.R. Butyrate and propionate protect against diet-induced obesity and regulate gut hormones via free fatty acid receptor 3-independent mechanisms. *PLoS ONE* **2012**, *7*, e35240. [CrossRef] [PubMed]
52. Schneider, S.M.; Girard-Pipau, F.; Anty, R.; van der Linde, E.G.; Philipsen-Geerling, B.J.; Knol, J. Effects of total enteral nutrition supplemented with a multi-fibre mix on faecal short-chain fatty acids and microbiota. *Clin. Nutr.* **2006**, *25*, 82–90. [CrossRef] [PubMed]
53. Clarkson, T.B. Soy, soy phytoestrogens and cardiovascular disease. *J. Nutr.* **2002**, *132*, 566S–569S. [CrossRef] [PubMed]
54. Lichtenstein, A.H.; Jalbert, S.M.; Adlercreutz, H.; Goldin, B.R.; Rasmussen, H.; Schaefer, E.J. Lipoprotein response to diets high in soy or animal protein with and without isoflavones in moderately hypercholesterolemic subjects. *Arterioscler. Thromb. Vasc. Biol.* **2002**, *22*, 1852–1858. [CrossRef] [PubMed]
55. Matsumoto, K.; Watanabe, Y.; Yokoyama, S.I. Okara, soybean residue, prevents obesity in a diet-induced murine obesity model. *Biosci. Biotechnol. Biochem.* **2007**, *71*, 720–727. [CrossRef] [PubMed]
56. Otieno, D.O.; Shah, N.P. Endogenous β-glucosidase and β-galactosidase activities from selected probiotic micro-organisms and their role in isoflavone biotransformation in soymilk. *J. Appl. Microbiol.* **2007**, *103*, 910–917. [CrossRef] [PubMed]
57. Suzuki, T.; Hara, H. Role of flavonoids in intestinal tight junction regulation. *J. Nutr. Biochem.* **2011**, *22*, 401–408. [CrossRef] [PubMed]
58. Kim, M.H.; Park, J.S.; Jung, J.W.; Byun, K.W.; Kang, K.S.; Lee, Y.S. Daidzein supplementation prevents non-alcoholic fatty liver disease through alternation of hepatic gene expression profiles and adipocyte metabolism. *Int. J. Obes.* **2011**, *35*, 1019. [CrossRef] [PubMed]
59. Begley, M.; Gahan, C.G.; Hill, C. The interaction between bacteria and bile. *FEMS Microbiol. Rev.* **2005**, *29*, 625–651. [CrossRef] [PubMed]
60. Kakiyama, G.; Pandak, W.M.; Gillevet, P.M.; Hylemon, P.B.; Heuman, D.M.; Daita, K. Modulation of the fecal bile acid profile by gut microbiota in cirrhosis. *J. Hepatol.* **2013**, *58*, 949–955. [CrossRef] [PubMed]
61. Ridlon, J.M.; Kang, D.J.; Hylemon, P.B.; Bajaj, J.S. Bile acids and the gut microbiome. *Curr. Opin. Gastroenterol.* **2014**, *30*, 332. [CrossRef] [PubMed]
62. Islam, K.S.; Fukiya, S.; Hagio, M.; Fujii, N.; Ishizuka, S.; Ooka, T. Bile acid is a host factor that regulates the composition of the cecal microbiota in rats. *Gastroenterology* **2011**, *141*, 1773–1781. [CrossRef] [PubMed]
63. Zhang, M.; Hang, X.; Fan, X.; Li, D.; Yang, H. Characterization and selection of Lactobacillus strains for their effect on bile tolerance, taurocholate deconjugation and cholesterol removal. *World J. Microbiol. Biotechnol.* **2008**, *24*, 7–14. [CrossRef]
64. Begley, M.; Hill, C.; Gahan, C.G. Bile salt hydrolase activity in probiotics. *Appl. Environ. Microbiol.* **2006**, *72*, 1729–1738. [CrossRef] [PubMed]
65. Nagata, Y.; Ishiwaki, N.; Sugano, M. Studies on the mechanism of antihypercholesterolemic action of soy protein and soy protein-type amino acid mixtures in relation to the casein counterparts in rats. *J. Nutr.* **1982**, *112*, 1614–1625. [CrossRef] [PubMed]
66. El-Gawad, I.A.A.; El-Sayed, E.M.; Hafez, S.A.; El-Zeini, H.M.; Saleh, F.A. The hypocholesterolaemic effect of milk yoghurt and soy-yoghurt containing bifidobacteria in rats fed on a cholesterol-enriched diet. *Int. Dairy J.* **2005**, *15*, 37–44. [CrossRef]
67. Imaizumi, K.; Hirata, K.; Zommara, M.; Sugano, M.; Suzuki, Y. Effects of cultured milk products by Lactobacillus and Bifidobacterium species on the secretion of bile acids in hepatocytes and in rats. *J. Nutr. Sci. Vitaminol.* **1992**, *38*, 343–351. [CrossRef] [PubMed]

68. Gudbrandsen, O.A.; Wergedahl, H.; Liaset, B.; Espe, M.; Berge, R.K. Dietary proteins with high isoflavone content or low methionine-glycine and lysine-arginine ratios are hypocholesterolaemic and lower the plasma homocysteine level in male Zucker fa/fa rats. *Br. J. Nutr.* **2005**, *94*, 321–330. [CrossRef] [PubMed]
69. Ni, W.; Yoshida, S.; Tsuda, Y.; Nagao, K.; Sato, M.; Imaizumi, K. Ethanol-extracted soy protein isolate results in elevation of serum cholesterol in exogenously hypercholesterolemic rats. *Lipids* **1999**, *34*, 713–716. [CrossRef] [PubMed]
70. Cao, Y.; Ma, Z.; Zhang, H.; Jin, Y.; Zhang, Y.; Hayford, F. Phytochemical properties and nutrigenomic implications of yacon as a potential source of prebiotic: Current evidence and future directions. *Foods* **2018**, *7*, 59. [CrossRef] [PubMed]
71. Okarter, N.; Liu, R.H. Health benefits of whole grain phytochemicals. *Crit. Rev. Food Sci. Nutr.* **2010**, *50*, 193–208. [CrossRef] [PubMed]
72. Wang, C.Y.; Wu, S.J.; Fang, J.Y.; Wang, Y.P.; Shyu, Y.T. Cardiovascular and intestinal protection of cereal pastes fermented with lactic acid bacteria in hyperlipidemic hamsters. *Food Res. Int.* **2012**, *48*, 428–434. [CrossRef]
73. Lazaridou, A.; Biliaderis, C.G. Molecular aspects of cereal β-glucan functionality: Physical properties, technological applications and physiological effects. *J. Cereal Sci.* **2007**, *46*, 101–118. [CrossRef]
74. Ooi, L.G.; Liong, M.T. Cholesterol-lowering effects of probiotics and prebiotics: A review of in vivo and in vitro findings. *Int. J. Mol. Sci.* **2010**, *11*, 2499–2522. [CrossRef] [PubMed]
75. Bäckhed, F.; Ley, R.E.; Sonnenburg, J.L.; Peterson, D.A.; Gordon, J.I. Host-bacterial mutualism in the human intestine. *Science* **2005**, *307*, 1915–1920. [CrossRef] [PubMed]
76. Yusof, N.; Hamid, N.; Ma, Z.F.; Lawenko, R.M.; Mohammad, W.M.Z.W.; Collins, D.A.; Lee, Y.Y. Exposure to environmental microbiota explains persistent abdominal pain and irritable bowel syndrome after a major flood. *Gut Pathog.* **2017**, *9*, 75. [CrossRef] [PubMed]
77. Sáez, C. Gut Microbiota May Improve Sugar Metabolism in Humans. 2016. Available online: http://www.gutmicrobiotaforhealth.com/en/gut-microbiota-may-improve-sugar-metabolism-in-humans/ (accessed on 11 February 2016).
78. De Filippo, C.; Cavalieri, D.; Di Paola, M.; Ramazzotti, M.; Poullet, J.B.; Massart, S. Impact of diet in shaping gut microbiota revealed by a comparative study in children from Europe and rural Africa. *Proc. Natl. Acad. Sci. USA* **2010**, *107*, 14691–14696. [CrossRef] [PubMed]
79. Pan, X.D.; Chen, F.Q.; Wu, T.X.; Tang, H.G.; Zhao, Z.Y. Prebiotic oligosaccharides change the concentrations of short-chain fatty acids and the microbial population of mouse bowel. *J. Zhejiang Univ. Sci. B* **2009**, *10*, 258–263. [CrossRef] [PubMed]

8

The Effect of Diabetes-Specific Enteral Nutrition Formula on Cardiometabolic Parameters in Patients with Type 2 Diabetes

Omorogieva Ojo [1,*], Sharon Marie Weldon [1,2], Trevor Thompson [3], Rachel Crockett [4] and Xiao-Hua Wang [5]

1 Department of Adult Nursing and Paramedic Science, University of Greenwich, London SE9 2UG, UK
2 Barts Health NHS Trust, The Royal London Hospital, Whitechapel Rd, Whitechapel E1 1BB, UK
3 Department of Psychology, University of Greenwich, London SE10 9LS, UK
4 Division of Psychology, Faculty of Natural Sciences, University of Stirling, Scotland FK9 4LA, UK
5 The School of Nursing, Soochow University, Suzhou 215006, China
* Correspondence: o.ojo@greenwich.ac.uk

Abstract: Background: The prevalence of diabetes is on the increase in the UK and worldwide, partly due to unhealthy lifestyles, including poor dietary regimes. Patients with diabetes and other co-morbidities such as stroke, which may affect swallowing ability and lead to malnutrition, could benefit from enteral nutrition, including the standard formula (SF) and diabetes-specific formulas (DSF). However, enteral nutrition presents its challenges due to its effect on glycaemic control and lipid profile. Aim: The aim of this review was to evaluate the effectiveness of diabetes-specific enteral nutrition formula versus SF in managing cardiometabolic parameters in patients with type 2 diabetes. Method: This review was conducted in accordance with the preferred reporting items for systematic reviews and meta-analyses. Three databases (Pubmed, EMBASE, PSYCInfo) and Google scholar were searched for relevant articles from inception to 2 January 2019 based on Population, Intervention, Comparator, Outcomes and Study designs (PICOS) framework. Key words, Medical Subject Heading (MeSH) terms, and Boolean operators (AND/OR) formed part of the search strategy. Articles were evaluated for quality and risks of bias. Results: Fourteen articles were included in the systematic review and five articles were selected for the meta-analysis. Based on the findings of the review and meta-analysis, two distinct areas were evident: the effect of DSF on blood glucose parameters and the effect of DSF on lipid profile. All fourteen studies included in the systematic review showed that DSF was effective in lowering blood glucose parameters in patients with type 2 diabetes compared with SF. The results of the meta-analysis confirmed the findings of the systematic review with respect to the fasting blood glucose, which was significantly lower ($p = 0.01$) in the DSF group compared to SF, with a mean difference of −1.15 (95% CI −2.07, −0.23) and glycated haemoglobin, which was significantly lower ($p = 0.005$) in the DSF group compared to the SF group following meta-analysis and sensitivity analysis. However, in relation to the sensitivity analysis for the fasting blood glucose, differences were not significant between the two groups when some of the studies were removed. Based on the systematic review, the outcomes of the studies selected to evaluate the effect of DSF on lipid profile were variable. Following the meta-analysis, no significant differences ($p > 0.05$) were found between the DSF and SF groups with respect to total cholesterol, LDL cholesterol and triglyceride. The level of the HDL cholesterol was significantly higher ($p = 0.04$) in the DSF group compared to the SF group after the intervention, with a mean difference of 0.09 (95% CI, 0.00, 0.18), although this was not consistent based on the sensitivity analysis. The presence of low glycaemic index (GI) carbohydrate, the lower amount of carbohydrate and the higher protein, the presence of mono-unsaturated fatty acids and the different amounts and types of fibre in the DSF compared with SF may be responsible for the observed differences in cardiometabolic parameters in both groups.

Conclusion: The results provide evidence to suggest that DSF is effective in controlling fasting blood glucose and glycated haemoglobin and in increasing HDL cholesterol, but has no significant effect on other lipid parameters. However, our confidence in these findings would be increased by additional data from further studies.

Keywords: diabetes specific formula; standard formula; type 2 diabetes; enteral nutrition; enteral tube feeding; lipids; fasting blood glucose; glycated haemoglobin

---

1. Introduction

Diabetes is a metabolic condition which is characterised by chronic hyperglycaemia and is caused by a range of factors including genetic inheritance and environmental influences [1]. The prevalence of diabetes is on the increase in the UK and worldwide, partly due to the changes in lifestyle, including lack of physical activity and unhealthy diets, which lead to overweight and obesity [2–5]. In addition, improvements in technology and the greater awareness of the condition have meant that diabetes is now better detected and more people are engaging in screening programmes. About 90% of patients with diabetes are diagnosed with type 2 diabetes [6–8]. The impact of diabetes on the people living with the condition can be profound in terms of morbidity and mortality, as well as a cost burden to the National Health Service (NHS). Individuals with diabetes are more likely to be admitted to hospital and it can have a significant effect on the quality of life of patients [9,10]. Diabetes is a major risk factor for kidney dysfunction, lower limb amputations, retinopathy, cardiovascular disease and other co-morbidities such as stroke, which can lead to swallowing problems and malnutrition. Based on these issues, diabetes continues to be a major public health concern in the UK and globally, and strategies for managing the condition continue to evolve. Often, management relies on lifestyle modifications such as increased physical activity levels and the use of dietary interventions in order to prevent the onset of type 2 diabetes and ultimately reduce the possibility of diabetic complications [11]. However, in patients who are sedentary and immobile, the use of physical activity as a strategy for managing the condition is sometimes impracticable.

Therefore, individuals with diabetes and other conditions, such as stroke, which could affect mobility and swallowing ability, may benefit from enteral nutrition such as oral nutrition supplements and the use of a nasogastric feeding tube (for short-term feeding) or a percutaneous endoscopic gastrostomy tube for long-term intervention to deliver enteral feeds and formulas [12]. Usually, these individuals have functional guts and the essence is to provide adequate nutrition, hydration and medication to these patients in order to improve their nutritional status and clinical outcomes, including quality of life.

Why it is important to do this review:

The current review focuses mainly on patients with type 2 diabetes from a range of backgrounds, including those attending diabetes centre/outpatient diabetic clinics, rehabilitation departments, ambulatory patients, nursing homes and long-term care facilities, and intensive care units. Patients with diabetes are at a greater risk of developing stroke, peripheral vascular disease, renal impairment and dementia compared with those without the condition due to chronic hyperglycaemia [13]. The long-term complications of diabetes, including its co-morbidities, have implications for the length of hospital stay. Thus, while the average length of hospital stay in patients with diabetes as the primary diagnosis has been estimated to be 4.3 days, it is 8 days in patients with additional diagnoses and 3.1 days in all hospitalisations [14]. The use of enteral feeding in patients with diabetes can present a range of challenges in the control of blood glucose levels and other cardiometabolic parameters [15]. These parameters, including lipid profile, such as total cholesterol, high density lipoprotein cholesterol, low density lipoprotein cholesterol and triglyceride, are important biomarkers in patients with type 2 diabetes as they have implications for insulin resistance and cardiovascular mortality.

In patients with diabetes who are on enteral nutrition, the enteral feeds provided can be in the form of either Standard Formulas (SF) or Diabetes Specific Formulas (DSF). Enteral feeding formulas have a tendency to promote hyperglycaemia and insulinemic responses in patients with diabetes and in healthy subjects [16,17]. In addition, the effect of enteral nutrition on blood glucose parameters may be due to the fact that continuous enteral feeding is a source of continuous supply of glucose, providing 10–20 g of carbohydrates per hour, which is not the same during normal eating [15]. The absence of the normal postprandial glucose peak in patients with diabetes on enteral nutrition makes the management of hyperglycaemia difficult [15]. On the other hand, the effect of different types and amounts of fibre and mono-unsaturated fatty acids in various enteral feeds may influence lipid profile and other cardiometabolic parameters such as fasting blood glucose and glycated haemoglobin in patients with type 2 diabetes [18]. The role of the different enteral feeding formulas such as SF and DSF and their impact on cardiometabolic parameters in patients with diabetes continues to generate interest and controversy, and there appears to be no consensus among researchers on the most effective management strategy for these patients.

DSFs usually contain carbohydrates with low GI such as fructose and large amounts of monounsaturated fatty acids in varying amounts, which have effect on glycaemic control [17–20]. On the other hand, SFs are often high in carbohydrate and contain only low to moderate levels of lipids and do not have dietetic fibre [17].

Previous reviews on the use of enteral nutrition in patients with diabetes [16,17,21–23] either lacked consensus in the recommendations, were based only on glycaemic control or did not involve meta-analysis. In addition, concerns remain with the use of DSF in terms of the safety and tolerance of relatively high levels of fat and fructose with respect to lipid metabolism and lactic acidosis, despite its advantage in improving blood glucose compared with SFs [16,19]. Therefore, this review provides a quantitative assessment of the relative effectiveness of DSF compared with SF.

Aim: The aim was to evaluate the effectiveness of diabetes specific enteral nutrition formula versus SF in managing cardiometabolic parameters in patients with type 2 diabetes.

2. Methods

This study was conducted in accordance with the preferred reporting items for systematic reviews and meta-analyses (PRISMA) [24].

2.1. *Types of Studies and Participants*

Only randomised controlled studies were included in this review and participants were patients with type 2 diabetes.

Inclusion and Exclusion Criteria.

The criteria for considering studies for the review are outlined in Table 1.

Table 1. Criteria for considering studies for the review based on the Population, Intervention, Comparator, Outcomes and Study designs (PICOS) Structure.

	Inclusion Criteria	Exclusion Criteria
Population	Patients with type 2 diabetes and on enteral nutrition irrespective of type of feeding tube.	Patients with type 1 diabetes. Pregnant women with gestational diabetes. Healthy individuals without diabetes on enteral nutrition. Patients with diabetes on parenteral nutrition and parenteral plus enteral nutrition. Studies involving animals
Intervention	Diabetes specific formulas (Oral nutrition supplement or enteral tube feeding)	Parenteral nutrition, parenteral plus enteral nutrition.
Comparator	Standard formulas (Oral nutrition supplement or enteral tube feeding)	Parenteral nutrition and parenteral plus enteral nutrition.
Outcomes	Cardiometabolic parameters	Qualitative outcomes such as patient feelings.
Study Design:	Randomised Controlled Trials	Letters, comments, reviews, qualitative studies

2.2. *Type of Intervention*

The intervention for this review was based on diabetes-specific enteral formula, irrespective of the type of feeding tube, mode and rate of delivery of the enteral feed and clinical settings.

2.3. *Types of Outcome Measures*

The following were the outcome measures of interest;

- Blood glucose parameters—Fasting blood glucose and glycated haemoglobin.
- Lipid profile: Total cholesterol, low density lipoprotein (LDL) cholesterol, high density lipoprotein (HDL) cholesterol and triglycerides.

2.4. *Search Strategy*

Databases encompassing Pubmed, EMBASE, PSYCInfo and Google scholar were searched for relevant articles based on the Population (Patients with diabetes), Intervention (Diabetes Specific Formula), Comparator (Standard enteral formulas), Outcomes (outcome measures) and Study designs (Randomised controlled studies)—PICOS framework (Table 2) [25]. The use of key words, truncation symbols, Medical Subject Heading (MeSH) terms and Boolean operators (AND/OR) formed part of the search strategy. Searches were conducted from the date of inception of databases until 2 January 2019.

The screening of studies and the evaluation of their eligibility and inclusion were in line with PRISMA [24] guidelines (Figure 1). These procedures were conducted by five researchers (OO, SMW, TT, RC, X-HW) and differences were resolved through consensus.

Table 2. Search method for identification of studies.

Patient/Population	Intervention	Comparator	Study Designs	Combining Search Terms
Patients with type 2 diabetes	Diabetes specific formulas	Standard formulas	Randomised Controlled Trial	
Type 2 diabetes OR type 2 diabetes mellitus OR Diabetes complications OR diabetes mellitus, type 2	Diabetes specific formula OR Diabetes specific form* OR Enteral nutrition OR Enteral* OR Enteral feed OR Enteral feed* OR Enteral form* OR Diabetes formula OR tube feeding OR enteral feeding		Randomised Controlled Trial OR Randomized Controlled Trial OR Randomized Controlled study OR RCT OR Randomized* OR controlled clinical trial OR placebo OR randomly OR trial OR groups	Column 1 AND Column 2 AND Column 3

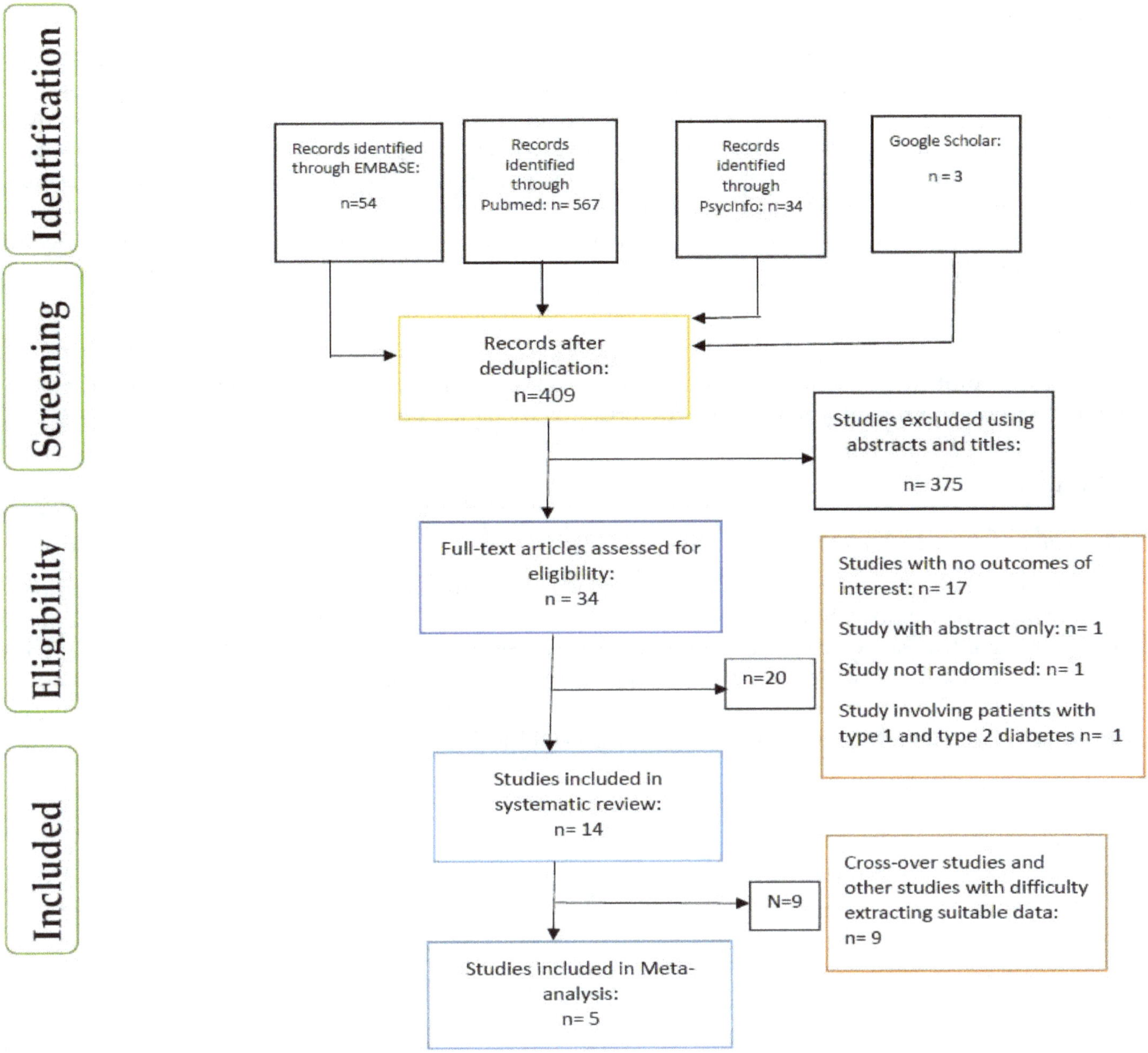

Figure 1. PRISMA flow chart on selection and inclusion of studies.

2.5. *Data Extraction*

All the articles from different databases were exported to ENDNote (Analytics, Philadelphia, PA, USA) for de-duplication. Data extraction was carried out by one researcher (OO) and cross-checked by the other four researchers (SMW, TT, RC, X-HW).

2.6. *Assessment of Risk of Bias and Evaluation of Quality*

A critical appraisal skills programme (CASP) tool was used to appraise the quality of the articles [26]. In addition, the researchers carried out an assessment of the risk of bias using the domain-based tool (random sequence generation, allocation concealment, blinding of participants, personnel and outcome assessment, reporting bias and selective reporting) to evaluate the studies included [27].

2.7. Statistical Analysis

Articles that met the inclusion criteria for meta-analysis were exported to RevMan (Review Manager, 5.3) [28] for data analysis. Therefore, cross-over studies and other studies which presented with difficulty in extracting suitable data were excluded from the meta-analysis. The data analysis included both meta-analysis and sensitivity analysis, the latter being conducted to test the consistency of the effect of DSFs on the different cardiometabolic paramters. The random effects model was used for the parameters of interest due to the high level of heterogeneity measured by the statistic I^2 with values ranging from 34% to 100%. A p value of 0.10 was used to determine the statistical significance of heterogeneity.

2.8. Effect Size

A forest plot was used to present the results of the meta-analysis and statistical significance for the overall effect of the intervention was determined by a p value of <0.05.

3. Results

3.1. Data Inclusion Decisions

Fasting blood glucose in the studies included was measured after overnight fasting, using standard measuring instruments. This is the standard method of measuring fasting blood glucose: the blood glucose concentrations were expressed as Means. However, the studies by Pohl et al. [29,30] were expressed as median and interquartile ranges and these were converted to means and standard deviations [27]. Fourteen studies were included in the systematic review (Table 3) while only five studies [29–33] were selected for the meta-analysis (Table 4).

Table 3. Characteristics of the articles included in this review ($n = 14$).

Citation	Country	Length of Study	Study Type/Design	Sample Size/Description	Age (Years)	Type of Enteral Formula/Feeding Method	Duration of Diabetes (Years)	Study Results/Conclusion
Ceriello et al. [18]	Netherlands	24 h	Randomized, controlled, double-blind, cross-over	$n = 11$	Mean ± SEM 67.2 ± 1.3	The DSF had 1 kcal/mL and low GI and/or slowly digestible CHO. The SF was isocaloric fibre containing formula. Bolus Feeding	Mean ± SEM 6.6 ± 1.4 years	Administration of DSF lowered glucose profiles. Using DSF resulted in significantly lower 24 h and postprandial glucose profiles than fibre-containing SF after bolus administration.
Buranapin et al. [20]	Thailand	180 min	Single centre, prospective, randomized, double blind, cross-over study. Administration of oral DSF and SF	$n = 30$	Mean ± SD 60.93 ± 11.71	55% CHO, 15% protein, 30% fat for DSF and SF. However, DSF substituted sucrose for combination of fructose, polydextrose and FOS. Bolus Feeding	More than 6 months.	DSF resulted in significantly lower postprandial blood glucose concentration than SF.
Pohl et al. [29]	Germany	12 weeks	Randomized, double-blind, controlled, multi-centre trial.	$n = 78$	Median (Range) Test group (DSF): 71 (42–86) Control group (SF): 72 (51–87)	DSF contained 37% energy as CHO, 45% as fat, 18% as protein, SF contained 52% energy as CHO, 30% of energy as total fat and 18% as protein. Continuous Feeding.	No data	DSF formula resulted in a more effective glycaemia control than SF, and was comparable in DSF significantly decreased triglycerides compared with SF, but differences were not significant in relation to total cholesterol, HDL and LDL cholesterols.
Pohl et al. [30]	Germany	84 days	Parallel design. Stage two of a randomized, prospective, double-blind, controlled, multicentre, parallel group study	$n = 97$	Median (Range) DSF: 74 (44–91) SF: 69 (53–86)	DSF contained 37% energy as CHO, 45% as fat, 18% as protein, SF contained 52% energy as CHO, 30% of energy as total fat and 18% as protein. Continuous Feeding.	No data	Compared to SF, DSF significantly lowered FBG and improved glycaemic control. There were no significant differences between the two groups with respect to TG, TC, HDL and LDL cholesterols.

Table 3. *Cont.*

Citation	Country	Length of Study	Study Type/Design	Sample Size/Description	Age (Years)	Type of Enteral Formula/Feeding Method	Duration of Diabetes (Years)	Study Results/Conclusion
Craig et al. [31]	USA–New York State	3 months	Randomized, double-blind, controlled, parallel group 3 months pilot trial.	$n = 34$	DSF: 82 ± 3 (range 52–94) 80 ± 2 (range-SF: 52–100)	Per 1000 mL, DSF contained 1000 kcal, 41.8 g protein, 93. 7 g CHO, 55.7 g fat. SF contained 1060 kcal, 44.4 g protein, 151.7 CHO, 35.9 g fat. Continuous or intermittent feeding.	No data	DSF resulted in lower fasting serum glucose and HbA1c than SF. No significant differences between the DSF and SF groups with respect to LDL cholesterol and TG 3 months post intervention, but the DSF group had significantly higher level of HDL cholesterol than the SF group.
Lansink et al. [32]	Netherlands	4 weeks	Randomized, controlled, double-blind, parallel-group study.	$n = 44$	Mean ± SD DSF: 65.2 ± 7.4 SF: 64.2 ± 5.9	DSF contained 1 kcal/mL, 47 Energy% CHO, 19 Energy% protein, 34 Energy% fat and 2 g fibres/100 mL. The SF contained 50 Energy% CHO, 16 Energy% protein, 34 Energy% fat and 1.5 g fibres/100 mL. Bolus Feeding	Mean (Range) DSF: 84 (18–216) months SF: 66 (10–504) months	DSF significantly lowered postprandial glucose compared with SF. Levels of TG, TC, HDL and LDL cholesterols were not significantly different between the two groups at baseline and 4 weeks post intervention.
Vaisman et al. [33]	No data	12 weeks	Randomized, controlled, double-blind, parallel group study.	$n = 25$	Total: 76.2 ± 12.8 years DSF: 73.0 ± 14.7 SF: 79.2 ± 10.4	DSF contained 100 kcal, 45 Energy% CHO, 38 Energy% fat, 17 Energy% protein and 1.5 g/100 kcal fibre. SF contained 100 kcal, 55 Energy% CHO, 30 Energy% fat, 15 Energy% protein, 2 g/100 kcal fibre. Bolus, Continuous or intermittent feeding.	Mean ± SD Total: 8.6 ± 7.6 years DSF: 5.0 ± 4.9 SF: 12.6 ± 8.4	The DSF significantly reduced HbA1c compared to SF. No significant effect was found with respect to fasting blood glucose. DSF significantly increased HDL cholesterol, but differences were not significant in relation to TG, TC and LDL cholesterol compared with SF.

Table 3. *Cont.*

Citation	Country	Length of Study	Study Type/Design	Sample Size/Description	Age (Years)	Type of Enteral Formula/Feeding Method	Duration of Diabetes (Years)	Study Results/Conclusion
Alish et al. [34]	USA	10 days	Randomized, double blind, two treatment, crossover design. DSF (Postprandial response protocol) vs. SF (Continuous glucose monitoring).	*n* = 12	Mean ± SEM Postprandial: 63.1 ± 1.9 Continuous feed: 74.1 ± 4.0	DSF had 1.2 kcal/mL, 114.5 g CHO, 17 g/L fibre, 60 g/L protein, 60 g/L fat. SF had 1.2 kcal/mL, 169.4 g CHO, 18 g/L fibre, 55.5 g/L protein, 39.3 g/L fat. Continuous Feeding.	NS	Use of DSF produced lower postprandial glycaemic and insulinemic responses, reduced glycaemic variability, and resulted in less hyperglycaemia, reduced short acting insulin requirements.
Gulati et al. [35]	India	8 months	Open-label, randomized, crossover, pilot single centre study.	*n* = 40	35–60 years	DSF administered was 55 g in 210 mL of water to make 250 mL at standard reconstitution (1 kcal/mL) which can be used as tube feed or oral nutrition supplement. The SF was isocaloric Meal. Bolus Feeding	No data	DSF demonstrated lower blood glucose and insulin post meal levels than SF. The level of HDL cholesterol was significantly higher in the DSF group compared with the SF group after intervention, but differences were not significant in relation to TG, TC and LDL cholesterol.
Hofman et al. [36]	Netherlands	360 min	Randomized, double blind, cross over study involving SF (A), DSF with moderate amount of carbohydrate and MUFA (B) and Test feed with low amount of carbohydrate and high amount of fat (C)	*n* = 12	63 ± 9.4 years	DSF (45 Energy% CHO, 26 Energy% MUFA), SF (49 Energy% CHO, 21 Energy% MUFA). Continuous Feeding.	No data	DSF showed significantly lower glucose levels compared with SF. With respect to TG level, the DSF B with a lower amount of fat showed significantly lower levels than test feed C.

Table 3. *Cont.*

Citation	Country	Length of Study	Study Type/Design	Sample Size/Description	Age (Years)	Type of Enteral Formula/Feeding Method	Duration of Diabetes (Years)	Study Results/Conclusion
Lansink et al. [37]	Netherlands	8 h	Randomized, controlled, double-blind cross-over study	$n = 24$	Mean ± SD 64.6 ± 10.7	The DSF had 1.5 kcal/mL, high protein, a mixture of 6 different dietary fibre and low GI CHO. SF was isocaloric fibre containing formula. Continuous Feeding.	Median (Minimum and Maximum) 76.5 months (13, 303)	Administration of a new, high-protein DSF during 4 h of continuous feeding resulted in lower glucose and insulin levels compared with a fiber-containing SF. DSF may contribute to lower glucose levels in these patients.
Mesejo et al. [38]	Spain	2 years	Prospective, open-label, randomized study	$n = 157$	Median (Q1–Q3) New generation DSF: 57 (43–70) SF: 60 (45–71) Control DSF: 58 (46–68)	Per 100 mL, DSF had 100 kcal, 5.7 g protein, 8.2 g CHO, 4.4 g fat. SF had 100 kcal, 5/7 g protein, 10.93/15.3 g CHO, 3.79/5.3 g fat. Continuous Feeding.	No data	DSFs lowered insulin requirements, improved glycaemic control and reduced the risk of acquired infections relative to SF. Plasma levels of cholesterol and TG were similar across the three treatment groups.
Voss et al. [39]	USA	240 min	Randomized cross over-study Double-blinded with three-treatments	$n = 48$	Mean ± SEM 56 ± 1.4 years	DSF had 1 kcal/mL, 47.8 g CHO, 7.2 g fibre, 20.9 g protein, 27.2 g fat. SF had 1.06 kcal/mL, 73 g CHO, 7.2 g fibre, 20.9 g protein, 16.4 g fat. Bolus Feeding		DSF resulted in lower postprandial blood glucose response compared with SF.
Vanschoonbeek et al. [40]	Netherlands	10 days	Randomized, double-blind, cross over study.	$n = 15$	Mean ± SEM 63 ± 1 years	Per 100 mL, DSF had 98 kcal, 1.44 g fibre and 5.44/50 (g/energy%) of fat. SF had 100 kcal, 1.4 g of fibre, 3.4/30 (g/energy%) of fat.), Bolus Feeding	Mean ± SEM 9 ± 2 years	DSF rich in lowly digestible carbohydrate sources can be equally effective in lowering the postprandial blood glucose response as low-carbohydrate, high-fat enteral formulas without elevating the plasma triglyceride response.

Abbreviations: NS (Not stated); DSF (Diabetes Specific Formula); CHO (Carbohydrate); FOS (Fructo-oligosaccharide); GI (Glycaemic Index); HbA1c (Glycated haemoglobin); SF (Standard Formula); LDL (low density lipoprotein) Cholesterol; HDL (high density lipoprotein)Cholesterol; MUFA (mono-unsaturated fatty acid); FBG (fasting blood glucose); TC (total cholesterol); TG (triglycerides); T2DM (type 2 diabetes mellitus).

Table 4. Blood glucose parameters among individuals with diabetes (Meta-analysis Data Extraction Table).

Study Reference	Interventions	Pre-and Post Intervention	Fasting Blood Glucose mmol/L Mean ± SD/Median (Quartiles)	Glycated Haemoglobin % Mean ± SD/Median (Quartiles)	Total Cholesterol mmol/L Mean ± SD/Median (Quartiles)	LDL Cholesterol mmol/L Mean ± SD/Median (Quartiles)	HDL Cholesterol mmol/L Mean ± SD/Median (Quartiles)	Triglycerides mmol/L Mean ± SD/Median (Quartiles)
Pohl. et al. [29]	DSF, $n = 39$	Change from baseline	** Δ−1.59 (−3.38 to −0.06)	** Δ−0.8 (−1.5 to −0.5)	** Δ−0.37 (−1.00 to 0.56)	** Δ−0.28 (−1.46 to 0.53)	** Δ0.08 (−0.06 to 0.28)	** Δ−0.37 (−0.36 to 0.38)
	SF, $n = 39$	Change from baseline	** Δ−0.08 (−1.34 to 0.79)	** Δ0.0 (−0.4 to 0.3)	** Δ−0.23 (−1.22 to 0.46)	** Δ−0.52 (−1.48 to 0.04)	** Δ0.05 (−0.10 to 0.32)	** Δ0.203 (−0.07 to 0.84)
Pohl et al. [30]	DSF, $n = 48$	Change from baseline	** Δ−2.17 (−2.55/−1.33)	** Δ−1.30 (−2.60/−0.10)	** Δ0.30 (−1.22/1.06)	** Δ0.27 (−0.71/1.40	** Δ0.03 (−0.26/0.4)	** Δ−0.45 (−1.65/0.27)
	SF, $n = 49$	Change from baseline	** Δ−0.67 (−0.90/−0.10)	** Δ−1.20 (−2.35/−0.55)	** Δ0.21 (−1.02/0.48)	** Δ−0.33 (−1.03/0.56)	** Δ0.00 (−0.22/0.28)	** Δ−0.70 (−1.50/1.73)
Craig et al. [31]	DSF, $n = 14$	Baseline	* 7.3 ± 0.4	* 6.9 ± 0.3	* 4.16 ± 0.31	* 2.66 ± 0.23	* 1.01 ± 0.05	* 0.97 ± 0.13
		Final	6.7 ± 0.7	6.5 ± 0.4	3.96 ± 0.31	2.51 ± 0.28	0.98 ± 0.05	0.91 ± 0.17g/L
	SF, $n = 13$	Baseline	* 6.9 ± 0.6	* 6.9 ± 0.5	* 4.21 ± 0.18	* 2.69 ± 0.15	* 0.98 ± 0.05	* 0.9 ± 0.07
		Final	8.3 ± 1.7	6.9 ± 0.14	3.96 ± 0.23	2.53 ± 0.21	0.83 ± 0.05	1.06 ± 0.12 g/L
Lansink et al. [32]	DSF, $n = 21$	Baseline	* 8.32 ± 0.33	No data	No data	No data	No data	No data
		Final	8.13 ± 0.33					
	SF, $n = 22$	Baseline	* 7.73 ± 0.22	No data	No data	No data	No data	No data
		Final	8.22 ± 0.26					
Vaisman et al. [33]	DSF, $n = 12$	Baseline	No data	*** 6.9 ± 0.3	No data	No data	*** 1.04 ± 0.08	No data
		Final		6.2 ± 0.4			1.23 ± 0.10	
	SF, $n = 13$	Baseline	No data	*** 7.9 ± 0.3	No data	No data	*** 1.06 ± 0.08	No data
		Final		8.7 ± 0.4			0.94 ± 0.09	

Abbreviations: NS (Not stated); SD (Standard deviation); SEM (Standard Error of Mean); Δ (Change from baseline) * Mean ± SD; ** Median (Quartiles); *** Mean ± SEM.

3.2. *Assessment of Risk of Bias in Included Studies*

Figure 2 shows the risk of bias summary of the various studies included in the meta-analysis. All the studies demonstrated low risk of bias in all the areas, except with respect to incomplete outcome data (attrition bias) where two studies [29,33] showed high risk of bias.

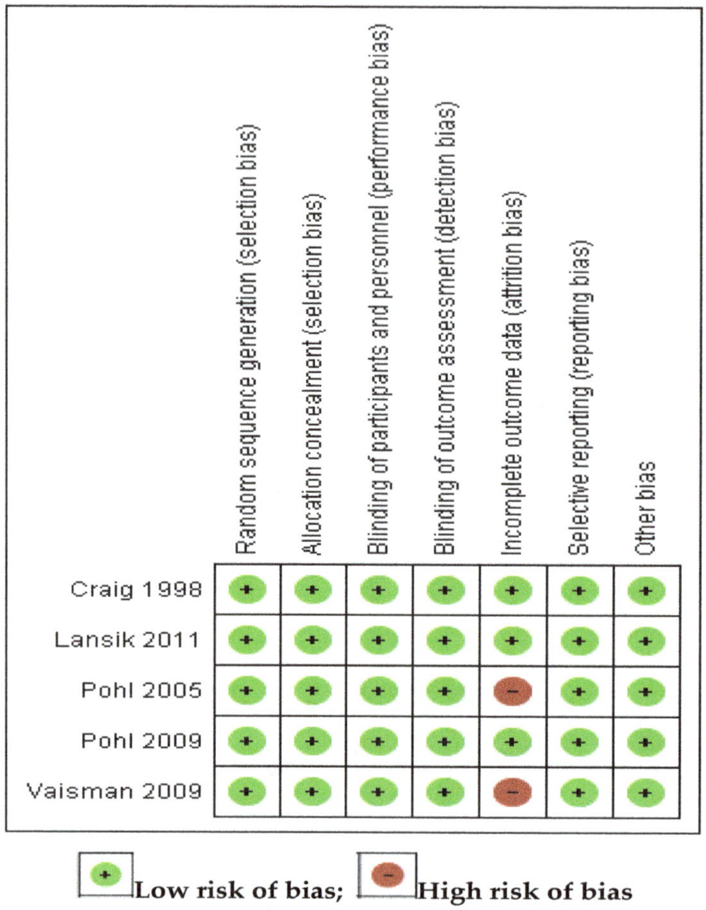

Figure 2. Risk of bias summary.

Based on the findings of the review and the meta-analysis, two distinct areas were evident: the effect of DSF on blood glucose parameters and the effect of DSF on lipid profile.

The effect DSF on blood glucose parameters:

All the fourteen studies included in the systematic review showed that DSF was effective in lowering blood glucose parameters in patients with type 2 diabetes compared with SF. In particular, DSF improved glycaemic control and lowered insulin requirements [18,29,31,35–39]. It provided better clinical outcomes, including reducing the risk of acquired infections and pressure ulcer, reduced body weight and was safer compared to SF [29,31,32]. In addition, the use of DSF was shown to be effective in lowering postprandial blood glucose levels compared to SF [20,32,34,40].

Pohl et al. [30] observed that long-term tube feeding with a DSF significantly lowered fasting blood glucose and improved glycaemic control. Similarly, Vaisman et al. [33] reported that DSF significantly improved longer-term glycaemic control in diabetic patients compared to SF. The results of the meta-analysis confirmed the findings of the systematic review. With respect to the fasting blood glucose, it was significantly lower ($p = 0.01$) in the DSF group compared to SF, with a mean difference of −1.15 (95% CI −2.07, −0.23) (Figure 3). However, in relation to the sensitivity analysis, there were no significant differences ($p > 0.05$) between the two groups with the removal of Pohl et al. [29,30] studies.

Study or Subgroup	Experimental Mean	Experimental SD	Experimental Total	Control Mean	Control SD	Control Total	Weight	Mean Difference IV, Random, 95% CI
Craig 1998	6.7	0.7	14	8.3	1.7	13	20.6%	-1.60 [-2.59, -0.61]
Lansik 2011	8.13	0.33	21	8.22	0.26	22	26.8%	-0.09 [-0.27, 0.09]
Pohl 2005	-1.59	0.86	39	-0.08	0.53	39	26.2%	-1.51 [-1.83, -1.19]
Pohl 2009	-2.17	0.97	48	-0.67	0.2	49	26.4%	-1.50 [-1.78, -1.22]
Total (95% CI)			**122**			**123**	**100.0%**	**-1.15 [-2.07, -0.23]**

Heterogeneity: Tau² = 0.81; Chi² = 104.62, df = 3 (P < 0.00001); I² = 97%
Test for overall effect: Z = 2.44 (P = 0.01)

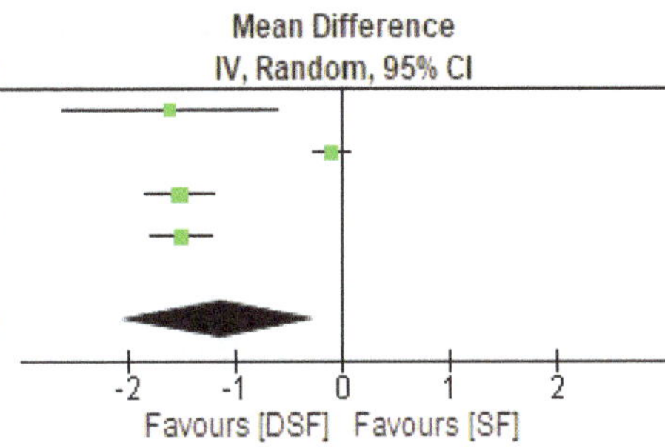

Figure 3. The effect of DSF on fasting blood glucose (mmol/L).

The glycated haemoglobin was significantly lower ($p = 0.005$) in the DSF group compared to the SF group following meta-analysis (Figure 4) and sensitivity analysis.

Study or Subgroup	Diabetes Specific Formula Mean	Diabetes Specific Formula SD	Diabetes Specific Formula Total	Standard Formula Mean	Standard Formula SD	Standard Formula Total	Weight	Mean Difference IV, Random, 95% CI
Craig 1998	6.5	0.4	14	6.9	0.14	13	29.0%	-0.40 [-0.62, -0.18]
Pohl 2005	-0.8	0.25	39	0	0.18	39	30.7%	-0.80 [-0.90, -0.70]
Pohl 2009	-1.3	0.63	48	-1.2	0.45	49	29.1%	-0.10 [-0.32, 0.12]
Vaisman 2009	6.2	1.39	12	8.7	1.44	13	11.2%	-2.50 [-3.61, -1.39]
Total (95% CI)			**113**			**114**	**100.0%**	**-0.67 [-1.14, -0.21]**

Heterogeneity: Tau² = 0.18; Chi² = 49.12, df = 3 (P < 0.00001); I² = 94%
Test for overall effect: Z = 2.83 (P = 0.005)

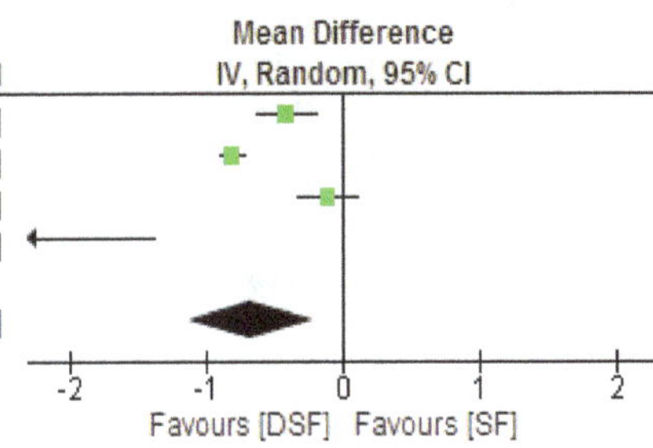

Figure 4. The effect of DSF on Glycated Haemoglobin %.

3.3. The Effect of DSF on Lipid Profile

Based on the systematic review, the outcomes of the studies selected to evaluate the effect of DSF on lipid profile were variable. Craig et al. [31] did not find significant differences with respect to LDL cholesterol and triglyceride between the DSF and the SF groups, but differences were significantly higher ($p < 0.05$) in the DSF group in relation to HDL cholesterol. In two other studies [33,35], the level of HDL cholesterol was significantly higher ($p < 0.05$) in the DSF group compared with the SF group after intervention, but differences were not significant ($p > 0.05$) in relation to triglycerides, total cholesterol and LDL cholesterols. Differences between DSF and SF were also not significant ($p > 0.05$) in terms of triglyceride, total cholesterol, HDL cholesterol and LDL cholesterol in other studies [30,32,38]. In contrast, Pohl et al. [29] reported that there was a significant difference ($p < 0.05$) between the DSF group and the SF group with respect to triglycerides, but differences were not significant ($p > 0.05$) in relation to total cholesterol, HDL and LDL cholesterol. Other studies [36,40] have also shown that DSF is effective in controlling plasma triglyceride.

Following meta-analysis, no significant differences ($p > 0.05$) were found between the DSF and SF groups with respect to total cholesterol, LDL cholesterol and triglyceride (Figures 5–7). However, the DSF group had a significantly higher level ($p = 0.04$) of HDL cholesterol compared to the SF group after the intervention, with a mean difference of 0.09 (95% CI, 0.00, 0.18) (Figure 8). The results of the sensitivity test for HDL cholesterol demonstrated no significant differences ($p > 0.05$) between the two groups when the Craig et al. [31] and Vaisman et al. [33] studies were removed from the analysis. In addition, the sensitivity analysis showed no significant differences ($p > 0.05$) between the two groups with respect to total cholesterol and triglyceride, while significant differences (<0.05) were observed in relation to LDL cholesterol when the Craig et al. [31] study was removed.

Study or Subgroup	Diabetes Specific Formula Mean	SD	Total	Standard Formula Mean	SD	Total	Weight	Mean Difference IV, Random, 95% CI
Craig 1998	3.96	0.31	14	3.96	0.23	13	30.4%	0.00 [-0.20, 0.20]
Pohl 2005	-0.37	0.39	39	-0.23	0.42	39	36.1%	-0.14 [-0.32, 0.04]
Pohl 2009	0.3	0.57	48	0.21	0.36	49	33.6%	0.09 [-0.10, 0.28]
Total (95% CI)			**101**			**101**	**100.0%**	**-0.02 [-0.16, 0.12]**

Heterogeneity: Tau² = 0.00; Chi² = 3.03, df = 2 (P = 0.22); I² = 34%
Test for overall effect: Z = 0.29 (P = 0.77)

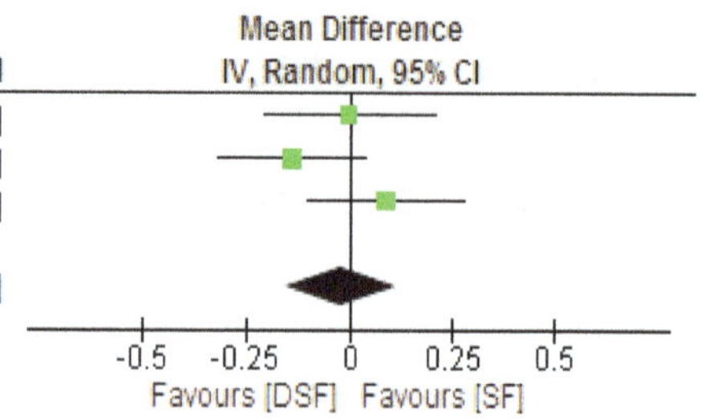

Figure 5. The effect of DSF on total cholesterol (mmol/L).

Study or Subgroup	Diabetes Specific Formula Mean	SD	Total	Standard Formula Mean	SD	Total	Weight	Mean Difference IV, Random, 95% CI
Craig 1998	2.51	0.28	14	2.53	0.21	13	33.5%	-0.02 [-0.21, 0.17]
Pohl 2005	-0.28	0.5	39	-0.52	0.38	39	33.1%	0.24 [0.04, 0.44]
Pohl 2009	0.27	0.53	48	-0.33	0.4	49	33.4%	0.60 [0.41, 0.79]
Total (95% CI)			**101**			**101**	**100.0%**	**0.27 [-0.09, 0.63]**

Heterogeneity: Tau² = 0.09; Chi² = 21.38, df = 2 (P < 0.0001); I² = 91%
Test for overall effect: Z = 1.49 (P = 0.14)

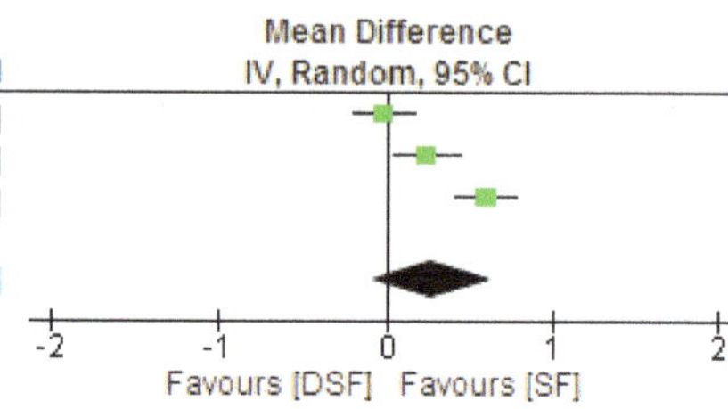

Figure 6. The effect of DSF on LDL cholesterol (mmol/L).

Study or Subgroup	Diabetes Specific Formula Mean	SD	Total	Standard Formula Mean	SD	Total	Weight	Mean Difference IV, Random, 95% CI
Craig 1998	1.03	0.19	14	1.12	0.14	13	34.2%	-0.09 [-0.22, 0.04]
Pohl 2005	-0.37	0.19	39	0.2	0.23	39	34.6%	-0.57 [-0.66, -0.48]
Pohl 2009	-0.45	0.48	48	-0.7	0.81	49	31.2%	0.25 [-0.01, 0.51]
Total (95% CI)			**101**			**101**	**100.0%**	**-0.15 [-0.59, 0.29]**

Heterogeneity: Tau² = 0.14; Chi² = 57.54, df = 2 (P < 0.00001); I² = 97%
Test for overall effect: Z = 0.67 (P = 0.50)

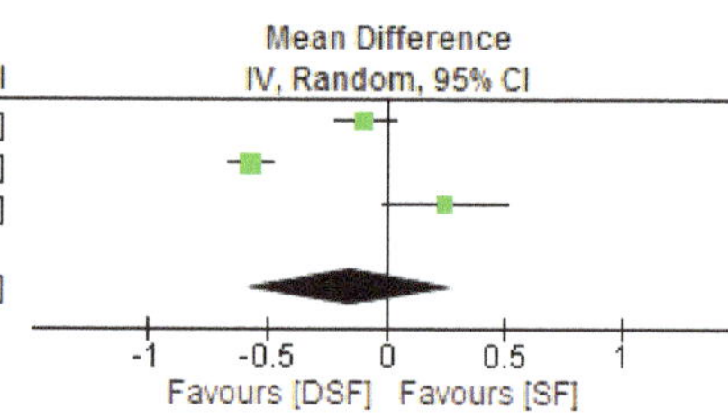

Figure 7. The effect of DSF on Triglycerides (mmol/L).

Study or Subgroup	Diabetes Specific Formula Mean	SD	Total	Standard Formula Mean	SD	Total	Weight	Mean Difference IV, Random, 95% CI
Craig 1998	0.98	0.05	14	0.83	0.05	13	33.4%	0.15 [0.11, 0.19]
Pohl 2005	0.08	0.09	39	0.05	0.11	39	32.7%	0.03 [-0.01, 0.07]
Pohl 2009	0.03	0.17	48	0	0.3	49	25.2%	0.03 [-0.07, 0.13]
Vaisman 2009	1.23	0.35	12	0.94	0.32	13	8.8%	0.29 [0.03, 0.55]
Total (95% CI)			**113**			**114**	**100.0%**	**0.09 [0.00, 0.18]**

Heterogeneity: Tau² = 0.01; Chi² = 20.14, df = 3 (P = 0.0002); I² = 85%
Test for overall effect: Z = 2.03 (P = 0.04)

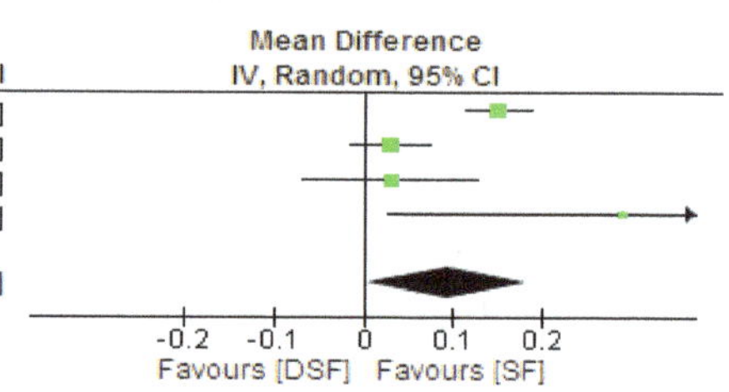

Figure 8. The effect of DSF on HDL cholesterol (mmol/L).

4. Discussion

The findings of the systematic review and meta-analysis revealed that DSF was effective in lowering blood glucose (fasting blood glucose and glycated haemoglobin) compared with SF in patients with type 2 diabetes. However, the sensitivity analysis for the fasting blood glucose did not demonstrate a significant difference ($p > 0.05$) with the removal of the Pohl et al. [29,30] studies. In addition, there were no significant differences ($p > 0.05$) between the DSF and SF groups with respect to total cholesterol, LDL cholesterol and triglyceride (although a few studies reported significant differences with respect to triglyceride). Differences in the outcomes of studies in the systematic review were observed with respect to the effect of DSF on HDL cholesterol and the meta-analysis also showed significantly higher levels for the DSF group compared with the SF group. The high level of heterogeneity in the studies included in the meta-analyses may explain why the results of the meta-analysis and the sensitivity analysis were not consistent with respect to HDL cholesterol and fasting blood glucose.

The presence of low glycaemic index (GI) carbohydrate in the form of isomaltulose, the lower amount of carbohydrate and the higher protein content in the DSF may have contributed to the findings of this review [37]. In addition, the presence of mono-unsaturated fatty acids (MUFA) and the different amounts and types of fibre in the DSF compared with SF may be responsible for the observed differences in the fasting blood glucose, glycated haemoglobin and lipid profiles in both groups [18,41]. DSFs are usually higher in fat (40–50% of energy with a significant portion of MUFA) and have a lower carbohydrate level (30–40% of energy) and about 15% of energy is derived from fructose and soluble fibre [20]. DSFs contain carbohydrates with low GI such as non-hydrolysed starches, disaccharides, fibre and fructose in varying amounts which are aimed at controlling postprandial glucose [17–20]. In contrast, SFs are high in carbohydrate (about 50%) and have low–moderate levels of lipids (about 30%) and do not contain dietetic fibre [17]. A study by Hofman et al. [42] demonstrated that, in 12 enteral formulas examined, the GI ranged from 12 for DSFs up to 61 for SFs. The GI of food is a measure of how quickly the food is digested and the glucose reaches the blood stream [22,43]. Foods with high GI rapidly increase blood glucose and insulin responses after consumption [43,44]. The results from meta-analysis showed that the intake of a low GI diet was associated with reductions in blood glucose parameters [35,43]. In addition, high soluble fibre-containing foods can improve glycaemic control partly due to delayed absorption [36].

Therefore, DSFs may improve glycaemic control through delay in gastric emptying, delayed intestinal absorption of carbohydrate and lower glycaemic response [20]. In the study by Alish et al. [34], the blend of DSF was made up of low glycaemic and slowly digestible carbohydrates, resistant maltodextrin, isomaltulose, sucromalt and prebiotic fibres, including fructo-oligosaccharides. These constituents collectively produce a slow and consistent release of glucose into the blood stream [34]. Isomaltulose is a naturally occurring low GI slowly digestible carbohydrate [18]. The slower hydrolysation of isomaltulose during digestion may be responsible for the slower rise in blood glucose in patients with diabetes on DSF [18]. In addition, the higher protein content of the DSF may have contributed to the lowering of blood glucose parameters by delaying gastric emptying [18].

The use of high fat content, including MUFA, in the DSF may slow the transit time in the gastrointestinal tract and slow the absorption of sugars which could help improve glycaemic control [35,41]. Diets that are high in MUFA have been shown to increase HDL cholesterol and reduce other components of the lipid profiles [35,41]. HDL cholesterol is useful for reducing the risk of cardiovascular disease [35]. The result of the meta-analysis of the current review confirmed the positive role of DSF in increasing HDL cholesterol. However, the sensitivity tests did not demonstrate consistency in terms of the effect of DSF on HDL cholesterol, which could explain why researchers may be reluctant to recommend the use of high fat content in DSF due to the risk of alterations in lipid profiles [41]. This may also be due to the fact that there have been differences in the outcomes of studies on the effect of DSF on lipid profile [41].

5. Limitation

The limitation of this review was that only five studies were included in the meta-analysis. In particular, there were fewer studies included for lipid outcomes (three for several parameters) and there was substantial variability in the studies. Therefore, the differences between the meta-analysis and the sensitivity analysis in some of the parameters suggest that those results were not quite consistent, which may be due to the high level of heterogeneity of the studies. Therefore, more studies are needed to address this problem.

6. Conclusions

The results provide evidence to suggest that DSF is effective in controlling fasting blood glucose and glycated haemoglobin. In addition, DSF was effective in increasing HDL cholesterol but had no significant effect on other lipid parameters. However, our confidence in these findings would be increased by additional data from further studies. Additional research would also provide the opportunity to refine our understanding of the effect of DSF on cardiometabolic parameters.

Author Contributions: Conceptualization, O.O., S.M.W., T.T., R.C., X.-H.W.; methodology, O.O., S.M.W., T.T., R.C., X.-H.W.; validation, O.O., S.M.W., T.T., R.C., X.-H.W.; formal analysis, O.O. and reviewed by S.M.W., T.T., R.C., X.-H.W.; writing—original draft preparation, O.O.; writing—review and editing, O.O., S.M.W., T.T., R.C., X.-H.W.

References

1. DeFronzo, R.A.; Ratner, R.E.; Han, J.; Kim, D.D.; Fineman, M.S.; Baron, A.D. Effects of exenatide (exendin-4) on glycemic control and weight over 30 weeks in metformin-treated patients with type 2 diabetes. *Diabetes Care* **2005**, *28*, 1092–1100. [CrossRef] [PubMed]
2. Jansink, R.; Braspenning, J.; Laurant, M.; Keizer, E.; Elwyn, G.; Weijden, T.D.; Grol, R. Minimal improvement of nurses' motivational interviewing skills in routine diabetes care one year after training: A cluster randomized trial. *BMC Fam. Pract.* **2013**, *14*, 44. [CrossRef] [PubMed]
3. National Collaborating Centre for Chronic Conditions (NCCCC). *Type 2 Diabetes: National Clinical Guideline for Management in Primary and Secondary Care (Update)*; Royal College of Physicians: London, UK, 2008.
4. Public Health England. 3.8 Million People in England Now Have Diabetes. 2016. Available online: https://www.gov.uk/government/news/38-million-people-in-england-now-have-diabetes (accessed on 1 February 2019).
5. National Health Service (NHS) Digital and Healthcare Quality Improvement Partnership. National diabetes audit, 2015–2016 Report 1: Care Processes and Treatment Targets. 2017. Available online: http://www.content.digital.nhs.uk/catalogue/PUB23241/nati-diab-rep1-audi-2015-16.pdf (accessed on 1 February 2019).
6. Diabetes UK. State of the Nation Report. 2015. Available online: https://www.diabetes.org.uk/Documents/About%20Us/What%20we%20say/State%20of%20the%20nation%202014.pdf (accessed on 1 February 2019).
7. Holman, N.; Young, B.; Gadsby, R. What is the current prevalence of diagnosed and yet to be diagnosed diabetes in the UK. *Diabetes Med.* **2014**, *31*, 510–511. [CrossRef] [PubMed]
8. Diabetes UK. Diabetes in the UK 2012: Key Statistics on Diabetes. 2012. Available online: http://tinyurl.com/owcyr7b (accessed on 1 February 2019).
9. Holmes, C.; Dyer, P. Diabetes training for nurses: The effectiveness of an inpatient diabetes half-day workshop. *J. Diabetes Nurs.* **2013**, *17*, 86–94.
10. Pereira, D.A.; da Silva Campos Costa, N.M.; Lima Sousa, A.L.; Veiga Jardim, P.B.; de Oliveira Zanini, C.R. The effect of educational intervention on the disease knowledge of diabetes mellitus patients. *Rev. Lat. Am. De Enferm.* **2012**, *20*, 478–485. [CrossRef] [PubMed]
11. Wyness, L. Understanding the role of diet in type 2 diabetes prevention. *Br. J. Commun. Nurs.* **2009**, *14*, 374–379. [CrossRef] [PubMed]
12. Ojo, O. The role of nutrition and hydration in disease prevention and patient safety. *Br. J. Nurs.* **2017**, *26*, 1020–1022. [CrossRef] [PubMed]
13. Arinzon, Z.; Shabat, S.; Shuval, I.; Peisakh, A.; Berner, Y. Prevalence of diabetes mellitus in elderly patients received enteral nutrition long-term care service. *Arch. Gerontol. Geriatr.* **2008**, *47*, 383–393. [CrossRef]
14. Wong, V.W.; Manoharan, M.; Mak, M. Managing hyperglycaemia in patients with diabetes on enteral nutrition: The role of a specialized diabetes team. *Eur. J. Clin. Nutr.* **2014**, *68*, 1305–1308. [CrossRef]
15. Oyibo, S.; Sagi, S.; Home, C. Glycaemic control during enteral tube feeding in patients with diabetes who have had a stroke: A twice-daily insulin regimen. *Pract. Diabetes* **2012**, *29*, 135–139. [CrossRef]
16. Elia, M.; Ceriello, A.; Laube, H.; Sinclair, A.J.; Engfer, M.; Stratton, R.J. Enteral nutritional support and use of diabetes specific formulas for patients with diabetes. *Diabetes Care* **2005**, *28*, 2267–2279. [CrossRef] [PubMed]
17. Sanz-Paris, A.; Álvarez Hernández, J.; Ballesteros-Pomar, M.D.; Botella-Romero, F.; León-Sanz, M.; Martín-Palmero, Á.; Olveira, G. Evidence-based recommendations and expert consensus on enteral nutrition in the adult patient with diabetes mellitus or hyperglycemia. *Nutrition* **2017**, *41*, 58–67. [CrossRef] [PubMed]
18. Ceriello, A.; Lansink, M.; Rouws, C.H.F.C.; van Laere, K.M.J.; Frost, G.S. Administration of a new diabetes specific enteral formula results in an improved 24 h glucose profile in type 2 diabetic patients. *Diabetes Res. Clin. Pract.* **2009**, *84*, 259–266. [CrossRef] [PubMed]
19. Hise, M.E.; Fuhrman, M.P. *The Effect of Diabetes Specific Enteral Formulae on Clinical and Glycaemic Indicators*; Parrish, C.R., Ed.; Nutrition Issues in Gastroenterology Series 74; Shugar Publishing: New York, NY, USA, 2009; pp. 20–36.
20. Buranapin, S.; Siangruangsang, S.; Chantapanich, V.; Hengjeerajarus, N. The comparative study of diabetic specific formula and standard formula on postprandial plasma glucose control in type 2 DM patients. *J. Med. Assoc. Thail.* **2014**, *97*, 582–588.

21. McMahon, M.M.; Nystrom, E.; Braunschweig, C.; Miles, J.; Compher, C. The American Society of Parenteral and Enteral Nutrition (ASPEN) Clinical Guidelines: Nutrition support of adult patients with hyperglycaemia. *J. Parenter. Enter. Nutr.* **2013**, *37*, 23–36. [CrossRef] [PubMed]
22. Ojo O and Brooke J Evaluation of the role of enteral nutrition in managing patients with Diabetes: A systematic review. *Nutrients* **2014**, *6*, 5142–5152. [CrossRef]
23. Jones, S.; Honnor, M.; Castro, E.; Alsmadi, A. Management of people with diabetes receiving artificial nutrition: A review. *J. Diabetes Nurs.* **2017**, *21*, 179–183.
24. Moher, D.; Liberati, A.; Tetzlaff, J.; Altman, D.G.; Prisma, G. Preferred reporting items for systematic reviews and meta-analyses: The PRISMA statement. *BMJ* **2009**, *339*, b2535. [CrossRef]
25. Methley, A.M.; Campbell, S.; Chew-Graham, C.; McNally, R.; Cheraghi-Sohi, S. PICO, PICOS and SPIDER: A comparison study of specificity and sensitivity in three search tools for qualitative systematic reviews. *BMC Health Serv. Res.* **2014**, *14*, 579. [CrossRef]
26. Critical Appraisal Skills Programme (CASP) Case Control Study Checklist. Available online: http://docs.wixstatic.com/ugd/dded87_afbfc99848f64537a53826e1f5b30b5c.pdf (accessed on 29 January 2019).
27. Higgins, J.P.T.; Green, S. *Cochrane Handbook for Systematic Reviews of Interventions*; Wiley-Blackwell: Hoboken, NJ, USA, 2009.
28. The Nordic Cochrane Centre. Review Manager (RevMan). In *Computer Program*; Version 5.3; The Nordic Cochrane Centre, The Cochrane Collaboration: Copenhagen, Denmark, 2014.
29. Pohl, M.; Mayr, P.; Mertl-Roetzer, M.; Lauster, F.; Lerch, M.; Eriksen, J.; Haslbeck, M.; Rahlfs, V.W. Glycaemic control in type II diabetic tube-fed patients with a new enteral formula low in carbohydrates and high in monounsaturated fatty acids: A randomised controlled trial. *Eur. J. Clin. Nutr.* **2005**, *59*, 1221–1232. [CrossRef]
30. Pohl, M.; Mayr, P.; Mertl-Roetzer, M.; Lauster, F.; Haslbeck, M.; Hipper, B.; Steube, D.; Tietjen, M.; Eriksen, J.; Rahlfs, V.W. Glycemic control in patients with type 2 diabetes mellitus with a disease-specific enteral formula: Stage II of a randomized, controlled multicenter trial. *J. Parenter. Enter. Nutr.* **2009**, *33*, 37–49. [CrossRef] [PubMed]
31. Craig, L.D.; Nicholson, S.; Silverstone, F.A.; Kennedy, R.D.; Coble Voss, A.; Allison, S. Use of a reduced-carbohydrate, modified-fat enteral formula for improving metabolic control and clinical outcomes in long-term care residents with type 2 diabetes: Results of a pilot trial. *Nutrition* **1998**, *14*, 529–534. [CrossRef]
32. Lansink, M.; van Laere, K.M.; Vendrig, L.; Rutten, G.E. Lower postprandial glucose responses at baseline and after 4 weeks use of a diabetes-specific formula in diabetes type 2 patients. *Diabetes Res. Clin. Pract.* **2011**, *93*, 421–429. [CrossRef] [PubMed]
33. Vaisman, N.; Lansink, M.; Rouws, C.H.; van Laere, K.M.; Segal, R.; Niv, E.; Bowling, T.E.; Waitzberg, D.L.; Morleyf, J.E. Tube feeding with a diabetes-specific feed for 12 weeks improves glycaemic control in type 2 diabetes patients. *Clin. Nutr.* **2009**, *28*, 549–555. [CrossRef] [PubMed]
34. Alish, C.J.; Garvey, W.T.; Maki, K.C.; Sacks, G.S.; Hustead, D.S.; Hegazi, R.A.; Mustad, V.A. A diabetes-specific enteral formula improves glycemic variability in patients with type 2 diabetes. *Diabetes Technol. Ther.* **2010**, *12*, 419–425. [CrossRef] [PubMed]
35. Gulati, S.; Misra, A.; Nanda, K.; Pandey, R.M.; Garg, V.; Ganguly, S.; Cheung, L. Efficacy and tolerance of a diabetes specific formula in patients with type 2 diabetes mellitus: An open label, randomized, crossover study. *Diabetes Metab. Syndr. Clin. Res. Rev.* **2015**, *9*, 252–257. [CrossRef] [PubMed]
36. Hofman, Z.; Lansink, M.; Rouws, C.; van Drunen, J.D.E.; Kuipers, H. Diabetes specific tube feed results in improved glycaemic and triglyceridaemic control during 6 h continuous feeding in diabetes patients. *e-SPEN* **2007**, *2*, 44–50. [CrossRef]
37. Lansink, M.; Hofman, Z.; Genovese, S.; Rouws, C.H.F.C.; Ceriello, A. Improved Glucose Profile in Patients with Type 2 Diabetes with a New, High-Protein, Diabetes-Specific Tube Feed During 4 Hours of Continuous Feeding. *JPEN J. Parenter. Enter. Nutr.* **2017**, *41*, 968–975. [CrossRef]
38. Mesejo, A.; Montejo-Gonzalez, J.C.; Vaquerizo-Alonso, C.; Lobo-Tamer, G.; Zabarte-Martinez, M.; Herrero-Meseguer, J.I.; Escirbano, J.A.; Malpica, A.B.; Lozano, F.M. Diabetes-specific enteral nutrition formula in hyperglycemic, mechanically ventilated, critically ill patients: A prospective, open-label, blind-randomized, multicenter study. *Crit. Care* **2015**, *19*, 390. [CrossRef]

39. Voss, A.C.; Maki, K.C.; Garvey, W.T.; Hustead, D.S.; Alish, C.; Fix, B.; Mustad, V.A. Effect of two carbohydrate-modified tube-feeding formulas on metabolic responses in patients with type 2 diabetes. *Nutrition* **2008**, *24*, 990–997. [CrossRef]
40. Vanschoonbeek, K.; Lansink, M.; van Laere, K.M.; Senden, J.M.; Verdijk, L.B.; van Loon, L.J. Slowly digestible carbohydrate sources can be used to attenuate the postprandial glycemic response to the ingestion of diabetes-specific enteral formulas. *Diabetes Educ.* **2009**, *35*, 631–640. [CrossRef] [PubMed]
41. Vahabzadeh, D.; Valizadeh Hasanloei, M.A.; Vahdat Shariatpanahi, Z. Effect of high-fat, low-carbohydrate enteral formula versus standard enteral formula in hyperglycemic critically ill patients: A randomized clinical trial. *Int. J. Diabetes Dev. Ctries* **2019**, *39*, 173–180. [CrossRef]
42. Hofman, Z.; van Drunen, J.D.E.; de Later, C.; Kuipers, H. The Glycaemic index of standard and diabetes specific enteral formulas. *Asia Pac. J. Clin. Nutr.* **2006**, *15*, 412–417. [PubMed]
43. Ojo, O.; Ojo, O.O.; Adebowale, F.; Wang, X.H. The Effect of Dietary Glycaemic Index on Glycaemia in Patients with Type 2 Diabetes: A Systematic Review and Meta-Analysis of Randomized Controlled Trials. *Nutrients* **2018**, *10*, 373. [CrossRef] [PubMed]
44. Chang, K.T.; Lampe, J.W.; Schwarz, Y.; Breymeyer, K.L.; Noar, K.A.; Song, X.; Neuhouser, M.L. Low Glycemic Load Experimental Diet More Satiating Than High Glycemic Load Diet. *Nutr. Cancer* **2012**, *64*, 666–673. [CrossRef] [PubMed]

9

Maternal Low-Protein Diet Modulates Glucose Metabolism and Hepatic MicroRNAs Expression in the Early Life of Offspring

Jia Zheng, Xinhua Xiao *, Qian Zhang, Tong Wang, Miao Yu and Jianping Xu

Department of Endocrinology, Key Laboratory of Endocrinology, Ministry of Health, Peking Union Medical College Hospital, Diabetes Research Center of Chinese Academy of Medical Sciences & Peking Union Medical College, Beijing 100730, China; zhengjiapumc@163.com (J.Z.); rubiacordifolia@yahoo.com (Q.Z.); tongtong0716@sina.com (T.W.); yumiao@mendmail.com.cn (M.Y.); jpxuxh@163.com (J.X.)

* Correspondence: xiaoxinhua@medmail.com.cn

† Parts of this study were presented in abstract form at the American Diabetes Association's 76th Scientific Sessions, 10–14 June 2016 in New Orleans, Louisiana.

Abstract: Emerging studies revealed that maternal protein restriction was associated with increased risk of type 2 diabetes mellitus in adulthood. However, the mechanisms of its effects on offspring, especially during early life of offspring, are poorly understood. Here, it is hypothesized that impaired metabolic health in offspring from maternal low-protein diet (LPD) is associated with perturbed miRNAs expression in offspring as early as the weaning age. We examined the metabolic effects on the C57BL/6J mice male offspring at weaning from dams fed with LPD or normal chow diet (NCD) throughout pregnancy and lactation. Maternal LPD feeding impaired metabolic health in offspring. Microarray profiling indicated that mmu-miR-615, mmu-miR-124, mmu-miR-376b, and mmu-let-7e were significantly downregulated, while, mmu-miR-708 and mmu-miR-879 were upregulated in LPD offspring. Bioinformatic analysis showed target genes were mapped to inflammatory-related pathways. Serum tumor necrosis factor-α (TNF-α) levels were higher and interleukin 6 (IL-6) had a tendency to be elevated in the LPD group. Finally, both mRNA and protein levels of IL-6 and TNF-α were significantly increased in the LPD group. Our findings provide novel evidence that maternal LPD can regulate miRNAs expression, which may be associated with chronic inflammation status and metabolic health in offspring as early as the weaning age.

Keywords: maternal low-protein diet; metabolic health; microRNAs; inflammation; early life; offspring

---

1. Introduction

The prevalence of type 2 diabetes mellitus (T2DM) is increasing significantly throughout the world. However, the pathogenesis of diabetes has not been clearly demonstrated. Traditionally, it is generally believed that genes and adult lifestyle are critical factors of some metabolic diseases. Recently, several epidemiological studies of human populations highlighted that maternal nutrition, including over-nutrition and under-nutrition, may strongly influence the risks of developing metabolic diseases in adult life [1–3]. The mechanism underlying the increased susceptibility of T2DM in offspring of maternal malnutrition is poorly determined.

Recently, it seems as though epigenetic modifications may be one of the major mechanisms explaining the association between early life malnutrition and late-onset diseases, such as obesity, insulin resistance, impaired glucose tolerance, and T2DM [4–7]. MicroRNAs (miRNAs) have emerged as important epigenetic modifications in recent years. They are a major class of small non-coding RNAs with about 20–22 nucleotides, which can mediate posttranscriptional regulation of gene expressions.

miRNAs can specifically bind to the 3′-untranslated regions (3′-UTR) of target genes, resulting in translation inhibition [8]. Numerous studies show that miRNAs play critical roles in the pathogenesis of diabetes, such as glucose uptake, transport, and insulin secretion [9].

Human studies have revealed that poor intrauterine environment elicited by maternal dietary insufficiency or imbalance increased the risk for intrauterine growth restriction (IUGR) and led to metabolic diseases in the offspring during adulthood, such as insulin resistance, impaired glucose tolerance, and T2DM [3,10]. The maternal protein restriction model, with 5%–9% protein, as compared to 20% protein in normal diet, has been one of the most extensively studied models [11]. However, these studies were confined to long-term influences in offspring of a maternal low-protein diet (LPD) with varying durations range from 1 to 18 months (adulthood to aging) [12–14], yet the metabolic health in the early life of offspring, such as at weaning, has not been well documented. Furthermore, little information is known about the role of miRNAs between maternal low-protein diet (LPD) and glucose metabolism in the early life of offspring, such as at weaning. It is noted that computational predictions of miRNA targets based on several databases exhibits that one single miRNA can affect a gamut of different genes, ranging from several to hundreds, suggesting that a large proportion of the transcriptome is subjected to miRNA modulation [15]. Thus, using a trans-generational mouse model of maternal protein restriction and microarray platform, we address the hypothesis that impaired metabolic health in offspring from LPD-fed dams is associated with perturbation of the programmed expression of key miRNAs in offspring as early as at weaning age.

2. Materials and Methods

2.1. Animals and Diets

The seven-week-old C57BL/6J female and male mice were purchased from the Institute of Laboratory Animal Science, Chinese Academy of Medical Sciences and Peking Union Medical College (Beijing, China). All of the mice were maintained under controlled conditions with room temperature at 22 ± 2 °C and 12-h light/dark cycle. The mice were fed a normal chow diet (NCD) (D02041001, Research Diets, New Brunswick, NJ, USA) for one week for acclimatization. Then, mating was performed by housing males with females together (male:female = 1:2) until a vaginal plug was detected, which was considered day 0.5 of pregnancy. Pregnant females were single-housed and were randomly assigned to either isocaloric LPD (9.6% protein, 80.2% carbohydrate, and 10.2% fat as kcal%, D02041002, Research Diets, New Brunswick, NJ, USA) or NCD (23.5% protein, 66.3% carbohydrate, and 10.2% fat as kcal%, D02041001, Research Diets, New Brunswick, NJ, USA) during pregnancy and lactation. Thus, offspring were divided into two groups according to maternal diets as the LPD group and the NCD group. At day 1 after birth, all of the litters were adjusted to six pups each to ensure no litter was nutritionally biased. Birth weight was measured by calculating the average of one litter. All offspring were weaned at 21 days postnatal. At weaning, only one male offspring was randomly selected from one litter and was sacrificed in each group (one mouse per litter, $n = 6$ to 8 per group). The female offspring were not examined in our present study in order to prevent confounding factors related to their hormone profile and estrus cycle. Blood samples were taken from the intraorbital retrobulbar plexus after 12-h of fasting in anesthetized mice, and the liver samples were quickly removed, snap frozen in liquid nitrogen, and stored at −80 °C for further analysis. Body weight in offspring and food intake of dams were monitored weekly. All of the animal experiments were conducted in accordance with the Guide of the Care and Use of Laboratory Animals (NIH Publication No. 86-23, revised 1996) and were approved by the Animal Care and Use Committee of the Peking Union Medical College Hospital (Beijing, China, MC-07-6004).

2.2. Glucose Tolerance Tests

The tolerance test was performed as described previously [16]. Mice were overnight-fasted (12–16 h) and fasted blood glucose was measured in tail vein blood samples. Mice were injected intraperitoneally with glucose (2 g/kg body weight), and blood glucose was measured at 30 min, 60 min, and 120 min following injection using a glucometer (Bayer, Beijing, China). Blood glucose response to glucose tolerance tests was calculated as the area under the glucose curve for each mouse according to the trapezoidal method, as previously described [17].

2.3. Measurement of Serum Insulin and Inflammatory Factors

Serum insulin levels were measured using the mouse ultrasensitive insulin enzyme-linked immunosorbent assay (ELISA) kit (80-INSMSU-E01, ALPCO Diagnostics, Salem, NH, USA). Serum interleukin 6 (IL-6) and tumor necrosis factor-α (TNF-α) concentrations were measured by mouse ELISA kits (ab100712 and ab108910, Abcam, MA, USA), respectively.

2.4. Microarray Profiling of MiRNAs in Offspring

Because of financial constraints, we could not perform a whole genome array for each mouse in the LPD and NCD groups. Thus, in order to obtain a relatively reliable estimate of the mean gene expression, each group contained three biological replicates, which were randomly selected from each group. We performed the microarray with pooled RNA samples, a method that has been shown to be appropriate and statistically valid for efficient microarray experiments, according to previous studies [18,19]. As our study previously described [20], total RNA was extracted from the liver tissues in LPD and NCD offspring using Trizol reagent (Life Technologies Inc., Carlsbad, CA, USA), according to the manufacturer's instructions. MiRNAs expressions in livers were detected by GeneChip microRNA 3.0 Array (Affymetrix, Inc., Santa, CA, USA), which provides for 100% miRBase v17 coverage [21,22].

2.5. Differential MiRNAs Expression Analysis in Offspring

Robust Multi-array Analysis (RMA) was utilized to convert raw data into recognizable miRNA expression data. Then it was followed by median normalization and $\log_2$ transformation using Affy package [23]. Differentially-expressed miRNAs between the LPD and NCD groups were analyzed by the Limma package of R language [23], which is based on the combined two criteria for true positive differences: (1) $|\text{FC (fold change)}| \geq 2$ and (2) p value < 0.05 [21], which is a relatively robust cutoff point.

2.6. Bioinformatics Analysis of Predicted Targets for MiRNAs in Offspring

All of the microarray data were also pooled for further analysis. According to our previously published work [24], target genes of differentially expressed miRNAs between the two groups were identified using the miRWalk database [25], which can provide validated target genes information on miRNAs for mouse [26]. To further reveal the potential biological functions and pathways of the target genes, the target genes were analyzed with the Kyoto Encyclopedia of Genes and Genomes (KEGG) pathways [27] using Database for Annotation, Visualization and Integrated Discovery (DAVID) [28]. p value < 0.05 was the criterion for significant KEGG pathway terms.

2.7. Validation of Differentially Expressed MiRNAs in Offspring

In order to validate the expressions of differential miRNAs, quantitative real-time PCR (qRT-PCR) were utilized to detect the relative expression of differentially-expressed miRNAs, with samples enlarged in each group (n = 6 to 8 per group) using the TaqMan detection system (Life Technologies, Foster City, CA, USA). All of the mice in each group were included for the validation. Total RNA was reversely transcribed using the TaqMan MicroRNA Reverse Transcription kit (Applied Biosystems, Life Technologies, Foster City, CA, USA). All of the miRNA-specific reverse-transcription primers were provided with the TaqMan MicroRNA Assay and purchased from Life Technologies Corporation (Applied Biosystems, Life Technologies, Foster City, CA, USA). The primers were mmu-miR-615

(ID 2353), mmu-miR-124 (ID 2197), mmu-miR-376b (ID 2452), mmu-let-7e (ID 2407), mmu-miR-708 (ID 1643), and mmu-miR-879 (ID 2473). U6 small nuclear RNA (ID 1973) was used as an endogenous control. Gene expression was quantified by qRT-PCR and performed on an ABI prism Vii7 Sequence Detection System platform (ABI Prism® Vii7, Applied Biosystems, Life Technologies, Foster City, CA, USA). Data were analyzed and the fold change was calculated using the comparative Ct method. All reactions were carried out with three biological replicates, and each analysis consisted of three technical replicates.

2.8. Target Gene Expression by Quantitative Real-Time PCR

For the validation of miRNA target genes, mRNA expressions of target genes were performed using SYBR Green. Prior to PCR, total RNA of each sample was processed with Rnase-free Dnase (Qiagen, New York, NY, USA). The RNA was reverse transcribed by 1 μg of total RNA from each sample using the Power cDNA Synthesis kit (A3500, Promega BioSciences LLC, Sunnyvale, CA, USA). We used Oligo 7.0 software (Molecular Biology Insights, Inc., Cascade, CO, USA) to design the sequences of the primers for IL-6, TNF-α, and housekeeping gene β-actin. The sequences of the primers are as following: IL-6, forward 5′-CCAAGAGGTGAGTGCTTCCC-3′, reverse 5′-CTGTTGTTCAGACTCTCTCCCT-3′; TNF-α, forward 5′-CCCACGTCGTAGCAAACCA-3′, reverse 5′-ACAAGGTACAACCCATCGGC-3′; MAPK1, forward 5′-AATTGGTCAGGACAAGGGCT-3′, reverse 5′-GAGTGGGTAAGCTGAGACGG-3′; β-actin, forward 5′-TGTTACCAACTGGGACGACA-3′ reverse 5′-GGGGTGTTGAAGGTCTCAAA-3′. The reaction production was accurately measured by the ABI prism Vii7 Sequence Detection System (ABI Prism® Vii7, Applied Biosystems, Life Technologies, Foster City, CA, USA). Data were analyzed and quantified using the comparative Ct method, as described in the preceding section.

2.9. Immunohistochemical Staining

The liver tissues from offspring mice were rapidly dissected. Then, they were fixed overnight in a freshly-prepared 10% buffered formaldehyde solution. The tissue samples were ethanol-dehydrated and embedded in paraffin wax. Serial 5 μm paraffin embedded tissue sections were mounted on slides. Then, the slides were stained with the primary antibodies overnight at 4 °C, which were IL-6 (1:300; ab83339, Abcam, Cambridge, MA, USA) and TNF-α (1:50, ab6671, Abcam, Cambridge, MA, USA), while negative controls were incubated with phosphate-buffered saline (PBS). The slices were then washed and incubated for 1 h at 37 °C with secondary antibodies (1:1000, Cell Signaling, Danvers, MA, USA). Then, the slides were stained with 3, 3′-diaminobenzidine (DAB) and hematoxylin. Brownish yellow granular or linear deposits were identified as positive. Image-Pro Plus 5.0 (Media Cybernetics, Silver Spring, MD, USA) was used for semi-quantitative analysis.

2.10. Statistical Analysis

Results are expressed as the mean ± SEM. Statistical analyses were performed with Student's *t*-tests of unpaired samples. The comparisons of glucose tolerance tests were analyzed with a two-way ANOVA. Fisher's exact test was used for KEGG pathway analysis. A p value < 0.05 was considered statistically significant. Prism version 6.0 (GraphPad Software Inc., San Diego, CA, USA) was used for statistical analysis.

3. Results

3.1. Effects of Diets on Body Weight and Glucose Tolerance in Dams

By the end of lactation, there was no significant difference in maternal body weight between the dams (noted as F0) fed with LPD and NCD (Figure 1a). Glucose tolerance testing showed that blood glucose was indistinguishable between the two groups, as well as with the area under the curve (AUC) (Figure 2b,c). There was no significant difference in food intake between dams fed with LPD and NCD.

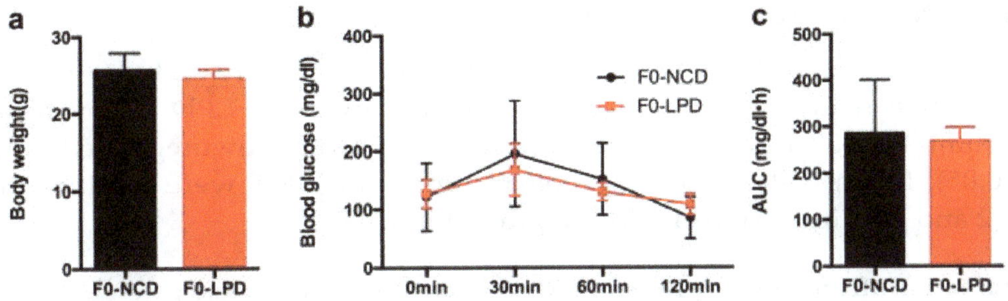

Figure 1. Effects of diets during pregnancy and lactation on metabolic phenotype in dams. (**a**) Body weight; (**b**) intraperitoneal glucose tolerance tests; and (**c**) area under the curve (AUC) of glucose tolerance tests. Data represented as the mean ± SEM (n = 6 to 8, per group). Dams were noted as F0; LPD, low-protein diet; NCD, normal chow diet.

3.2. Effects of Maternal Diet on Metabolic Profile in Offspring at Weaning

At birth, newborns whose mother was fed with LPD during pregnancy and lactation showed lower body weight compared to offspring of control diet mothers ($p < 0.05$, Figure 2a). No significant difference was found in litter size between LPD and NCD groups (Figure 2b). At weaning, the male offspring of LPD-fed dams exhibited significantly lower body weight, compared with the offspring of dams fed a control diet ($p < 0.05$, Figure 2c). There was no difference of fasted blood glucose in the LPD and NCD male offspring at weaning. However, the blood glucose of the male offspring in LPD group was higher at 30 min ($p < 0.05$) after intraperitoneal glucose administration (Figure 2d). Consistently, the area under the curve (AUC) of the glucose tolerance test was greater in LPD offspring ($p < 0.05$, Figure 2e). We further examined insulin concentration of the male offspring. As consistent with previous studies [15,29], LPD offspring showed lower fasted insulinemia at weaning, compared to control offspring (Figure 2f), which may be caused by aberrant insulin secretion due to intrauterine growth restriction.

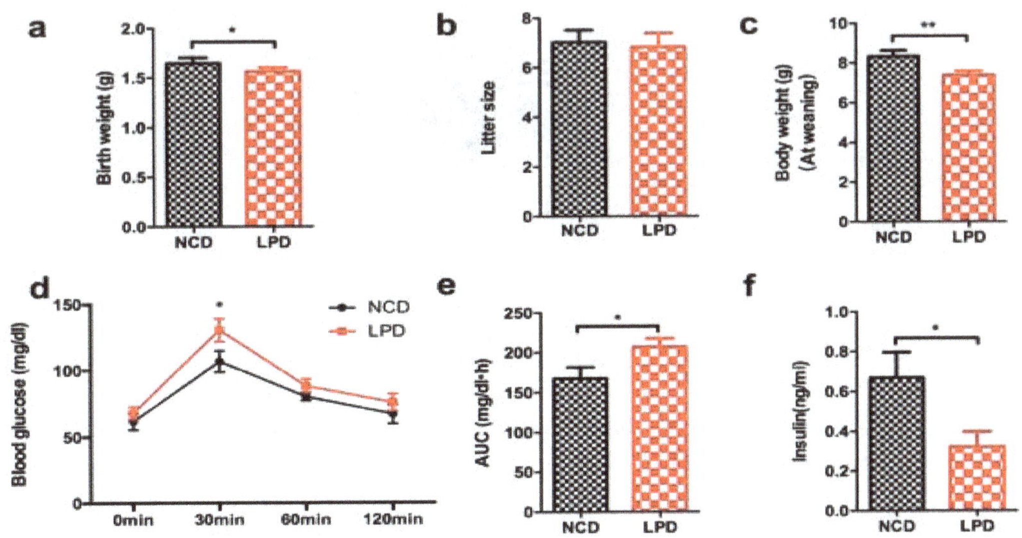

Figure 2. Metabolic profile and serum insulin concentration in offspring at weaning. (**a**) Birth weight; (**b**) litter size; (**c**) body weight at weaning; (**d**) intraperitoneal glucose tolerance test; (**e**) area under curve (AUC) of glucose tolerance test; and (**f**) serum insulin level. Data represented as the mean ± SEM (n = 6 to 8, per group). * $p < 0.05$, ** $p < 0.01$ vs. the NCD group. LPD, low-protein diet; NCD, normal chow diet.

3.3. Differential MiRNAs Expression in Offspring

Six miRNAs were shown to be significantly differentially expressed (|fold change| ≥ 2 and p value < 0.05) between LPD and NCD groups. In the livers of LPD offspring, mmu-miR-615, mmu-miR-124, mmu-miR-376b, and mmu-let-7e were significantly downregulated (fold change ≤ -2 and p value < 0.05). Meanwhile, mmu-miR-708 and mmu-miR-879 were significantly upregulated (fold change ≥ 2 and p value < 0.05) (Table 1, Figure 3).

Table 1. Differentially-expressed miRNA (|fold change| ≥ 2 and p-value < 0.05).

Probe Set ID	Fold Change	*p* Value	Sequence Length	Sequence
mmu-miR-615	−7.61	0.004	22	GGGGGUCCCCGGUGCUCGGAUC
mmu-miR-124	−4.37	0.014	22	CGUGUUCACAGCGGACCUUGAU
mmu-miR-376b	−3.81	0.016	21	AUCAUAGAGGAACAUCCACUU
mmu-let-7e	−2.60	0.000	22	CUAUACGGCCUCCUAGCUUUCC
mmu-miR-708	3.89	0.007	23	AAGGAGCUUACAAUCUAGCUGGG
mmu-miR-879	10.05	0.034	22	GCUUAUGGCUUCAAGCUUUCGG

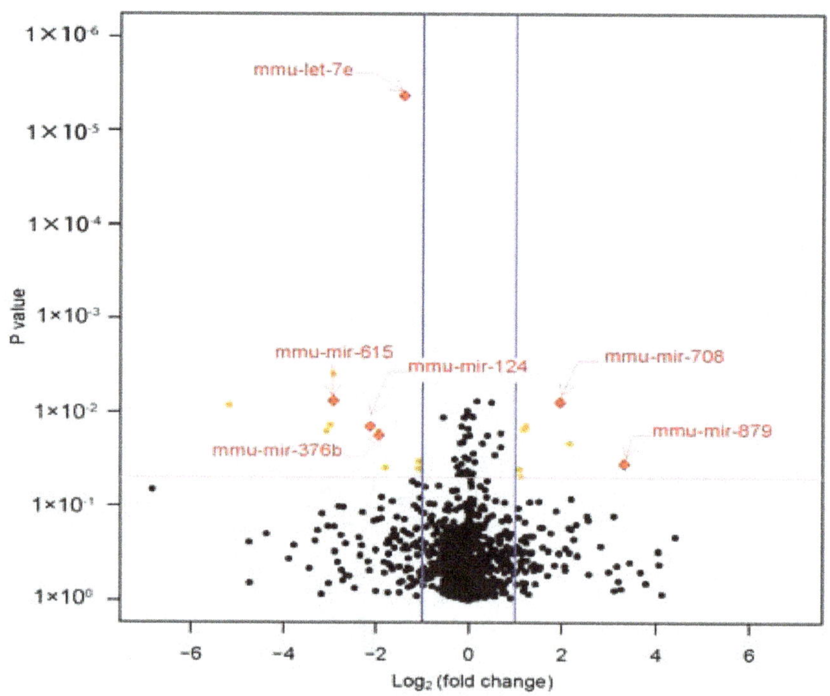

Figure 3. The volcano plot of the miRNA array. This graph shows $\log_2$ (fold change) in the expression miRNAs and p value from the t-test between LPD and NCD offspring. The vertical blue line indicates that the threshold of |$\log_2$ (fold change)| is 1. The horizontal red line indicates that the p value threshold is 0.05. It showed six miRNAs were significantly differentially expressed (|fold change| ≥ 2 and p value < 0.05) between LPD and NCD offspring. LPD, Low-protein diet; NCD, normal chow diet.

3.4. Validation of Differentially Expressed MiRNAs

To verify the results of microRNA array, all the six differentially-expressed miRNAs were validated by increasing the quantity of samples in LPD and NCD groups using qRT-PCR (n = 6 to 8, per group). It showed that the expression levels of all the six miRNA were consistent with the results of microRNA array analysis, which were analyzed and quantified by qRT-PCR (Figure 4).

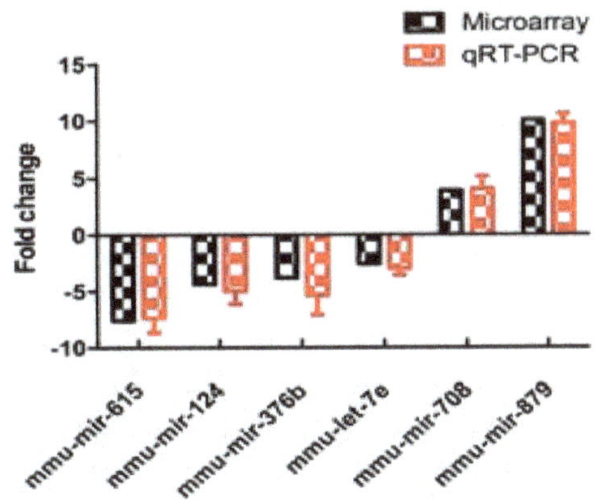

Figure 4. Differentially-expressed miRNAs were detected by miRNA array and validated by qRT-PCR. Data represented as the mean ± SEM (n = 6 to 8, per group). The fold change was calculated using the comparative Ct method. qRT-PCR: quantitative real time-PCR.

3.5. Functional Enrichment Analysis for Target Genes by Bioinformatics Analysis

Furthermore, target genes of these six differentially-expressed miRNAs were identified by the miRWalk database. The six miRNAs, including mmu-miR-615, mmu-miR-124, mmu-miR-376b, mmu-let-7e, mmu-miR-708, and mmu-miR-879 had a total of 349 validated target genes in the miRWalk database (Table 2). By utilizing the Database for Annotation, Visualization and Integrated Discovery (DAVID) and Kyoto Encyclopedia of Genes and Genomes (KEGG) databases, the functional enrichment analysis of these 349 validated genes were mapped in the MAPK signaling pathway, TGF-beta signaling pathway, Jak-STAT signaling pathway, cytokine-cytokine receptor interaction, chemokine signaling pathway, adipocytokine signaling pathway, and Toll-like receptor signaling pathway (Table 3), which are all associated with inflammation responses.

Table 2. Validated targeted genes for differentially-expressed miRNAs.

MiRNA	Count	Target Genes
mmu-miR-615	6	*Msx2, Hoxa7, Mbp, Lin28, Cdkn2a, Igf2*
mmu-miR-124	87	*Dll1, Sox9, Camk2g, Zic2, Fabp7, Hod, Pou5f1, Dicer1, Fgf8, Fgf10, H1foo, Bmp4, Lin28, Tcfap2b, Calb2, Btg2, Dcx, Pax6, Ifitm3, Dppa3, Mapk14, Evi1, Nr4a2, Mtpn, Nefm, Eomes, Cpeb1, Ctdspl, Mstn, Gata1, Stmn2, Rest, Trpm3, Mbp, Hprt1, Th, Oog4, Des, Uchl1, Foxp2, Rho, Eif2c3, Efnb1, Dnmt3b, Dbh ,H2afx, Npy, Med13, Prkca, Eif2c2, Fgf21, Phox2a, Mos, Gbx2, Emx1, Myh6, Mt1, Eif2c1, L1cam, Phox2b, Ctdsp1, Lmx1b, Tbr1, Nppa, Ccne1, Ccnb2, Eif2c4, Casp3, Tcfap2a, Sycp1, Gja1, Zp3, Rfpl4, Cdh1, Vax2, Slc6a3, Dlk1, Ntrk2, Pou3f3, Myh7, Sycp3, H2afz, Stat3, Wnt1, Foxa2, Ntrk3, Gja5*
mmu-miR-376b	28	*Hprt1, Oog4, Dnmt3b, H2afx, Fgf21, Mos, Dlk1, Mt1, Mbp, Ccne1, Ccnb2, Lin28, Zp3, Rfpl4, Gpr172b, Sycp3, H2afz, Timp4, Camk2g, Dicer1, Atg4c, Pou5f1, H1foo, Frap1, Ifitm3, Dppa3, Cpeb1, Ctdspl*
mmu-let-7e	217	*Lin28, Casp3, Ptch1, Zfp106, Mov10, Fgf16, E2f6, Fgf21, Ptges, Akt1, Scpep1, Rad52, Mgst1, Cdc34, Git1, Ebp, Mos, Kras, Il6, Capn10, Col1a1, Smad4, Hace1, Igfbp3, Fas, Hmga2, Fgfr1, Sox2, Irf4, Mt1, Kcnj16, Socs1, Mmp9, Prl, Nr2e1, Sp1, Il10, Trim71, Notch1, Nrip1, Lamc1, Acvr2a, Smox, Igf2, Cdkn1a, Egr1, Ccne1, Tagln, Akt1, Ccnb2, Vsnl1, Spp1, Egfr, Syne1, Mdk, Hnf4a, Msi1, Dnmt3a, Cd4, Sparcl1, Hspd1, Tppp3, Vim, Smad3, Tnf, Cyp2b10, Gtf2h4, Zp3, Hyou1, E2f2, Csf1r, Rfpl4, Akap6, Stat3, Golph3, Snai1, Arc, Scamp2, bp1, Mov10, Nanog, Clock, Acvr1, Wnt1, Bcl2l1, BC060632, Cdkn2a, Trp53, Fn1, Sycp3, Tpm1, Scpep1, Lpar1, H2afz, Gmfb, Pten, Arc, Snai1, Dync1i1, Mapre1, Dcn, Bcl2, Scpep1, Hras1, Igf1, E2f6, Grb2, Camk2g, Ogt, Pgc, Ctcf, Dicer1, Mapk1, Scpep1, Cxcr4, Rcan1, Clu, Dut, Piwil2, Ifng, Mtpn, Dclk1, Igfbp3, , Igf1r, Akt1, Kdr, Nanog, Hras1, Neurod1, Dppa3, H1foo, Bmpr2, Ebp, Hmox1, Gpd1, Cyp2b10, Socs3, Inha, Eif2c2, Epb4.1l3, Serpina1c, Ssr3, E2f2, Dicer1, Mstn, Pten, Ifitm3, Dhcr24, Racgap1, Dppa3, Gad1, Ccr4, Ddit3, Nr4a1, Hmga1, Ppargc1a, Bcl2, Nr6a1, Gadd45a, Scpep1, Ptp4a2, Nanog, Runx2, Zeb1, Bak1, Ghr, Birc2, Sall4, Cpeb1, Capn8, Il23r, Ctdspl, Ptges3, Ephb2, Rpe, Syt4, Trim32, Foxp1, Scpep1, Mmp14, Bcl2, Gnb1, Madd, Pgc, Gnrh1, Hmox1, Myc, Mycn, Socs1, Jarid1b, Hprt1, Cyp2b10, Oog4, Pdzd7, Cdkn1a, Cebpb, Aqp4, Rdx, Mbp, Hand1, Bcl2, Lancl1, Mapk3, Casp9, Fmr1, Klf15, Dnmt3b, Adora1, Stx1a, Kitl, Cd34, H2afx, Itgb1, Smad5, Pou5f1*
mmu-miR-708	9	*Foxo3, Cd34, Mbp, Lin28, Stat5a, Cd34, E2f6, Aqp1, Bmi1*
mmu-miR-879	2	*Mbp, Lin28*

Table 3. Validated target genes enriched by the Kyoto Encyclopedia of Genes and Genomes (KEGG) pathway.

KEGG ID	Term	Count	%	p Value	Genes
mmu04010	MAPK signaling pathway	24	9.7	2.8×10^{-8}	*Egfr, Prkca, Trp53, Fgfr1, Fgf8,* ***Tnf****, Grb2, Fgf16, Fgf10, Nr4a1, Fgf21, Ddit3, Hras1, Akt1, Mapk1, Casp3, Kras, Mapk14, Ntrk2, Mapk3, Mos, Fas, Myc, Gadd45a*
mmu04350	TGF-beta signaling pathway	14	5.7	7.3×10^{-8}	*Bmp4,* ***Tnf****, Smad5, Bmpr2, Smad4, Smad3, Dcn, Mapk1, Acvr2a, Sp1, Ifng, Mapk3, Myc, Acvr1*
mmu04630	Jak-STAT signaling pathway	14	5.7	4.4×10^{-5}	***Il6****, Il23r, Socs3, Grb2, Stat5a, Socs1, Bcl2l1, Stat3, Il10, Akt1, Ifng, Myc, Prl, Ghr*
mmu04060	Cytokine-cytokine receptor interaction	17	6.9	1.4×10^{-4}	*Egfr,* ***Il6****,* ***Tnf****, Il23r, Bmpr2, Kitl, Il10, Kdr, Acvr2a, Ccr4, Cxcr4, Ifng, Fas, Prl, Acvr1, Ghr, Csf1r*
mmu04062	Chemokine signaling pathway	11	4.5	9.3×10^{-3}	*Akt1, Mapk1, Kras, Ccr4, Gnb1, Cxcr4, Grb2, Mapk3, Foxo3, Stat3, Hras1*
mmu04920	Adipocytokine signaling pathway	6	2.4	1.9×10^{-2}	*Akt1,* ***Tnf****, Npy, Socs3, Ppargc1a, Stat3*
mmu04620	Toll-like receptor signaling pathway	7	2.8	2.7×10^{-2}	*Akt1, Mapk1,* ***Il6****,* ***Tnf****, Mapk14, Mapk3, Spp1*

MAPK: mitogen-activated protein kinase; TGF: transforming growth factor; Jak-STAT: janus kinase-signal transducer and activator of transcription. *Il-6* and *Tnf* were marked as bold.

3.6. Effects of Maternal Diet on Serum Pro-Inflammatory Cytokines in Offspring

Our functional enrichment analysis indicated that target genes of our six differentially-expressed miRNAs were mapped in inflammatory pathways (Tables 2 and 3). *IL-6* and *Tnf* were two important target genes, which were located in several pathways (marked as bold in Table 3). Therefore, we first measured two important pro-inflammatory cytokines (serum IL-6 and TNF-α) in male offspring of dams fed with LPD and NCD, to determine whether maternal diets modulated the levels of inflammatory markers in the early life of offspring. It showed there was a tendency to be higher of serum IL-6 level in LPD male offspring ($p = 0.07$) (Figure 5a), and it also showed the level of serum TNF-α was significantly elevated in LPD male offspring at weaning ($p < 0.05$) (Figure 5b). However, no difference of MAPK1 expression was observed in offspring (data not shown).

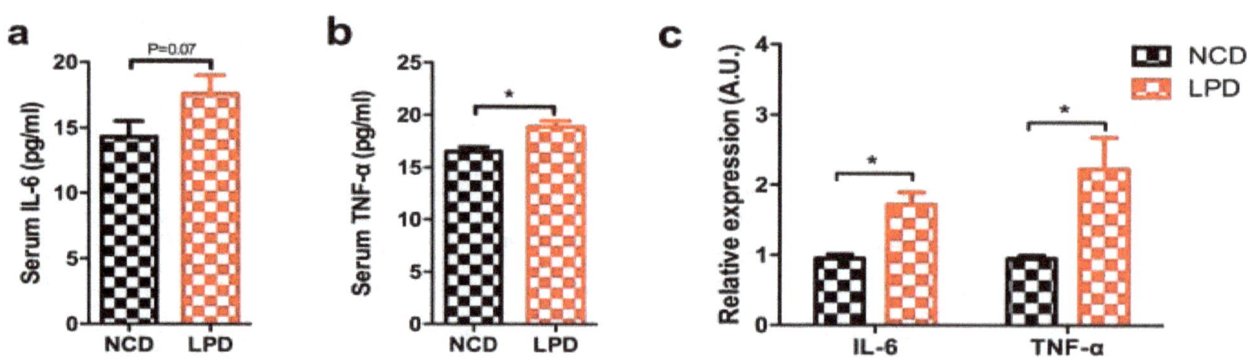

Figure 5. Effect of maternal LPD on serum IL-6 and TNF-α concentrations and mRNA expression in the offspring at weaning. (**a**) Serum IL-6; (**b**) serum TNF-α; and (**c**) IL-6 and TNF-α mRNA expression in the livers of offspring. Data represented as the mean ± SEM ($n = 6$ to 8, per group). * $p < 0.05$, vs. the NCD group. LPD, low-protein diet; NCD, normal chow diet; IL-6: interleukin-6; TNF-α: tumor necrosis factor-α.

3.7. Differential Expression of Pro-Inflammatory Markers in Offspring

Next, we measured *Il-6* and *TNF-α* expression in liver samples of male offspring of LPD- and NCD-fed dams using qRT-PCR. It indicated that *IL-6* and *TNF-α* expression were significantly increased in the LPD group, and the fold change of IL-6 and TNF-α expression is about 1.8 and 2.2, respectively ($p < 0.05$, Figure 5c). To further determine whether the protein expressions of *IL-6* and *TNF-α* in offspring were modulated by maternal LPD, the protein expressions of these two genes were examined by immunohistochemistry. As shown in Figure 6, there was a statistically significant increase in the immunoreactivities of *IL-6* and *TNF-α* in the early life of offspring exposed to maternal LPD during pregnancy and lactation, compared to offspring of NCD-fed dams ($p < 0.05$).

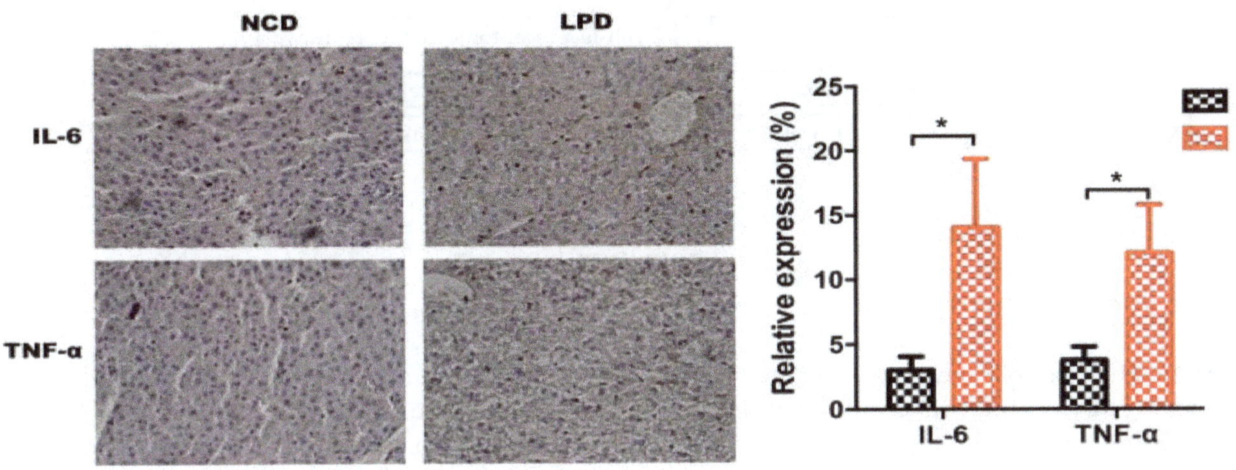

Figure 6. Immunohistochemistry for *IL-6* and *TNF-α* expression and semi-quantitative assessments. (**left**) *IL-6* and *TNF-α* staining in NCD and LPD groups. (**right**) Semi-quantitative scores of *IL-6* and *TNF-α*. Data represented as the mean ± SEM (n = 6 to 8, per group). * $p < 0.05$, vs. the NCD group. LPD, low-protein diet; NCD, normal chow diet; IL-6: interleukin-6; TNF-α: tumor necrosis factor-α.

4. Discussion

Epidemiological studies and animal experiments have indicated that adverse maternal nutriture influence organ development and metabolism of progeny, which may increase the susceptibility of developing diabetes in later life, and even in the following generation [30,31]. Maternal nutrition has long-term metabolic effects on offspring, which was known as the "fetal programming hypothesis" [32]. Here, our findings demonstrate that the exposure of LPD feeding during pregnancy and lactation resulted in low birth weight, impaired glucose tolerance, and lower insulin secretion in offspring, at as early as weaning age. We also observed that offspring from LPD-fed dams showed perturbation of the programmed expression of some key miRNAs in offspring at weaning. Thus, using microarray profiling, bioinformatics approaches, and functional enrichment analysis, all of the target genes of misexpressed miRNAs were mapped in seven inflammatory-related pathways. Finally, we showed that that serum levels of pro-inflammatory cytokines IL-6 and TNF-α were also increased in offspring from LPD-fed dams. Furthermore, the mRNA expression and protein levels of IL-6 and TNF-α were significantly increased in offspring from maternal LPD feeding. Therefore, these results show that maternal LPD consumption may regulate the expression of miRNAs, which may be associated with chronic inflammation status and glucose intolerance in offspring as early as weaning age (Figure 7).

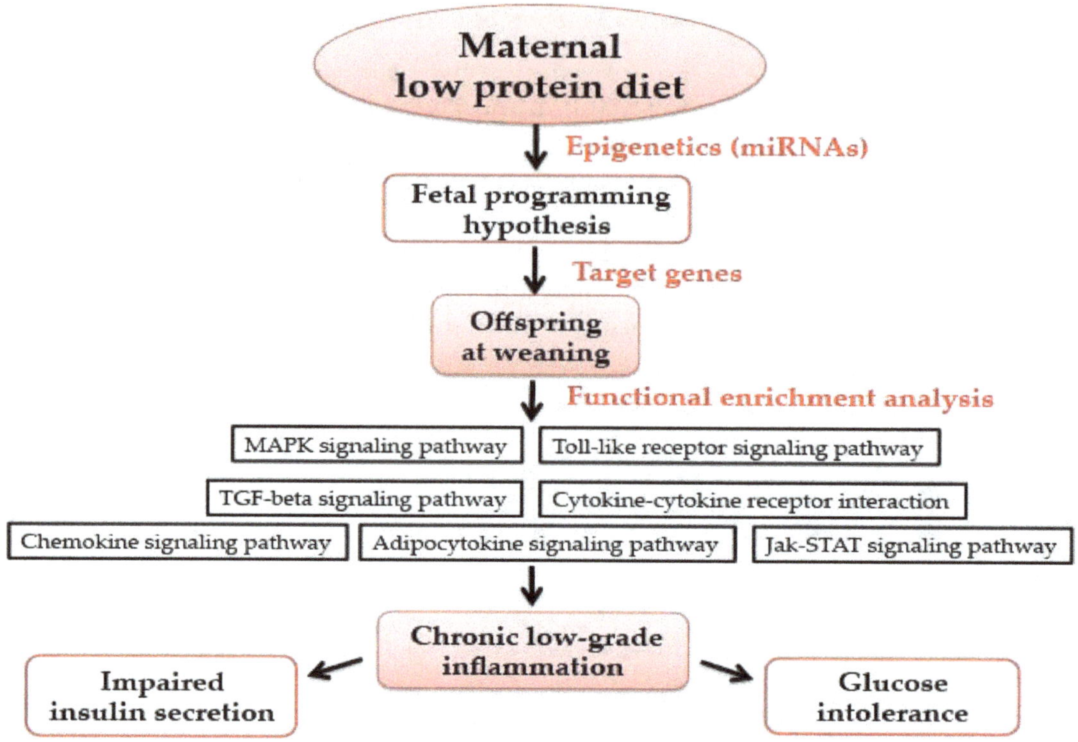

Figure 7. The possible mechanism of maternal low-protein diet during pregnancy and lactation on offspring at weaning. Maternal nutrition has long-term metabolic effects on offspring, which is known as the "fetal programming hypothesis". Epigenetics (such as miRNAs) has been deemed as an important molecular basis of maternal nutrition and metabolic health in offspring. Using functional enrichment analysis, the target genes of differentially-expressed miRNAs were mapped into seven pathways, which are all associated with inflammation. Thus, it may be related to chronic low-grade inflammation, which may cause impaired insulin secretion and glucose intolerance. MAPK: mitogen-activated protein kinase; TGF: transforming growth factor; Jak-STAT: Janus kinase-signal transducer and activator of transcription.

Obesity, insulin resistance, and diabetes mellitus are associated with chronic low-grade inflammation [33–35]. One recent review summarized that chronic inflammation is characterized by increased levels of pro-inflammatory cytokines in response to physiological and environmental stimuli that can arrest the immune system in a low-level activation state [36]. Our study demonstrates that maternal protein restriction diet during pregnancy and lactation may induce an inflammatory state in offspring at weaning age. Similar to our study, one recent study showed that male Wistar rats exposed to a low-protein (8%) diet in utero that had a low birth weight, but then underwent postnatal catch-up growth exhibited higher indexes of inflammatory, with increased hepatic expression of interleukin-6 (IL-6) levels, tumor necrosis factor α (TNF-α), and monocyte chemotactic protein-1 (MCP-1) at 12 months of age [37]. Sílvia et al. also showed that maternal low-protein (6%) diet during pregnancy and lactation showed increased transcription of nuclear factor kappa B (NF-κB) and IL-6, with reduced transcription of interleukin-6 (IL-10) (an anti-inflammatory cytokine) at 90 days of age in offspring [38]. However, the inflammatory state of offspring was examined at an adult or even older age in the aforementioned studies. Here our findings demonstrate that maternal LPD feeding during pregnancy and lactation can induce an inflammatory state in the offspring as early as weaning age. In our previous study, we found that a maternal high-calorie diet is associated with altered hepatic microRNA expression and impaired metabolic health in offspring at weaning age [20]. The composition of the high-calorie diet is 16.4% protein, 25.6% carbohydrate, and 58% fat as the kcal%. However, we found that both of the two studies showed that maternal nutrition are associated with inflammation in offspring. We cannot draw a conclusion that the same biological mechanisms are at play in these two studies because our study is very preliminary, which needs further experimentation and validation. However, we can speculate that maternal malnutrition (whether over-nutrition or under-nutrition) may be associated with aberrant metabolic health and inflammation status in offspring at weaning.

Increasing evidence showed that epigenetic information could be inherited as a trans-generational carrier between generations. It showed that nutrient-dependent regulation of miRNAs may trigger disease susceptibility and metabolic complications in offspring [39]. One clinical study indicated that placental expression of miR-210 increased in preeclampsia and was inversely related to birth weight and gestational age [40]. It showed that a maternal low-protein diet exhibited impaired glucose tolerance and suppressed pancreatic β-cell proliferation in mouse offspring via miR-15b at 12 weeks of age [41]. In addition to maternal nutrition, the advanced fetal programming hypothesis proposes that maternal genetic variants may influence the offspring's phenotype indirectly via epigenetic modification. Hocher et al. showed that altered expression of hepatic microRNA was observed in offspring of female eNOS −/+ mice, demonstrating that a maternal genetic defect can epigenetically alter the phenotype of the offspring, without inheritance of the defect itself [42]. Recently, inflammatory signaling has been identified as an epigenetic mediator and increasing evidence has shown the epigenetics can regulate inflammatory gene expression, which can ultimately result in multiple adverse physiological consequences [43]. Our study shows that validated target genes of differentially-expressed miRNAs in offspring from LPD-fed dams are part of inflammatory signaling pathways. *IL-6* and *TNF* are two validated target genes of let-7e. Recent findings offer a putative role of non-coding RNAs, especially miRNAs, in the progression and management of the inflammatory response [44]. The let-7 family of miRNAs is highly conserved across diverse animal species, and plays critical roles in the regulation of cell proliferation and differentiation [45]. In addition to cancer, an altered expression of let-7 has been reported in inflammation. Let-7 miRNAs demonstrated to be repressed in inflammation, which resulted in increased expression of pro-inflammatory cytokines and increased inflammatory status [46], which is consistent with our results. One clinical study showed that let-7e target genes were predicted to be associated with ulcerative colitis susceptibility [47]. In addition, several miRNAs, such as miR-126, miR-132, miR-146, miR-155, and miR-221 have also emerged as important transcriptional regulators of some inflammation-related mediators [44]. Therefore, we propose that maternal protein restriction diet induce altered hepatic microRNA expression, which may be associated with enhanced inflammatory responses in offspring as early as at weaning age.

To the best of our knowledge, our study provides the first evidence that maternal LPD feeding may regulate the expression of miRNA, which may be associated with chronic inflammation status and glucose intolerance in offspring as early as weaning age. However, some limitations should be considered in our study. First, we agree with the reviewer that our data is preliminary and cannot exclude the possibility that the association between miRNAs and markers of inflammation is due to a state of chronic systemic inflammation causing altered hepatic miRNA, rather than the other way around. Second, our present study focused on the mechanisms between maternal protein restriction and its detrimental effects on offspring during early life of offspring and there was no data on long-term effects in adulthood of our model. Our further research will be focused on the miRNAs expression and inflammation status in older mice offspring to examine the long-term effects in adulthood of our model. Third, the function of miRNA analysis, which showed to be related to inflammation, is mainly based on microarray profiling, bioinformatics analysis, and some preliminary molecular biology experiments. Therefore, using in vivo and in vitro experiments, further studies should be investigated to demonstrate the role of perturbed miRNA expression on glucose metabolism and inflammation status. A fourth limitation is that it is unknown when the critical time window of maternal LPD consumption is; during the gestation period or lactation period, or both periods. Our undergoing work aims to determine the effects of LPD in the dams on glucose metabolism in offspring in specific time window. Furthermore, recent reviews showed that paternal nutritional challenges can also cause programming of glucose impairment in the offspring and alterations of noncoding sperm micro-RNAs, histone acetylation, and targeted, as well as global, DNA methylation seem to be particularly involved in paternal programming of offspring's diseases in later life [48,49]. Therefore, our future study will be interested in examining the underlying epigenetic mechanism linking paternal nutrition and its programming effect on offspring.

In conclusion, here we demonstrated that maternal protein restriction diet with IUGR predisposes to impaired glucose tolerance in the offspring as early as weaning age. This study contributes to the current knowledge on the putative role of miRNAs between maternal low-protein diet and metabolic health in offspring, which are likely to be associated with inflammatory responses. A better understanding of the function of these miRNAs might open the way to the development of new strategies for the early prevention of diabetes. Thus, further studies in the field of trans-generational effects to clarify the underlying mechanisms are urgently warranted.

Acknowledgments: This work was supported by the National Natural Science Foundation of China (No. 81570715 and No. 81170736), National Key Research and Development Program of China (No. 2016YFA0101002), National Natural Science Foundation for Young Scholars of China (No. 81300649), and the National Key Program of Clinical Science and Peking Union Medical College Hospital.

Author Contributions: Xinhua Xiao conceived and designed the experiments. Qian Zhang, Jia Zheng and Tong Wang carried out the experiments. Miao Yu and Jianping Xu analysed data. All authors were involved in writing the paper and had final approval of the submitted and published versions.

References

1. Curhan, G.C.; Willett, W.C.; Rimm, E.B.; Spiegelman, D.; Ascherio, A.L.; Stampfer, M.J. Birth weight and adult hypertension, diabetes mellitus, and obesity in US men. *Circulation* **1996**, *94*, 3246–3250. [CrossRef] [PubMed]
2. Gniuli, D.; Calcagno, A.; Caristo, M.E.; Mancuso, A.; Macchi, V.; Mingrone, G.; Vettor, R. Effects of high-fat diet exposure during fetal life on type 2 diabetes development in the progeny. *J. Lipid Res.* **2008**, *49*, 1936–1945. [CrossRef] [PubMed]
3. De Rooij, S.R.; Painter, R.C.; Phillips, D.I.; Osmond, C.; Michels, R.P.; Godsland, I.F.; Roseboom, T.J. Impaired insulin secretion after prenatal exposure to the Dutch famine. *Diabetes Care* **2006**, *29*, 1897–1901. [CrossRef] [PubMed]
4. Gluckman, P.D.; Hanson, M.A.; Buklijas, T.; Low, F.M.; Beedle, A.S. Epigenetic mechanisms that underpin metabolic and cardiovascular diseases. *Nat. Rev. Endocrinol.* **2009**, *5*, 401–408. [CrossRef] [PubMed]
5. Stefan, M.; Zhang, W.; Concepcion, E.; Yi, Z.; Tomer, Y. DNA methylation profiles in type 1 diabetes twins point to strong epigenetic effects on etiology. *J. Autoimmun.* **2014**, *50*, 33–37. [CrossRef] [PubMed]
6. Waddington, C.H. The epigenotype. 1942. *Int. J. Epidemiol.* **2012**, *41*, 10–13. [CrossRef] [PubMed]
7. Januar, V.; Desoye, G.; Novakovic, B.; Cvitic, S.; Saffery, R. Epigenetic regulation of human placental function and pregnancy outcome: Considerations for causal inference. *Am. J. Obstet. Gynecol.* **2015**, *213* (Suppl. 4), S182–S196. [CrossRef]
8. Reddy, M.A.; Natarajan, R. Epigenetic mechanisms in diabetic vascular complications. *Cardiovasc. Res.* **2011**, *90*, 421–429. [CrossRef] [PubMed]
9. Deiuliis, J.A. MicroRNAs as regulators of metabolic disease: Pathophysiologic significance and emerging role as biomarkers and therapeutics. *Int. J. Obes. (Lond.)* **2016**, *40*, 88–101. [CrossRef] [PubMed]
10. Kahn, H.S. Glucose tolerance in adults after prenatal exposure to famine. *Lancet* **2001**, *357*, 1798–1799. [CrossRef]
11. Zohdi, V.; Lim, K.; Pearson, J.T.; Black, M.J. Developmental programming of cardiovascular disease following intrauterine growth restriction: Findings utilising a rat model of maternal protein restriction. *Nutrients* **2014**, *7*, 119–152. [CrossRef] [PubMed]
12. Jousse, C.; Parry, L.; Lambert-Langlais, S.; Maurin, A.C.; Averous, J.; Bruhat, A.; Jockers, R. Perinatal undernutrition affects the methylation and expression of the leptin gene in adults: Implication for the understanding of metabolic syndrome. *FASEB J.* **2011**, *25*, 3271–3278. [CrossRef] [PubMed]
13. Erhuma, A.; Salter, A.M.; Sculley, D.V.; Langley-Evans, S.C.; Bennett, A.J. Prenatal exposure to a low-protein diet programs disordered regulation of lipid metabolism in the aging rat. *Am. J. Physiol. Endocrinol. Metab.* **2007**, *292*, E1702–E1714. [CrossRef] [PubMed]

14. Watkins, A.J.; Ursell, E.; Panton, R.; Papenbrock, T.; Hollis, L.; Cunningham, C.; Eckert, J.J. Adaptive responses by mouse early embryos to maternal diet protect fetal growth but predispose to adult onset disease. *Biol. Reprod.* **2008**, *78*, 299–306. [CrossRef] [PubMed]
15. Dumortier, O.; Hinault, C.; Gautier, N.; Patouraux, S.; Casamento, V.; van Obberghen, E. Maternal protein restriction leads to pancreatic failure in offspring: Role of misexpressed microRNA-375. *Diabetes* **2014**, *63*, 3416–3427. [CrossRef] [PubMed]
16. Zheng, J.; Xiao, X.; Zhang, Q.; Yu, M.; Xu, J.; Wang, Z. Maternal high-fat diet modulates hepatic glucose, lipid homeostasis and gene expression in the PPAR pathway in the early life of offspring. *Int. J. Mol. Sci.* **2014**, *15*, 14967–14983. [CrossRef] [PubMed]
17. Purves, R.D. Optimum numerical integration methods for estimation of area-under-the-curve (AUC) and area-under-the-moment-curve (AUMC). *J. Pharmacokinet. Biopharm.* **1992**, *20*, 211–226. [CrossRef] [PubMed]
18. Peng, X.; Wood, C.L.; Blalock, E.M.; Chen, K.C.; Landfield, P.W.; Stromberg, A.J. Statistical implications of pooling RNA samples for microarray experiments. *BMC Bioinform.* **2003**, *4*, 26. [CrossRef] [PubMed]
19. Bruce, K.D.; Cagampang, F.R.; Argenton, M.; Zhang, J.; Ethirajan, P.L.; Burdge, G.C.; McConnell, J.M. Maternal high-fat feeding primes steatohepatitis in adult mice offspring, involving mitochondrial dysfunction and altered lipogenesis gene expression. *Hepatology* **2009**, *50*, 1796–1808. [CrossRef] [PubMed]
20. Zheng, J.; Zhang, Q.; Mul, J.D.; Yu, M.; Xu, J.; Qi, C.; Xiao, X. Maternal high-calorie diet is associated with altered hepatic microRNA expression and impaired metabolic health in offspring at weaning age. *Endocrine* **2016**, *54*, 70–80. [CrossRef] [PubMed]
21. Luo, Y.; Zhang, C.; Tang, F.; Zhao, J.; Shen, C.; Wang, C.; Chen, R. Bioinformatics identification of potentially involved microRNAs in Tibetan with gastric cancer based on microRNA profiling. *Cancer Cell Int.* **2015**, *15*, 115. [CrossRef] [PubMed]
22. The miRBase Sequence Database. Release 21. Available online: http://www.mirbase.org (accessed on 24 June 2014).
23. Methods for Affymetrix Oligonucleotide Arrays. Available online: http://www.bioconductor.org/packages/release/bioc/html/affy.html (accessed on 24 June 2015).
24. Zhang, Q.; Xiao, X.; Li, M.; Li, W.; Yu, M.; Zhang, H.; Xiang, H. Acarbose Reduces Blood Glucose by Activating miR-10a-5p and miR-664 in Diabetic Rats. *PLoS ONE* **2013**, *8*, e79697. [CrossRef] [PubMed]
25. MiRWalk2.0 Database. Available online: http://www.umm.uni-heidelberg.de/apps/zmf/mirwalk/ (accessed on 29 April 2015).
26. Dweep, H.; Gretz, N. miRWalk2.0: A comprehensive atlas of microRNA-target interactions. *Nat. Methods* **2015**, *12*, 697.
27. Kyoto Encyclopedia of Genes and Genomes (KEGG) Database. Release 74.0. Available online: http://www.kegg.jp/ (accessed on 1 April 2015).
28. Database for Annotation, Visualization and Integrated Discovery (DAVID) Database. Available online: https://david.ncifcrf.gov (accessed on 1 April 2015).
29. Petrik, J.; Reusens, B.; Arany, E.; Remacle, C.; Coelho, C.; Hoet, J.J.; Hill, D.J. A low protein diet alters the balance of islet cell replication and apoptosis in the fetal and neonatal rat and is associated with a reduced pancreatic expression of insulin-like growth factor-II. *Endocrinology* **1999**, *140*, 4861–4873. [CrossRef] [PubMed]
30. Hales, C.N.; Barker, D.J. Type 2 (non-insulin-dependent) diabetes mellitus: The thrifty phenotype hypothesis. *Diabetologia* **1992**, *35*, 595–601. [CrossRef] [PubMed]
31. Jimenez-Chillaron, J.C.; Isganaitis, E.; Charalambous, M.; Gesta, S.; Pentinat-Pelegrin, T.; Faucette, R.R.; Patti, M.E. Intergenerational transmission of glucose intolerance and obesity by in utero undernutrition in mice. *Diabetes* **2009**, *58*, 460–468. [CrossRef] [PubMed]
32. Kermack, A.J.; van Rijn, B.B.; Houghton, F.D.; Calder, P.C.; Cameron, I.T.; Macklon, N.S. The "Developmental Origins" Hypothesis: Relevance to the obstetrician and gynecologist. *J. Dev. Orig. Health Dis.* **2015**, *6*, 415–424. [CrossRef] [PubMed]
33. Verdile, G.; Keane, K.N.; Cruzat, V.F.; Medic, S.; Sabale, M.; Rowles, J.; Newsholme, P. Inflammation and Oxidative Stress: The Molecular Connectivity between Insulin Resistance, Obesity, and Alzheimer's Disease. *Mediat. Inflamm.* **2015**, *2015*, 105828. [CrossRef] [PubMed]

34. Chen, H. Cellular inflammatory responses: Novel insights for obesity and insulin resistance. *Pharmacol. Res.* **2006**, *53*, 469–477. [CrossRef] [PubMed]
35. Samuel, V.T.; Shulman, G.I. The pathogenesis of insulin resistance: Integrating signaling pathways and substrate flux. *J. Clin. Investig.* **2016**, *126*, 12–22. [CrossRef] [PubMed]
36. Davinelli, S.; Maes, M.; Corbi, G.; Zarrelli, A.; Willcox, D.C.; Scapagnini, G. Dietary phytochemicals and neuro-inflammaging: From mechanistic insights to translational challenges. *Immun. Ageing* **2016**, *13*, 16. [CrossRef] [PubMed]
37. Tarry-Adkins, J.L.; Fernandez-Twinn, D.S.; Hargreaves, I.P.; Neergheen, V.; Aiken, C.E.; Martin-Gronert, M.S.; Ozanne, S.E. Coenzyme Q10 prevents hepatic fibrosis, inflammation, and oxidative stress in a male rat model of poor maternal nutrition and accelerated postnatal growth. *Am. J. Clin. Nutr.* **2016**, *103*, 579–588. [CrossRef] [PubMed]
38. Reis, S.R.; Feres, N.H.; Ignacio-Souza, L.M.; Veloso, R.V.; Arantes, V.C.; Kawashita, N.H.; Latorraca, M.Q. Nutritional recovery with a soybean diet after weaning reduces lipogenesis but induces inflammation in the liver in adult rats exposed to protein restriction during intrauterine life and lactation. *Mediat. Inflamm.* **2015**, *2015*, 781703. [CrossRef] [PubMed]
39. Ferland-McCollough, D.; Fernandez-Twinn, D.S.; Cannell, I.G.; David, H.; Warner, M.; Vaag, A.A.; Siddle, K. Programming of adipose tissue miR-483-3p and GDF-3 expression by maternal diet in type 2 diabetes. *Cell Death Differ.* **2012**, *19*, 1003–1012. [CrossRef] [PubMed]
40. Lee, D.C.; Romero, R.; Kim, J.S.; Tarca, A.L.; Montenegro, D.; Pineles, B.L.; Mittal, P. miR-210 targets iron-sulfur cluster scaffold homologue in human trophoblast cell lines: Siderosis of interstitial trophoblasts as a novel pathology of preterm preeclampsia and small-for-gestational-age pregnancies. *Am. J. Pathol.* **2011**, *179*, 590–602. [CrossRef] [PubMed]
41. Su, Y.; Jiang, X.; Li, Y.; Li, F.; Cheng, Y.; Peng, Y.; Wang, W. Maternal Low Protein Isocaloric Diet Suppresses Pancreatic beta-Cell Proliferation in Mouse Offspring via miR-15b. *Endocrinology* **2016**, *157*, 4782–4793. [CrossRef] [PubMed]
42. Hocher, B.; Haumann, H.; Rahnenführer, J.; Reichetzeder, C.; Kalk, P.; Pfab, T.; Püschel, G.P. Maternal eNOS deficiency determines a fatty liver phenotype of the offspring in a sex dependent manner. *Epigenetics* **2016**, *11*, 539–552. [CrossRef] [PubMed]
43. Zhou, D.; Pan, Y.X. Pathophysiological basis for compromised health beyond generations: Role of maternal high-fat diet and low-grade chronic inflammation. *J. Nutr. Biochem.* **2015**, *26*, 1–8. [CrossRef] [PubMed]
44. Marques-Rocha, J.L.; Samblas, M.; Milagro, F.I.; Bressan, J.; Martínez, J.A.; Marti, A. Noncoding RNAs, cytokines, and inflammation-related diseases. *FASEB J.* **2015**, *29*, 3595–3611. [CrossRef] [PubMed]
45. Pasquinelli, A.E.; Reinhart, B.J.; Slack, F.; Martindale, M.Q.; Kuroda, M.I.; Maller, B.; Spring, J. Conservation of the sequence and temporal expression of let-7 heterochronic regulatory RNA. *Nature* **2000**, *408*, 86–89. [PubMed]
46. Iliopoulos, D.; Hirsch, H.A.; Struhl, K. An epigenetic switch involving NF-kappaB, Lin28, Let-7 MicroRNA, and IL6 links inflammation to cell transformation. *Cell* **2009**, *139*, 693–706. [CrossRef] [PubMed]
47. Coskun, M.; Bjerrum, J.T.; Seidelin, J.B.; Troelsen, J.T.; Olsen, J.; Nielsen, O.H. miR-20b, miR-98, miR-125b-1*, and let-7e* as new potential diagnostic biomarkers in ulcerative colitis. *World J. Gastroenterol.* **2013**, *19*, 4289–4299. [CrossRef] [PubMed]
48. Li, J.; Yang, X.; Hocher, B. Paternal programming of offspring cardiometabolic diseases in later life. *J. Hypertens.* **2016**, *34*, 2111–2126. [CrossRef] [PubMed]
49. Reichetzeder, C.; Dwi Putra, S.E.; Li, J.; Hocher, B. Developmental Origins of Disease—Crisis Precipitates Change. *Cell. Physiol. Biochem.* **2016**, *39*, 919–938. [CrossRef] [PubMed]

10

How Does Diet Change with a Diagnosis of Diabetes? Protocol of the 3D Longitudinal Study

Emily Burch [1], Lauren T. Williams [1], Harriet Makepeace [1], Clair Alston-Knox [2] and Lauren Ball [1,*]

[1] Menzies Health Institute Queensland, Griffith University, Gold Coast 4215, Australia; emily.burch@griffithuni.edu.au (E.B.); lauren.williams@griffith.edu.au (L.T.W.); harriet.makepeace@griffithuni.edu.au (H.M.)

[2] Office of the Pro-Vice Chancellor, Arts, Education and Law, Griffith University, Mount Gravatt Campus, Brisbane 4222, Australia; c.alston-knox@griffith.edu.au

* Correspondence: l.ball@griffith.edu.au

Abstract: Diet quality influences glycemic control in people with type 2 diabetes (T2D), impacting their risk of complications. While there are many cross-sectional studies of diet and diabetes, there is little understanding of the extent to which people with T2D change their diet after diagnosis and of the factors that impact those changes. This paper describes the rationale for and design of the 3D longitudinal Study which aims to: (i) describe diet quality changes in the 12 months following T2D diagnosis, (ii) identify the demographic, physical and psychosocial predictors of sustained improvements in diet quality and glycemic control, and (iii) identify associations between glycemic control and diet quality in the 12 months following diagnosis. This cohort study will recruit adults registered with the Australian National Diabetes Services Scheme who have been recently diagnosed with T2D. Participants will be involved in five purposefully developed telephone surveys, conducted at 3 monthly intervals over a 12-month period. Diet quality will be determined using a 24-h dietary recall at each data collection point and the data will be scored using the Dietary Approaches to Stop Hypertension (DASH) diet-quality tool. This study is the first dedicated to observing how people newly diagnosed with T2D change their diet quality over time and the predictors of sustained improvements in diet and glycemic control.

Keywords: type 2 diabetes mellitus; nutrition; DASH; diet quality; diabetes management; dietary intake; longitudinal analysis; lifestyle management

---

1. Introduction

Diet quality plays a vital role in helping people with type 2 diabetes (T2D) to achieve and maintain optimal glycemic control, thereby lowering their risk of developing diabetes-related complications [1]. Diet quality can be described as the extent to which food intake complies with national or international dietary guidelines or a priori diet quality score [2]. Investigating diet quality based on dietary patterns, defined as multiple dietary components operationalized as a single exposure [3], provides valuable information, beyond analyzing specific nutrients (e.g., protein) or food groups (e.g., dairy) [4]. This is because dietary patterns closely reflect actual dietary behavior and have a stronger influence on disease risk than specific nutrients or foods [5]. Findings from dietary pattern analyses may facilitate the translation of useful recommendations to health professionals and the general population [5,6]. A dietary pattern rich in whole-grains, fruits, vegetables, legumes, and nuts; moderate in alcohol; and low in refined grains, red or processed meats, and sugar-sweetened beverages has been shown to improve glycemic control in people with T2D [7]. Consequently, a key feature of international T2D management recommendations is to eat healthy foods that provide a high-quality diet [8–10].

However, evidence has shown that people with T2D have low-quality diets, despite these recommendations [10–15]. Our recent systematic review identified that internationally, people with T2D do not adhere to food group recommendations outlined in dietary guidelines [15]. Qualitative studies examining lived experiences report that people with T2D find it challenging to adopt and maintain healthy dietary behaviors after diagnosis [13,14]. Our previous qualitative study that investigated the experiences and perceptions of Australian adults newly diagnosed with T2D found that while participants reported making immediate, widespread changes to dietary behaviors that led to improvements in diet quality initially, they found it challenging to maintain dietary change [13]. Participants described feeling restricted in food choice, being uncertain of ideal dietary behaviors and felt unheard and rushed when speaking about their diet with health professionals [13]. Similar results were obtained in a qualitative study in Mexico where people reported making only short-term adherence to improvements in dietary intake due to difficulties with controlling appetite and eating with others [14]. While these qualitative findings of experiences raise concerns, it is important to also investigate quantitative aspects of diet quality change following diagnosis.

Cross-sectional research has assessed the diet quality of people with T2D at a single-point in time [15], however, no research has quantitatively explored changes in diet quality after diagnosis. Consequently, there is no evidence as to whether diet quality remains fixed once an individual is diagnosed with T2D, or whether there are periods of marked increases or decreases in diet quality. Prospective, observational studies are valuable as they measure events in temporal sequence and can distinguish causes from effects [16,17]. Many factors influence diet quality. These include non-modifiable factors such as age and sex, and modifiable factors such as self-efficacy, perception of current diet, environmental factors such as marketing and food availability, and relationships with health professionals [11,13]. There is currently no data on the demographic and health characteristics influencing diet quality change for people with T2D [13,18]. There is a clear need to investigate how diet changes over time so targeted strategies can be developed to facilitate improved glycemic control.

This paper describes the methodological protocol of the 3D Longitudinal Study, so named because seeing something in three dimensions adds clarity. In this case it refers to the 3D's of Diet, after Diagnosis with Diabetes. The study aims are to:

(i) Describe diet quality changes in the 12 months following T2D diagnosis.
(ii) Identify the demographic, physical and psychosocial predictors of improvements in diet quality and glycemic control.
(iii) Identify associations between glycemic control and diet quality in the 12 months following diagnosis.

2. Theoretical Framework

The ability to predict and explain health-related behavior is important for developing strategies to change those behaviors [19]. The theory of planned behavior (TPB) is among the most influential and widely applied theories of the factors influencing health-related behavior [19]. According to the TPB, the single best predictor of a person's behavior is the intention to perform that behavior [20]. This is predicted by three constructs: attitude, subjective norm, and perceived behavioral control (PBC). The greater the PBC and more favorable the attitude and subjective norms, the stronger the intent will be to perform the behavior [20]. According to the TPB, people with T2D will intend to improve their diet quality to the extent that they believe the likely outcomes of consumption to be favorable, perceive social pressure from those who are important to them and feel capable of improving their diet quality without difficulty [21]. The constructs of the TPB are considered strong predictors of healthful eating and are commonly applied in the development of dietary behavior change interventions [21,22]. This study will integrate the TPB into its design in order to explore the factors that may serve as moderators in influencing the TPB constructs, thus affecting dietary behaviors and T2D management.

3. Materials and Methods

3.1. Study Design

The 3D Longitudinal Study is a prospective observational cohort study that will be conducted in Australia between 2018–2019. The study will recruit people newly diagnosed with T2D and monitor their dietary intake over 12 months. The Strengthening the Reporting of Observational Studies in Epidemiology (STROBE) checklist for cohort studies was used to guide the development of the research protocol [23]. The 3D Longitudinal Study is registered with the Australian New Zealand Clinical Trials Registry (ANZCTR) (ref: ACTRN12618000375257) and was approved by the Griffith University Human Research Ethics Committee (ref: 2017/951). Study results will be published in peer-reviewed journals and presented at scientific conferences.

3.2. Potential Participants

Eligible participants will be adults aged 18 years or older who have been recently diagnosed with T2D (<6 months prior to recruitment contact), are registered with the Australian National Diabetes Service Scheme (NDSS) and have indicated their willingness to be contacted for research purposes. The NDSS is an initiative of the Australian Government and is administered with the assistance of Diabetes Australia [24]. In 2017, there were approximately 1.1 million people registered with the NDSS [25]. Registration is part of usual care for people diagnosed with T2D, therefore this potential participant pool provides broad representation of the target population. People with T2D are authorized to register for free if they live in Australia or are visiting from a country with which Australia has a Reciprocal Health Care Agreement on an applicable visa [24]. Registering with the NDSS enables individuals to access a range of government approved diabetes-related products and information services [24]. All registrants have the option of consenting to being contacted for research purposes. Upon registration, patients are required to register their personal details on a form signed by a registered Australian medical practitioner, nurse practitioner or a credentialed diabetes educator [24]. The majority of T2D diagnoses in Australia are made by general practitioners (GPs), who are the usual coordinators of management [7]. A detailed participant inclusion and exclusion criteria is listed in Table 1.

Table 1. Inclusion and exclusion criteria for the 3D Longitudinal Study.

Inclusion Criteria	Exclusion Criteria
Adults aged >18 years	Individuals aged <18 years.
Diagnosed with T2D <6 months prior to recruitment contact	Diagnosed with LADA, T1D, gestational diabetes or pre-diabetes
Registered with the Australian NDSS and indicated their willingness to be contacted for research purposes.	Individuals who have been placed on a special diet due to a co-morbidity (e.g., renal disease)
Able to communicate in English	

LADA, Latent Autoimmune Diabetes in Adults; NDSS, National Diabetes Service Scheme; T1D, Type 1 diabetes; T2D, Type 2 diabetes.

3.3. Participant Recruitment and Screening

A convenience sample of all individuals registered with the NDSS with a new diagnosis of T2D over the previous 6-month period will be sent an initial invitation letter and a plain-language summary of the research project via email by Diabetes Australia. Interested individuals will be invited to contact the research team via email or telephone to confirm eligibility, provide informed consent and arrange data collection. Participants will be informed they can withdraw from the study at any stage. This recruitment method has been trialed in a feasibility study conducted in 2016–2017 (unpublished) which successfully recruited 22 participants from 1000 email invitees. Of these 22, 17 completed baseline data collection, six participants had left the study by 3 months, however all participants remaining at 3 months were retained to 12 months.

3.4. Data Collection

Data will be collected using a purpose-developed, interviewer-administered telephone surveys at five-time points; baseline, and then at 3, 6, 9, and 12 months after commencing the study. Surveys will be conducted by Accredited Practicing Dietitians (APDs). The feasibility study found each survey takes approximately 30 min to complete. A measuring tape will be posted to all participants within two working days of recruitment to provide enough time to measure their waist circumference before data collection begins. Strategies including contact and scheduling methods have been shown to improve cohort retention in longitudinal studies [26]. Participants will be contacted 2 weeks prior to their next anticipated data collection round to schedule a time. All participants will be sent a reminder via their preferred contact method (email or text message) one day prior to the date of their next survey. The recruitment and contact process is outlined in Figure 1.

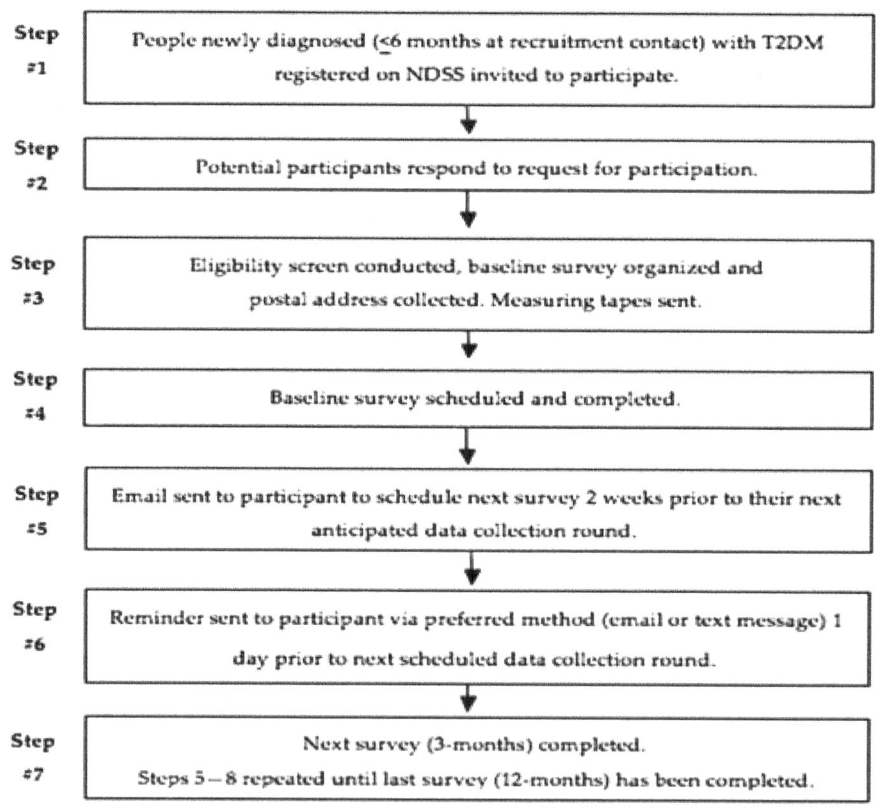

Figure 1. Recruitment and contact process for the 3D Longitudinal Study.

3.5. Survey Design

Data from all secondary outcome measures will be recorded in an online survey management system: www.limesurvey.org [27]. Item wording and response options were composed to align with the Australian Bureau of Statistics (ABS) 2016 Census and the Australian Longitudinal Study on Women's Health (ALSWH) to allow for comparison of outcomes [28,29]. Survey questions were generated using a developmental model [30] that employs five stages of questionnaire design and testing: conceptualization, design, testing, revision, and data collection. The feasibility study allowed testing of questions to ensure they were comprehendible, relevant and appropriate to participants and to confirm the survey length was suitable. Revisions were then made based on the feedback provided. For example, some participants in the feasibility study felt they were being asked the same question twice in the Healthy Eating Belief Scale. Therefore, the interviewer's scripted introduction and description of the Healthy Eating Belief Scale was modified to notify participants that there would be some repetition. The second draft was then pilot tested on three adults outside of the research team to ensure comprehensibility, suitability and flow.

3.6. Outcome Measures

Table 2 provides an overview of the primary (diet quality) and secondary outcomes and when they will be collected.

Table 2. Overview of data collection points in the 3D Longitudinal Study.

Data Collection Methods	Time Collected				
	0 Months	3 months	6 Months	9 Months	12 Months
Diet quality	✔	✔	✔	✔	✔
Glycemic control	✔	✔	✔	✔	✔
Medication use	✔	✔	✔	✔	✔
Baseline demographic factors	✔				
Physical factors	✔	✔	✔	✔	✔
Psychosocial factors	✔	✔	✔	✔	✔
Exposure to allied healthcare support	✔	✔	✔	✔	✔

3.6.1. Primary Outcome Measure: Change in Diet Quality (measured by DASH score)

Diet quality can be measured by a variety of purpose developed tools [31]. These are constructed by assigning higher scores within sub-scales based on more frequent or higher intakes of foods, nutrients or both [31]. Dietary Approaches to Stop Hypertension (DASH) is a dietary pattern high in whole-grains, fruits, and vegetables; moderate in low-fat dairy; and low in red and processed meats, added sugars, and sodium [32]. While originally developed to assist people in the prevention and management of hypertension, DASH is now recommended for the dietary management of T2D [18,33]. Adherence to DASH positively impacts on glycemic control, weight, and hypertension, which are key indicators of risk for diabetes-related complications [5,18,32]. A randomized controlled trial (RCT) conducted in adults with T2D showed that adherence to DASH improved glycated hemoglobin (HbA1c) (−1.2%), fasting blood glucose (−0.92 mmol/L), weight (−3 kg) and waist circumference (−4.8 cm) over 8 weeks when compared with a control diet [34,35]. Those following the DASH dietary pattern, also had a greater reduction in LDL cholesterol (difference from the control diet, −7.7 ± 3.3%).
A systematic review and meta-analysis of 20 RCTs found DASH significantly reduced systolic (−5·2 mmHg) and diastolic blood pressure (−2·6 mmHg) in adults with and without diabetes [36]. Another systematic review and meta-analysis of 13 RCTs revealed that adults without T2D who adhered to DASH achieved greater weight loss (−1.42 kg), reduced Body Mass Index (BMI) (−0.42 kg/m^2) and decreased waist circumference (−1.05 cm) compared with controls [37]. Considering the recognized impact on glycemic control, weight and hypertension, DASH was chosen as the dietary pattern used to assess diet quality in the present study. Participant DASH scores will be calculated using the DASH diet-quality tool which has been shown to have the highest correlation with health outcomes related to T2D compared to other tools that measure diet quality [38,39].

Change in DASH score from baseline to 3 months will be used to categorize participants as diet quality improvers or diet quality maintainers. Participants will be split into 2 groups; those who improved their DASH score by at least 3 DASH points (Diet quality improvers) and those who maintained their DASH score within 2.99 points or decreased their DASH score by at least 3 points (Diet quality maintainers). A change in DASH score of 3 points was selected based on findings from previous literature [40]. In a 20-year longitudinal study of over 40,000 adults, an average DASH score of 23.8 out of 40 was observed, and a change in score of approximately 3 points or more was sufficient to significantly influence long-term glycemic control [40].

Dietary intake data will be obtained through the Australian version of the Automated Self-Administered 24-h Dietary Assessment Tool (ASA-24). The ASA-24 is based on the validated Automated Multiple-Pass Method (AMPM) which is considered the optimal method for obtaining 24-h recall data due to its numerous probes, standardization of interviewer administration and validation against recovery biomarkers [41,42]. This method is also consistent with the methodology of the most recent population nutrition survey in Australia (the National Nutrition Survey) and has been shown to be a valid measure of dietary behavior at a given time point [43,44]. The ASA-24 is an online automated questionnaire that guides the individual through a system designed to maximize respondents' opportunities for remembering and reporting foods eaten in the previous 24 h [45]. The questionnaire is divided into five phases in line with published methodological guidelines; 'quick list', 'forgotten foods', 'time and occasion', 'detail cycle', and 'final probe' [45]. These phases encourage respondents to think about their intake in different ways and from several perspectives which has been shown to reduce bias in the estimation of dietary intake [45]. Once a specific food or beverage is reported, systematic questions are asked to capture more precise information about the food, cooking methods and quantity consumed. The ASA-24, usually a self-completed tool, will be adapted for use in a telephone survey; a researcher will ask the questions and enter the data. This will reduce participant burden and help decrease any bias associated with participant information technology literacy levels. This process was carried out successfully in a feasibility study with patients newly diagnosed with T2D. The data from the feasibility study was able to be used to assess changes in diet quality over a 12-month period.

Following data collection, participant 24-h dietary recall data will be sent from the ASA-24 program to the research team. This data will then be manually entered into FoodWorks by an experienced dietitian to allow determination of participant DASH scores. FoodWorks is a dietary analysis software program using standardized serve sizes that allows for quantification of specific food groups (e.g., vegetables) and nutrients (e.g., sodium) obtained from reported dietary intakes, recipes and meals [46]. FoodWorks draws on the national AUSNUT database [47]. AUSNUT was developed by Food Standards Australia and New Zealand and includes complete nutrient data sets of Australian foods designed specifically for nutrition surveys and is therefore suitable for use in this project [47].

DASH scores will be calculated using the standard scoring tool created by Fung et al [39]. Every tenth DASH score will be cross-checked by a second member of the research team to ensure accuracy. The standard scoring tool determines a score between 8 and 40 points, with 40 points representing optimal accordance with the DASH dietary pattern [39]. The DASH score is calculated by summing the number of daily servings of seven dietary components; fruits, vegetables, nuts and legumes, whole-grains, low-fat dairy, red and processed meats, added sugar, and sodium intake. For each of the components, participants are classified according to their intake ranking. Higher intakes of fruits, vegetables, low-fat dairy, whole-grains, and nuts and legumes receive higher scores. For example, quintile 1 is assigned 1 point and quintile 5 is assigned 5 points. Intake of sodium, red and processed meats and added sugars are scored in reverse as these are less desirable foods [39]. The lowest quintile is given a score of 5 points and the highest quintile is given a score of 1 point. The components scores are then summed to give an overall DASH score [39]. The scoring criteria for the DASH-style diet is outlined in Table 3.

Table 3. Dietary Approaches to Stop Hypertension (DASH) dietary pattern scoring criteria.

Component	Foods	Scoring Quintiles (Q) *
Fruits	All fruits and fruit juices	Q1 = 1 point
Vegetables	All vegetables except potatoes and legumes	Q2 = 2 points
Nuts and legumes	Nuts and peanut butter, dried beans, peas, tofu	Q3 = 3 points
Whole-grains	Brown rice, dark breads, cooked cereal, whole-grain cereal, other grains, popcorn, wheat germ, bran	Q4 = 4 points
Low-fat dairy	Skim milk, yogurt, cottage cheese	Q5 = 5 points
Sodium	Sum of sodium content of all foods	Q1 = 5 points
Red and processed meats	Beef, pork, lamb, deli meats, organ meats, hot dogs, bacon	Q2 = 4 points Q3 = 3 points
Added sugar	Foods and beverages with added sugars (i.e., sugar sweetened beverages)	Q4 = 2 points Q5 = 1 point

* Q1 represents low consumption and Q5 represents high consumption.

3.6.2. Secondary Outcome Measures

Secondary outcome measures will include: glycemic control, medication use, demographic factors, physical factors, psychosocial factors, and exposure to health provider support.

Glycemic Control

HbA1c reflects average plasma glucose over the previous six to eight-week period [48,49]. In Australia, it is best practice for GPs to conduct HbA1c testing on people with T2D every 3 months [8]. The test is subsidized by Medicare, the Australian Government's universal health scheme, up to four times in a 12-month period [50]. The GP on the research team will retrospectively obtain participants' HbA1c results over the 12-month study period from the relevant pathology laboratory. Other blood results collected will include; fasting blood glucose, high-density lipoprotein cholesterol, low-density lipoprotein cholesterol, and C-reactive protein.

Medication Use

Information on all medication use (name of medication and dosage) will be collected, including over-the-counter, and complementary medicines.

Demographic Factors

Demographic factors collected at baseline including; age, gender, highest education level, living arrangement, self-selected social class, household income, ability to manage on income, and smoking status. Response options will be dichotomous (e.g., gender), continuous (e.g., age) or categorical (e.g., highest educational level), consistent with categories used in the national consensus by the ABS.

Age and Gender

Participants' age at last birthday and gender will be collected. Sex response options will include three categories in line with the ABS 2016 Census; male, female and other [51].

Highest Education Level

Collecting data on highest educational level helps generate a single measure of an individual's overall educational attainment, whether it be a school or non-school qualification [51]. Participants will be asked to report their highest education level from eight categories in line with the ABS 2016 Census; postgraduate degree, graduate diploma and graduate certificate, bachelor degree, advanced diploma, diploma, certificate, year 12, or year 11 and below [51].

Living Arrangement

Data on participants' current living arrangement will be collected. In line with the ALSWH, response options will include; no one, partner/spouse, own children, someone else's children, parents, or other adults [29].

Self-Selected Social Class

Requesting information on self-selected social class allows class designation to be meaningful to participants and is more likely to reflect their actual class identity [52]. Participants will be asked to self-select their social class from one of four response options in line with the ALWHS; 'upper class', 'middle class', 'working class', or 'don't know' [52].

Household Income and Ability to Manage on Income

Gross income refers to the sum of income received from all sources before any deductions (income tax, the Medicare Levy or salary sacrificed amounts) are taken out [51]. Participants will be asked to report their average yearly gross household income from six response options in line with the ALSWH; less than $20,000, $20,001–$30,000, $30,001–$50,000, $50,001–$100,000, more than $100,000 or 'don't know/would rather not say'. Details on participants' ability to manage on their current income will also be collected. Seven response options in line with the ALSWH will include; 'impossible', 'difficult', 'always difficult', 'sometimes difficult', 'not too bad', 'easy', or 'not sure' [53].

Smoking Status

Participants will be asked to report their smoking status. Wording of the question has been developed to correspond with the ABS 2016 Census and response categories will include 'yes' or 'no' [51].

Physical Factors

Self-reported anthropometric data is valid and recommended for monitoring prevalence of obesity, particularly for large-scale studies because of its simplicity and low cost [54–56]. Physical factors will include; self-reported waist circumference, weight, and height. All response options will be continuous.

Waist Circumference

Waist circumference is a better indicator of central obesity than BMI or waist-to-hip ratio and is more strongly correlated with intra-abdominal fat content and cardiovascular risk factors [57]. Participants will be asked to self-report their waist circumference to the nearest centimeter. Participants will be asked to report results of two measures at each round of data collection, which will be averaged during data analysis. Measuring instructions adapted from the ALSWH will be provided to participants in the postal envelope [58]. Instructions will request participants to measure mid-central adiposity using the tape to measure at the level of the mid-point between the lower costal border and the iliac crest [58].

Weight

Weight will be self-reported at each data collection point to the nearest decimal point. If the participant can only report the amount in stones and pounds, a conversion factor of 2.203 will be used to convert pounds into kilograms in line with the ALSWH [52]. Participants will be asked to describe where and how their weight was measured to assess the accuracy of the information.

Height

Height will be self-reported to the nearest centimeter at baseline only. If the participant can only report the information in feet or inches, a factor of 2.54 will be used to convert inches to centimeters in line with the ALSWH [52].

BMI

BMI provides the most useful population-level measure of obesity [58,59]. Participants' BMI will be calculated after each round of data collection using the standard equation (weight (kg)/height (m)^2) [58]. Participants will be grouped into BMI categories for analysis according to the World Health Organization guidelines; underweight (<18.50 kg/m^2), normal weight (18.50–24.99 kg/m^2), overweight ($\geq$25.00 kg/m^2) and obese ($\geq$30.00 kg/m^2) [59].

Physical Activity

Regular physical activity is a key feature of international T2D management guidelines [9,60]. This is because it has been shown to improve glycemic control (regardless of whether weight loss has occurred), lipid levels, and blood pressure in people with T2D [61–63]. Participants' physical activity levels will be measured through the IPAQ-SF which is one of the most widely used physical activity assessment questionnaires and has been shown to be a valid measure of obtaining internationally comparable physical activity data [64,65]. It measures self-reported physical activity in the previous seven days and includes seven items that collect information on walking time, moderate and vigorous physical activity time and sitting time [66]. Data obtained in the IPAQ-SF will be used to estimate total metabolic equivalent (MET)-minutes per week for each participant [67].

Psychosocial Factors

Healthful Eating Beliefs

Healthy eating beliefs will be investigated at each of the five data collection points to better understand their beliefs, attitudes and intentions towards making positive dietary behaviors and how these impact on diet quality change over time. Participants' healthy eating beliefs will be assessed through the Healthful Eating Beliefs Scale. This scale is based on the TPB [68]. Standardized questions have been selected from previous Healthful Eating Beliefs Scales to suit the current study. Table 4 provides an outline of the rationale for investigation behind the questions and modes of responses. Participant scores will be generated for each of the seven subscales of the Healthful Eating Beliefs Scale by calculating the mean of the 5-point Likert scale items, with higher scores representing more positive beliefs, attitudes, and intentions towards improving dietary behaviors.

Mental Health

Mental health data will be collected at baseline, 6 and 12 months using the internationally validated K10 questionnaire [69]. This 10-item questionnaire yields a global measure of distress based on questions about anxiety and depressive symptoms experienced in the most recent four-week period [70]. It is scored using a five-level response scale based on the frequency of symptoms reported for each question. One is the minimum score for each item (none of the time) and five is the maximum score (all of the time). The maximum score is 50 indicating severe distress, the minimum score is 10 indicating no distress [70].

Table 4. Healthful Eating Beliefs Scale rationale for investigation and modes of responses.

Category	Rationale for Investigation	Area of Enquiry	Standardized Questions and Response Options	Source
Healthful Eating Beliefs Scale	To better understand healthy eating beliefs among participants and determine if they change over time.	Behavioral intention	"I intend to eat a healthful diet each day in the next 2 months," 5-pt Likert "I will try to eat a healthful diet each day in the next 2 months," 5-pt Likert "I plan to eat a healthful diet each day in the next 2 months," 5-pt Likert	[68]
		Perceived behavioral control	"I have the self-discipline to eat a healthful diet" 5-pt Likert "I have the ability to eat a healthful diet" 5-pt Likert "Me eating a healthful diet would be easy/difficult" 5-pt Likert "Whether I do or do not follow the recommendations for my diet is entirely up to me" 5-pt Likert	[71]
		Subjective norm	"People important to me think I should not/I should eat a healthful diet" 5-pt Likert "Other people expect me to follow the daily recommendations for diet" 5-pt Likert "People important to me want me to eat a healthful diet" 5-pt Likert "Other people with diabetes follow the daily recommendations for diet" 5-pt Likert	[71,72]
		Attitudes towards self-care	"Following the recommendations for my diet would be harmful/beneficial" 5-pt Likert "It would be worthless/valuable for me to follow the daily recommendations for my diet" 5-pt Likert "Following daily recommendations for diet is unnecessary/necessary" 5-pt Likert Following daily recommendations for diet is unpleasant/pleasant" 5-pt Likert	[72]

Exposure to GP and Allied Healthcare Support

Interactions with health professionals may help facilitate positive changes in dietary behaviors [73]. At each data collection point, participants will be asked about their concurrent and previous exposure to healthcare provider support (e.g., dietitian, diabetes educator). Participants will also be asked to report how useful they found the advice on a 5-point Likert scale (1 being 'not at all useful', 2 being 'slightly useful', 3 being 'neutral', 4 being 'somewhat useful' and 5 being 'extremely useful'). Question wording has been modified from previously conducted qualitative research that explored the experiences of dietary change in people with T2D [13].

3.7. *Participant Confidentiality*

All study related information will be de-identified and stored securely online with password-protected access systems. Daily back-ups of all electronic data will occur to minimize any risk of lost data. Only members of the research team who need to contact study patients, enter data or perform data quality control will have access to participant information.

3.8. *Statistical Modeling and Sample Size*

The longitudinal aspect of diet quality change will be analyzed using regression models [74]. Diet quality at 12 months (measured by the DASH score) will be the primary outcome, with glycemic control, interim diet changes (primarily at 3 months), medication use, demographic measures, physical measures, psychosocial measures, and exposure to healthcare provider support as the explanatory variables. This model will determine the relative importance of diet quality change both immediately after diagnosis and in the medium term with regards to a 12-month outcome towards sustained healthy eating.

Sample size calculations, such as those provided in Diggle et al. [74] are not readily computed for complex regression models and assessment using simulation studies would be more appropriate [75]. However, due to the relatively small participation rate in the feasibility study (22 participants/1000 invited) credible model parameters are currently unable to be formulated, and the effect differences over time cannot be reliably inferred. Additionally, current research of diet quality change post diabetes is lacking [15], therefore effects cannot be competently elicited. As a result, rather than determining an initial sample size for the study, a Bayesian updating procedure will be used to collect data. In this manner, sample size will be calculated during the early stages of data collection to yield an idea of how many samples should be collected. Additionally, using a Bayesian framework, the parameter estimates of the mixed model will be sequentially updated as batches of data are obtained, a process known as Bayesian learning [76,77].

4. Discussion

The study described in this paper, the 3D Longitudinal Study, will be the first to observe changes in diet quality in people with T2D after diagnosis and the factors (demographic, physical, and psychosocial) that influence those changes. Longitudinal studies help highlight differences or changes in the values of one or more variables between different time periods, describe participants' intra-individual and inter-individual changes over time and monitor the magnitude and patterns of those changes [78]. This is important for the proposed research because it is necessary to understand the extent to which people change their diet after a T2D diagnosis and why some people are able to sustain these changes over time and others are not. Understanding this will help to develop targeted strategies and facilitate enhanced dietary behavior support important to assist all people with T2D to have long-term success in improving their diet quality and help reduce the risk of complications. The results of this study will significantly add to the body of literature on the diet quality changes of people diagnosed with T2D, which is an under-researched area.

Limitations of the 3D Longitudinal Study are acknowledged. Recruitment through the NDSS is the most suitable way to access a large number of potential participants with T2D, however selection bias cannot be excluded as registration is voluntary, so participants may have greater diabetes self-management motivation. Self-reported dietary intake data and physical measurements may introduce misreporting bias and social desirability responses. Measurement errors associated with dietary assessment methods are also acknowledged. However, use of the ASA-24 h dietary recall (Australian version) which is a validated tool specifically designed for the Australian population, reduces risk of bias [43]. A feasibility study for this project has already determined that its recruitment capability, data collection and analysis procedures are achievable and appropriate.

Author Contributions: E.B., L.B., H.M. and L.T.W. identified the research question. All authors developed the research protocol. All authors have been involved in drafting the manuscript and revising it critically for intellectual content. All authors read and approved the final manuscript.

References

1. Coppell, K.J.; Kataoka, M.; Williams, S.M.; Chisholm, A.W.; Vorgers, S.M.; Mann, J.I. Nutritional intervention in patients with type 2 diabetes who are hyperglycaemic despite optimised drug treatment—Lifestyle Over and Above Drugs in Diabetes (LOADD) study: Randomised controlled trial. *BMJ* **2010**, *341*, c3337. [CrossRef] [PubMed]
2. Leech, R.M.; Worsley, A.; Timperio, A.; McNaughton, S.A. Understanding meal patterns: Definitions, methodology and impact on nutrient intake and diet quality. *Nutr. Res. Rev.* **2015**, *28*, 1–21. [CrossRef] [PubMed]
3. Lockheart, M.S.K.; Steffen, L.M.; Rebnord, H.M.; Fimreite, R.L.; Ringstad, J.; Thelle, D.S.; Pedersen, J.I.; Jacobs, D.R., Jr. Dietary patterns, food groups and myocardial infarction: A case–control study. *Br. J. Nutr.* **2007**, *98*, 380–387. [CrossRef] [PubMed]

4. Drehmer, M.; Odegaard, A.O.; Schmidt, M.I.; Duncan, B.B.; Cardoso, L.D.; Matos, S.M.A.; Molina, M.D.C.B.; Barreto, S.M.; Pereira, M.A. Brazilian dietary patterns and the dietary approaches to stop hypertension (DASH) diet-relationship with metabolic syndrome and newly diagnosed diabetes in the ELSA-Brasil study. *Diabetol. Metab. Syndr.* **2017**, *9*. [CrossRef]
5. Sievenpiper, J.L.; Dworatzek, P.D.N. Food and dietary pattern-based recommendations: An emerging approach to clinical practice guidelines for nutrition therapy in diabetes. *Can. J. Diabetes* **2013**, *37*, 51–57. [CrossRef] [PubMed]
6. Mozaffarian, D.; Ludwig, D.S. Dietary guidelines in the 21st century–A time for food. *JAMA* **2010**, *304*, 681–682. [CrossRef]
7. Ley, S.H.; Hamdy, O.; Mohan, V.; Hu, F.B. Prevention and management of type 2 diabetes: Dietary components and nutritional strategies. *Lancet* **2014**, *383*, 1999–2007. [CrossRef]
8. The Royal Australian College of General Practitioners (RACGP). *General Practice Management of Type 2 Diabetes: 2016–2018*; RACGP: East Melbourne, VIC, Australia, 2016.
9. National Institute for Health and Care Excellence (NICE). *Type 2 Diabetes in Adults: Management United Kingdom*; NICE: London, UK, 2017.
10. Vitolins, M.Z. Action for Health in Diabetes (Look AHEAD) trial: Baseline evaluation of selected nutrients and food group intake. *J. Am. Diet Assoc.* **2009**, *109*, 1367–1375. [CrossRef]
11. Nelson, K.M.; Reiber, G.; Boyko, E.J. Diet and exercise among adults with type 2 diabetes: Findings from the third national health and nutrition examination survey (NHANES III). *Diabetes Care* **2002**, *25*, 1722–1728. [CrossRef]
12. Jarvandi, S.; Gougeon, R.; Bader, A.; Dasgupta, K. Differences in food intake among obese and nonobese women and men with type 2 diabetes. *J. Am. Coll. Nutr.* **2011**, *30*, 225–232. [CrossRef]
13. Ball, L.; Davmor, R.; Leveritt, M.; Desbrow, B.; Ehrlich, C.; Chaboyer, W. Understanding the nutrition care needs of patients newly diagnosed with type 2 diabetes: A need for open communication and patient-focussed consultations. *Aust J Prim Health* **2016**, *22*, 416–422. [CrossRef] [PubMed]
14. Castro-Sanchez, A.E.; Avila-Ortiz, M.N. Changing dietary habits in persons living with type 2 diabetes. *J. Nutr. Educ. Behav.* **2013**, *45*, 761–766. [CrossRef] [PubMed]
15. Burch, E.; Ball, L.; Somerville, M.; Williams, L.T. Dietary intake by food group of individuals with type 2 diabetes mellitus: A systematic review. *Diab. Res. Clin. Prac.* **2018**, *10*, 160–172. [CrossRef] [PubMed]
16. Mann, C.J. Observational research methods. Research design II: Cohort, cross sectional, and case-control studies. *Emerg. Med. J.* **2003**, *20*, 54–60. [CrossRef] [PubMed]
17. Mariani, A.W.; Pego-Fernandes, P.M. Observational studies: Why are they so important? *Sao Paulo Med. J.* **2014**, *132*, 1–2. [CrossRef] [PubMed]
18. Evert, A.B.; Boucher, J.L.; Cypress, M.; Dunbar, S.A.; Franz, M.J.; Mayer-Davis, E.J.; Neumiller, J.J.; Nwankwo, R.; Verdi, C.L.; Urbanski, P.; et al. Nutrition therapy recommendations for the management of adults with diabetes. *Diabetes Care* **2013**, *36*, 3821–3842. [CrossRef] [PubMed]
19. McEachan, R.R.C.; Conner, M.T.; Taylor, N.J.; Lawton, R. Prospective prediction of health-related behaviors with Theory of Planned Behavior: A meta-analysis. *Health Psych. Rev.* **2011**, *5*, 97–144. [CrossRef]
20. Ajzen, I. The theory of planned behavior. *Organ. Behav. Hum. Decis. Process* **1991**, *50*, 179–211. [CrossRef]
21. Kothe, E.J.; Mullan, B.A. Interaction effects in the theory of planned behavior: Predicting fruit and vegetable consumption in three prospective cohorts. *Br. J. Health Psych.* **2015**, *20*, 549–562. [CrossRef]
22. Hardeman, W.; Johnston, M.; Johnston, D.W.; Bonetti, D.; Wareham, N.; Kinmonth, A.L. Application of the theory of planned behavior in behavior change interventions: A systematic review. *Psych. Health* **2002**, *17*, 123–158. [CrossRef]
23. von Elm, E.; Altman, D.G.; Egger, M.; Pocock, S.J.; Gotzsche, P.C.; Vandenbroucke, J.P.; STROBE Initiative. The Strengthening the Reporting of Observational Studies in Epidemiology (STROBE) Statement: Guidelines for reporting observational studies. *Int. J. Surg.* **2014**, *12*, 1495–1499. [CrossRef]
24. National Diabetes Service Scheme (NDSS): Registration. Available online: https://www.ndss.com.au/registration (accessed on 20 May 2018).
25. National Diabetes Services Scheme (NDSS): Type 2 Diabetes. Available online: https://www.ndss.com.au/data-snapshots (accessed on 1 July 2018).

26. Abshire, M.; Victor, D.D.; Cajita, M.I.A.; Eakin, M.N.; Needham, D.M.; Himmelfarb, C.D. Participant retention practices in longitudinal clinical research studies with high retention rates. *BMC Med. Res. Method* **2017**, *17*, 1–10. [CrossRef]
27. LimeSurvey Organisation. Available online: https://www.limesurvey.org/ (accessed on 1 September 2018).
28. Australian Bureau of Statistics (ABS). Available online: http://www.abs.gov.au/ausstats/abs@.nsf/Lookup/bySubject/2008.0~{}2016~{}MainFeatures~{}Age~{}99 (accessed on 1 September 2018).
29. Elstgeest, L.E.M.; Mishra, G.D.; Dobson, A.J. Transitions in living arrangements are associated with changes in dietary patterns in young women. *J. Nutri.* **2012**, *142*, 1561–1567. [CrossRef] [PubMed]
30. Brancato, G.; Macchia, S.; Murgia, M.; Signore, M.; Simeoni, G.; Blanke, K.; Körner, T.; Nimmergut, A.; Lima, P.; Paulino, R.; et al. *Handbook of Recommended Practices for Questionnaire Development and Testing in the European Statistical System*; Eurostat: Luxembourg city, Luxembourg, 2004.
31. Collins, C.E.; Burrows, T.L.; Rollo, M.E.; Boggess, M.M.; Watson, J.F.; Guest, M.; Duncanson, K.; Pezdirc, K.; Hutchesson, M.J. The comparative validity and reproducibility of a diet quality index for adults: The Australian recommended food score. *Nutrients* **2015**, *7*, 785–798. [CrossRef] [PubMed]
32. Campbell, A.P. DASH eating plan: An eating pattern for diabetes management. *Diabetes Spectrum* **2017**, *30*, 76. [CrossRef] [PubMed]
33. Clark, A.L. Use of the Dietary Approaches to Stop Hypertension (DASH) eating plan for diabetes management. *Diabetes Spectrum* **2012**, *25*, 244–252. [CrossRef]
34. Salehi-Abargouei, A.; Maghsoudi, Z.; Shirani, F.; Azadbakht, L. Effects of Dietary Approaches to Stop Hypertension (DASH)-style diet on fatal or nonfatal cardiovascular diseases-incidence: A systematic review and meta-analysis on observational prospective studies. *Nutrition* **2013**, *29*, 611–618. [CrossRef]
35. Azadbakht, L.; Surkan, P.J.; Esmaillzadeh, A.; Willett, W.C. The dietary approaches to stop hypertension eating plan affects C-reactive protein, coagulation abnormalities, and hepatic function tests among type 2 diabetic patients. *J. Nutr.* **2011**, *141*, 1083–1088. [CrossRef]
36. Siervo, M.; Lara, J.; Chowdhury, S.; Ashor, A.; Oggioni, C.; Mathers, J.C. Effects of the Dietary Approach to Stop Hypertension (DASH) diet on cardiovascular risk factors: A systematic review and meta-analysis. *Brit. J. Nutri.* **2015**, *113*, 1–15. [CrossRef]
37. Soltani, S.; Shirani, F.; Chitsazi, M.J.; Salehi-Abargouei, A. The effect of dietary approaches to stop hypertension (DASH) diet on weight and body composition in adults: A systematic review and meta-analysis of randomized controlled clinical trials. *Obesi. Rev.* **2016**, *17*, 442–454. [CrossRef]
38. Alkerwi, A.; Vernier, C.; Crichton, G.E.; Sauvageot, N.; Shivappa, N.; Hebert, J.R. Cross-comparison of diet quality indices for predicting chronic disease risk: Findings from the Observation of Cardiovascular Risk Factors in Luxembourg (ORISCAV-LUX) study. *Briti. J. Nutri.* **2015**, *113*, 259–269. [CrossRef] [PubMed]
39. Fung, T.T.; Chiuve, S.E.; McCullough, M.L.; Rexrode, K.M.; Logroscino, G.; Hu, F.B. Adherence to a DASH-Style diet and risk of coronary heart disease and stroke in women. *Arch. Intern. Med.* **2008**, *168*, 713–720. [CrossRef] [PubMed]
40. de Koning, L.; Chiuve, S.E.; Fung, T.T.; Willett, W.C.; Rimm, E.B.; Hu, F.B. Diet-quality scores and the risk of type 2 diabetes in men. *Diabetes Care* **2011**, *34*. [CrossRef]
41. National Institute of Health (NIH). Available online: https://epi.grants.cancer.gov/asa24/respondent/validation.html (accessed on 1 June 2018).
42. Moshfegh, A.J.; Rhodes, D.G.; Baer, D.J.; Murayi, T.; Clemens, J.C.; Rumpler, W.V.; Paul, D.R.; Sebastian, R.S.; Kuczynski, K.J.; Ingwersen, L.A.; et al. The US department of agriculture automated multiple-pass method reduces bias in the collection of energy intakes. *Amer. J. Clin. Nutri.* **2008**, *88*, 324–332. [CrossRef] [PubMed]
43. Kirkpatrick, S.I.; Subar, A.F.; Douglass, D.; Zimmerman, T.P.; Thompson, F.E.; Kahle, L.L.; George, S.M.; Dodd, K.W.; Potischman, N.; et al. Performance of the automated self-administered 24-hour recall relative to a measure of true intakes and to an interviewer-administered 24-h recall. *Amer. J. Clin. Nutri.* **2014**, *100*, 233–240. [CrossRef] [PubMed]
44. Thompson, F.E.; Dixit-Joshi, S.; Potischman, N.; Dodd, K.W.; Kirkpatrick, S.I.; Kushi, L.H.; Alexander, G.L.; Coleman, L.A.; Zimmerman, T.P.; Sundaram, M.E.; et al. Comparison of interviewer-administered and automated self-administered 24-hour dietary recalls in 3 diverse integrated health systems. *Amer. J. Epidem.* **2015**, *181*, 970–978. [CrossRef]

45. Australian Bureau of Statistics (ABS). Available online: http://www.abs.gov.au/ausstats/abs@.nsf/mf/4363.0.55.001 (accessed on 31 May 2018).
46. Xyris Software: FoodWorks 9 Professional. Available online: https://xyris.com.au/products/foodworks-9-professional/ (accessed on 1 June 2018).
47. Food Standard Australia New Zealand (FSANZ): Food Nutrient Database FSANZ. Available online: http://www.foodstandards.gov.au/science/monitoringnutrients/ausnut/foodnutrient/Pages/default.aspx (accessed on 1 May 2018).
48. Nathan, D.M.; Turgeon, H.; Regan, S. Relationship between glycated haemoglobin levels and mean glucose levels over time. *Diabetologia* **2007**, *50*, 2239–2244. [CrossRef]
49. Schifreen, R.; Hickingbotham, J.M.; Bowers, G.N. Accuracy, precision and stability in measurement of hemoglobin A1c by "high-performance" cation-exchange chromatography. *Clin. Chem.* **1980**, *26*, 466.
50. Australian Government: Medicare Benefits Schedule online. Available online: http://www.mbsonline.gov.au (accessed on 15 June 2018).
51. Australian Bureau of Statistics (ABS). Available online: http://www.abs.gov.au/ausstats/abs@.nsf/mf/2901.0 (accessed on 28 May 2018).
52. Williams, L.; Germov, J.; Young, A. The effect of social class on mid-age women's weight control practices and weight gain. *Appetite* **2011**, *56*, 719–725. [CrossRef]
53. Australian Longitudinal Study on Women's Health (ALSWH). *Australian Longitudinal Study on Women's Health, 1946–1951 Cohort Summary 1996–2013*; ALSWH: New South Wales, Australia, 2015.
54. Spencer, E.A.; Appleby, P.N.; Davey, G.K.; Key, T.J. Validity of self-reported height and weight in 4808 EPIC–Oxford participants. *Public Health Nutri.* **2002**, *5*, 561–565. [CrossRef]
55. Booth, M.L.; Hunter, C.; Gore, C.J.; Bauman, A.; Owen, N. The relationship between body mass index and waist circumference: Implications for estimates of the population prevalence of overweight. *Intern. J. Obesity* **2000**, *24*, 1058–1061. [CrossRef]
56. Chan, N.P.T.; Choi, K.C.; Nelson, E.A.S.; Sung, R.Y.T.; Chan, J.C.N.; Kong, A.P.S. Self-reported waist circumference: A screening tool for classifying children with overweight/obesity and cardiometabolic risk factor clustering: Self-reported waist circumference. *Pediatr. Obesity* **2012**, *7*, 110–120. [CrossRef] [PubMed]
57. Ma, W.Y.; Yang, C.Y.; Shih, S.R.; Hsieh, H.J.; Hung, C.S.; Chiu, F.C.; Lin, M.S.; Liu, P.H.; Hua, C.H.; Hsein, Y.C.; et al. Measurement of Waist Circumference: Midabdominal or iliac crest? *Diabetes Care* **2013**, *36*, 1660–1666. [CrossRef] [PubMed]
58. Williams, L.; Hollis, J.; Collins, C.; Morgan, P. The 40-Something randomized controlled trial to prevent weight gain in mid-age women. *BMC Public Health* **2013**, *13*, 1007. [CrossRef]
59. World Health Organization (WHO). *Obesity: Preventing and Managing the Global Epidemic*; WHO: Geneva, Switzerland, 2000.
60. International Diabetes Federation (IDF). *IDF Clinical Practice Recommendations for Managing Type 2 Diabetes in Primary Care*; IDF: Brussels, Belgium, 2017.
61. Colberg, S.R.; Sigal, R.J.; Fernhall, B.; Regensteiner, J.G.; Blissmer, B.J.; Rubin, R.R.; Chasan-Taber, L.; Albright, A.L.; Braun, B.; American College of Sports Medicine; et al. Exercise and type 2 diabetes: The American College of Sports Medicine and the American Diabetes Association: Joint position statement. *Diabetes Care* **2010**, *33*, e147–e167. [CrossRef] [PubMed]
62. Balducci, S.; Zanuso, S.; Nicolucci, A.; De Feo, P.; Cavallo, S.; Cardelli, P.; Fallucca, S.; Alessi, E.; Fallucca, F.; Pugliese, G.; et al. Effect of an intensive exercise intervention strategy on modifiable cardiovascular risk factors in subjects with type 2 diabetes mellitus. *Arch. Internal. Med.* **2010**, *20*, 1794–1803. [CrossRef] [PubMed]
63. Umpierre, D.; Ribeiro, P.A.; Kramer, C.K.; Leitão, C.B.; Zucatti, A.T.; Azevedo, M.J.; Gross, J.L.; Ribeiro, J.P.; Schaan, B.D. Physical activity advice only or structure exercise training and association with HbA1c levels in type 2 diabetes: A systematic review and meta-analysis. *JAMA* **2011**, *17*, 1790–1799. [CrossRef] [PubMed]
64. van Poppel, M.N.; Chinapaw, M.J.; Mokkink, L.B.; van Mechelen, W.; Terwee, C.B. Physical activity questionnaires for adults: A systematic review of measurement properties. *Sports Med.* **2010**, 565–600. [CrossRef]

65. Craig, C.L.; Marshall, A.L.; Sjostrom, M.; Bauman, A.E.; Booth, M.L.; Ainsworth, B.E. International Physical Activity Questionnaire: 12-country reliability and validity. *Med. Sci. Sports Exercise* **2003**, *35*, 1381–1395. [CrossRef]
66. International Physical Activity Group. Available online: https://sites.google.com/site/theipaq/questionnaire_links (accessed on 1 June 2018).
67. International Physical Activity Group. Available online: https://sites.google.com/site/theipaq/scoring-protocol (accessed on 1 June 2018).
68. Blue, C.L. Does the theory of planned behavior identify diabetes-related cognitions for intention to be physically active and eat a healthy diet? *Pub. Health Nurs.* **2007**, *24*, 141–150. [CrossRef]
69. Beyond Blue. Available online: https://www.beyondblue.org.au/the-facts/anxiety-and-depression-checklist-k10 (accessed on 1 June 2018).
70. Tan, L.S.; Khoo, E.Y.; Tan, C.S.; Griva, K.; Mohamed, A.; New, M.; Lee, Y.S.; Lee, J.; Tai, E.S.; Wee, H.L. Sensitivity of three widely used questionnaires. *Qual. Life Res.* **2015**, *24*, 153–162. [CrossRef] [PubMed]
71. Watanabe, T.; Berry, T.R.; Willows, N.D.; Bell, R.C. Assessing intentions to eat low-glycemic index foods by adults with diabetes using a new questionnaire based on the theory of planned behaviour. *Can. J. Diabetes* **2015**, *39*, 94–100. [CrossRef] [PubMed]
72. Gatt, S.; Sammut, R. An exploratory study of predictors of self-care behaviour in persons with type 2 diabetes. *Intern. J. Nursing Studies* **2008**, *45*, 1525–1533. [CrossRef] [PubMed]
73. Agborsangaya, C.B.; Gee, M.E.; Johnson, S.T.; Dunbar, P.; Langlois, M.F.; Leiter, L.A.; Pelletier, C.; Johnson, J.A. Determinants of lifestyle behavior in type 2 diabetes: Results of the 2011 cross-sectional survey on living with chronic diseases in Canada. *BMC Pub. Health* **2013**, *13*, 451. [CrossRef] [PubMed]
74. Diggle, P. *Analysis of Longitudinal Data*, 2nd ed.; Oxford University Press: New York, NY, USA, 2002.
75. Green, P.; MacLeod, C.J.; Nakagawa, S. SIMR: An R package for power analysis of generalized linear mixed models by simulation. *Methods Ecol. Evol.* **2016**, *7*, 493–498. [CrossRef]
76. Gill, J. *Bayesian Methods: A Social and Behavioral Sciences Approach*, 3rd ed.; CRC Press: Boca Raton, FL, USA, 2015.
77. Spiegelhalter, D.J.; Abrams, K.R.; Myles, J.P. *Bayesian Approaches to Clinical Trials and Health-Care Evaluation*, 1st ed.; John Wiley & Sons: Chichester, UK, 2004.
78. Ruspini, E. *Introduction to Longitudinal Research*, 1st ed.; Routledge: London, UK, 2002.

Reversing Type 2 Diabetes: A Narrative Review of the Evidence

Sarah J Hallberg [1,2,3,*], Victoria M Gershuni [4], Tamara L Hazbun [2,3] and Shaminie J Athinarayanan [1]

1 Virta Health, 535 Mission Street, San Francisco, CA 94105, USA; shaminie@virtahealth.com
2 Indiana University Health Arnett, Lafayette, IN 47904, USA; thazbun@iuhealth.org
3 Indiana University School of Medicine, Indianapolis, IN 46202, USA
4 Department of Surgery, Perelman School of Medicine University of Pennsylvania, Philadelphia, PA 19104, USA; victoriagershunimd@gmail.com
* Correspondence: sarah@virtahealth.com

Abstract: Background: Type 2 diabetes (T2D) has long been identified as an incurable chronic disease based on traditional means of treatment. Research now exists that suggests reversal is possible through other means that have only recently been embraced in the guidelines. This narrative review examines the evidence for T2D reversal using each of the three methods, including advantages and limitations for each. Methods: A literature search was performed, and a total of 99 original articles containing information pertaining to diabetes reversal or remission were included. Results: Evidence exists that T2D reversal is achievable using bariatric surgery, low-calorie diets (LCD), or carbohydrate restriction (LC). Bariatric surgery has been recommended for the treatment of T2D since 2016 by an international diabetes consensus group. Both the American Diabetes Association (ADA) and the European Association for the Study of Diabetes (EASD) now recommend a LC eating pattern and support the short-term use of LCD for weight loss. However, only T2D treatment, not reversal, is discussed in their guidelines. Conclusion: Given the state of evidence for T2D reversal, healthcare providers need to be educated on reversal options so they can actively engage in counseling patients who may desire this approach to their disease.

Keywords: diabetes; diabetes reversal; bariatric surgery; very-low-calorie; low-carbohydrate

---

1. Introduction

According to 2017 International Diabetes Federation (IDF) statistics, there are approximately 425 million people with diabetes worldwide [1]. In the United States, there are an estimated 30.3 million adults living with diabetes, and its prevalence has been rising rapidly, with at least 1.5 million new diabetes cases diagnosed each year [2]. Diabetes is a major public health epidemic despite recent advances in both pharmaceutical and technologic treatment options.

Type 2 diabetes (T2D) has long been identified as an incurable chronic disease. The best outcome that has been expected is amelioration of diabetes symptoms or slowing its inevitable progression. Approximately 50% of T2D patients will need insulin therapy within ten years of diagnosis [3] Although in the past diabetes has been called chronic and irreversible, the paradigm is changing [4,5].

The recent 2016 World Health Organization (WHO) global report on diabetes added a section on diabetes reversal and acknowledged that it can be achieved through weight loss and calorie restriction [4]. "Diabetes reversal" is a term that has found its way into scientific articles and the lay press alike; "remission" has also been used. While the exact criteria are still debated, most agree that a hemoglobin A1c (HbA1c) under the diabetes threshold of 6.5% for an extended period of time without the use of glycemic control medications would qualify [6]. Excluding metformin from the glycemic control medications list, as it has indications beyond diabetes, may also be a consideration [7,8]. Likewise, terms such as "partial" (HbA1c <6.5 without glycemic control medications for 1 year) or "complete" (HbA1c <5.7 without glycemic control medications for 1 year) remission have been defined by an expert panel as more evidence accumulates that points to the possibility of avoiding the presumably progressive nature of T2D [9]. It is important to note that the term "cure" has not been applied to T2D, as there does exist the potential for re-occurrence, which has been well documented in the literature.

Despite the growing evidence that reversal is possible, achieving reversal is not commonly encouraged by our healthcare system. In fact, reversal is not a goal in diabetes guidelines. Specific interventions aimed at reversal all have one thing in common: they are not first-line standard of care. This is important, because there is evidence suggesting that standard of care does not lead to diabetes reversal. This raises the question of whether standard of care is really the best practice. A large study by Kaiser Permanente found a diabetes remission rate of 0.23% with standard of care [10]. The status quo approach will not reverse the health crisis of diabetes.

A significant number of studies indicate that diabetes reversal is achievable using bariatric surgery, while other approaches, such as low-calorie diets (LCD) or carbohydrate restriction (LC), have also shown effectiveness in an increasing number of studies. This review will examine each of these approaches, identifying their beneficial effects, supporting evidence, drawbacks, and degree of sustainability.

2. Materials and Methods

A literature search was performed as appropriate for narrative reviews, including electronic databases of PubMed, EMBASE, and Google Scholar from 1970 through December 2018. We reviewed English-language original and review articles found under the subject headings diabetes, bariatric surgery, metabolic surgery, very low-calorie diet, calorie restriction, low carbohydrate diet, ketogenic diet, diabetes remission, and diabetes reversal. References of the identified publications were searched for more research articles to include in this review. Selected studies were reviewed and evaluated for eligibility for inclusion in this review based on their relevance for diabetes reversal and remission. Either remission or reversal needed to be discussed in the paper or the results were consistent with these terms for inclusion. Randomized clinical trials and intervention-based studies were given emphasis for inclusion.

A total of 99 original articles containing information pertaining to diabetes reversal or remission were included in this narrative review.

3. Results and Discussion

3.1. Bariatric Surgery

Bariatric surgery has long been recognized as a potential treatment for both morbid obesity and the metabolic processes that accompany it, specifically T2D. While the efficacy of T2D reversal depends on the choice of procedure, there is unilateral improvement in glycemia following operation [11], and bariatric surgery has been found to be superior to intensive T2D medical management. Accordingly, in 2016, the second Diabetes Surgery Summit (DSS-II) released recommendations, endorsed by 45 medical and scientific societies worldwide, to use bariatric surgery as a treatment for T2D (bariatric surgery is currently approved by the 2016 recommendations for adults with a body mass index (BMI) >40, or >35 kg/m^2 with obesity-related comorbidities) [12]. Of interest is the consistent finding that glycemic improvements occur rapidly, often within hours to days, and precede weight loss, which likely represents the enteroendocrine responses to altered flow of intestinal contents (i.e., bile acid signaling and changes in microbiota and their metabolome) [13–19].

The most commonly performed bariatric surgeries in the United States include laparoscopic and robotic Roux-en-Y Gastric Bypass (RYGB) or Sleeve Gastrectomy (SG). While surgical treatment is based on the principles of restriction and intestinal malabsorption, evidence suggests that there are more complex mechanisms at play. Bariatric surgery has consistently been shown to dramatically and rapidly improve blood glucose [20] while allowing decreased oral hypoglycemic medications and insulin use, effectively reversing diabetes in up to 80% of patients [21] in the short term. In addition to early post-operative improvement in blood glucose and insulin sensitivity, bariatric surgery has also been shown to cause alterations in GI hormone release, including ghrelin, leptin, cholecystokinin (CCK), peptide-tyrosine-tyrosine (PYY), and glucagon-like peptide 1 (GLP-1), that may impact feeding behavior via the gut–brain axis in addition to modulating euglycemia [22]. Furthermore, microbial changes in the human gut have been linked to obesity, and surgical alterations to gastrointestinal anatomy have been associated with dramatic changes in gut microbiota populations with reversion from an "obesogenic" to a lean bacterial population [13,14,16,19,23,24].

Long-term outcomes from bariatric surgery depend on multiple factors, including type of surgery performed, patient comorbidities, patient readiness for lifelong dietary change, and ongoing surveillance. While bariatric surgery has been demonstrated to be safe and effective overall, it is important to recognize that it is not without risks. Each patient must weigh the risks and benefits associated with untreated morbid obesity versus those associated with surgery or effective dietary management and choose accordingly. Surgery of any type can be associated with complications leading to morbidity or mortality; the complication rates have been stated to be as high as 13% and 21% for SG and RYGB, respectively. The postoperative mortality rate is 0.28–0.34% for SG and 0.35–0.79% for RYGB; in comparison, an elective laparoscopic cholecystectomy is associated with overall complication rates of 9.29% and with a 30-day mortality rate of 0.15–0.6%, depending on the series [25,26]. Significant complications include anastomotic leak or hemorrhage, post-operative readmission, need for reoperation, post-operative hypoglycemia, dumping syndrome, worsening acid reflux, marginal ulceration, and micronutrient deficiencies [25–29].

It is important to consider that while short-duration studies have shown early resolution of comorbidities following bariatric procedures, when followed for multiple decades, there may be decreased efficacy of disease resolution and increased incidence of hospital admission long-term. Long-term reversal of T2D and true glucose homeostasis remain uncertain. Weight loss after surgery is a significant predictor of a return to euglycemia post-operatively. Multiple studies have reported initial T2D remission rates as high as 80% [30,31], however, long-term remission is less durable. The five-year follow-up outcomes of the SLEEVEPASS RCT found complete or partial remission of T2D in 37% of SG and 45% of RYGB patients, which is similar to other studies showing long-term T2D remission in up to a third of patients [32]. In the large prospective cohort study Longitudinal Assessment of Bariatric Surgery 2 (LABS-2), the investigators found that long-term diabetes remission after RYGB was higher than predicted by weight loss alone, which suggests that the surgery itself impacts metabolic factors that contribute to disease management [31]. Similarly, the STAMPEDE trial—an RCT that followed 150 patients with T2D who were randomized to intensive medical intervention (IMT) versus IMT plus RYGB versus IMT plus SG for diabetes resolution (defined as HbA1c <6.0%) and followed for five years—revealed increased rates of T2D resolution with RYGB (29%) and SG (23%) compared to IMT alone (5%) (Figure 1). The surgery cohort also demonstrated greater weight loss and improvements in triglycerides, HDL, need for insulin, and overall quality of life [33–35].

Despite the likelihood of improved glycemic control, there are significant financial costs for the patient, health system, and insurance companies associated with bariatric surgery (U.S. average of $14,389) [36]. Despite the high initial cost of surgery, Pories and colleagues found that prior to surgery, patients spend over $10,000 per year on diabetes medications; after RYGB, the annual cost falls to less than $2000, which represents an $8000 cost savings at the individual level [30]. Furthermore, economic analyses show that surgery is likely to be cost-effective, especially in patients who are obese [37,38]. In a clinical effectiveness review of the literature that included 26 trials extracted from over 5000 references, Picot et al. found that bariatric surgery was a more effective intervention for weight loss than non-surgical options; however, there was extreme heterogeneity and questionable long-term adherence to the non-surgical interventions [39]. After surgery, metabolic syndrome improved, and there were higher rates of T2D remission compared to the non-surgical groups [39]. Further, while there were improvements in comorbidities after surgery independent of bariatric procedure, there was also an increased likelihood of adverse events. While the overall event rate remained low, major adverse events included medication intolerance, need for reoperation, infection, anastomotic leakage, and venous and thromboembolic events [39].

It is imperative to consider that one of the requirements of qualifying for bariatric surgery is demonstration of at least six months of unsuccessful attempts at weight loss using traditional dietary and exercise advice according to the 2016 Recommendations [12]. There are, however, no requirements as to what weight loss strategy is employed, which may represent a time point where dietary intervention, including low-calorie, ketogenic, or carbohydrate-restricted diets, should be utilized. At least two recent clinical trials have demonstrated safety and efficacy in pre-operative very low-carbohydrate ketogenic diets before bariatric surgery for increasing weight loss and decreasing liver volume [40,41].

Furthermore, despite technically adequate surgery, an alarming number of patients may still experience weight regain and/or recurrence of comorbid obesity-associated conditions. In these patients, effective strategies for dietary intervention are even more important. Approximately 10–15% of patients fail to lose adequate weight (failure defined as <50% of excess weight) or demonstrate significant weight regain after bariatric surgery without evidence of an anatomic or technical reason [42]. Additionally, in 25–35% of patients who undergo surgery, significant weight regain (defined as >15% of initial weight loss) occurs within two to five years post-operatively [43]. These patients often require further medical management with weight loss medications, further dietary and behavioral intervention, and, for some, reoperation. Reoperation can be for either revision for further weight loss (narrowing of the gastric sleeve, conversion of VSG to RYGB, and increasing the length of the roux limb) or reversal of RYGB due to health concerns, most commonly associated with malnutrition. A small cohort of patients (4%) may experience severe weight loss with significant malnutrition leading to hospitalization in over 50%, mortality rates of 18%, and need for reversal of RYGB anatomy. While the incidence of RYGB reversal is unknown, based upon a systematic review that included 100 patients spanning 1985–2015, the rate of reversal parallels the increasing rate of bariatric surgery [44].

In the short term, T2D reversal rates with surgery have been reported to be as high as 80%, with an additional 15% demonstrating partial improvement in T2D despite still requiring medication [17]. Within one week after RYGB, patients experience improved fasting hepatic insulin clearance, reduced basal de novo glucose production, and increased hepatic insulin sensitivity; by three months and one year after surgery, patients have improved beta-cell sensitivity to glucose, increased GLP-1 secretion from the gut, and improved insulin sensitivity in muscle and fat cells [45]. Over time, T2D remission rates remain high but do decline; Purnell and colleagues reported three-year remission rates of 68.7% after RYGB [29]. However, Pories published results from a 14-year prospective study with mean follow-up of 7.6 years, and found 10-year remission rates remained around 83% [46]. In a 10-year follow-up study of participants from the Swedish Obese Subjects (SOS) study that prospectively followed patients who underwent bariatric surgery, the authors reported a 72% (n = 342) and 36% (n = 118) recovery rate from T2D for RYGB at two years and 10 years, respectively [47].

The long-term metabolic impact and risk reduction from surgery remain high in a substantial number of patients and this route to reversal clearly has the most robust data to support its use. As evidenced by the dramatic improvements in metabolic state that precede weight loss, bariatric surgery is far more than merely a restrictive and/or malabsorptive procedure. Large shifts in bile acid signaling in the lumen of the small intestine, gut nutrient sensing, and changes in the microbiota community appear to greatly impact overall host health. Further research is ongoing using both basic and translational science models to identify the role of these various hormones and metabolites; perhaps there will be a way to one day harness the beneficial effects of bariatric surgery without the need for anatomic rearrangement.

3.2. Low-Calorie Diets (LCD)

As diabetes rates have risen to unprecedented levels [1,2], the number of studies examining diabetes reversal using non-surgical techniques has increased. A handful of studies have reported successful weight loss with decreased insulin resistance, plasma glucose, and medication use following a LCD. As early as 1976, Bistrian et al. [48] reported that a very low-calorie protein-sparing modified fast allowed for insulin elimination in all seven obese patients with T2D. The average time to insulin discontinuation was only 6.5 days, and the longest was 19 days. In a study by Bauman et al., a low-calorie diet of 900 kcal, including 115 g of protein, led to significant improvement in glycemic control that was mainly attributed to improvements in insulin sensitivity [49]. Furthermore, a study conducted in obese T2D patients found that a LCD and gastric bypass surgery were equally effective in achieving weight loss and improving glucose and HbA1c levels in the short term [50]. Weight loss, however, persisted in the diet-treated patients only for the first three months, indicating difficulty with long-term maintenance [47]. Similarly, other studies also reported similar pattern of early blood glucose normalization without medication use, but the improvements were not sustained long-term [51–53]. Likewise, the study by Wing et al., even though reported significant and greater improvements of HbA1c at 1 year in the intermittently delivered very low-calorie diet, the HbA1c improvement was not significantly different than what was reported in the patients receiving low-calorie diet (LCD) throughout the one year period [54]. Furthermore, the glycemic improvements observed at 1 year were not maintained through 2-years, even though the group with intermittent very low-calorie diet had less medication requirement than the group in the LCD arm at 2 years [54]. Lastly, micronutrient deficiencies with the use of calorie restricted diets has been shown and supplementation and monitoring for deficiencies is a consideration with their use [55,56].

While these previous studies were not assessing diabetes remission or reversal rate per se, they demonstrated the effectiveness of calorie restriction in achieving weight loss and improved glycemic control, which are the core goals of reversal. In 2003, the Look AHEAD trial randomized 5145 overweight or obese patients with T2D to an intervention group that received either an intensive lifestyle intervention (ILI) including calorie restriction and increased physical activity or to a control group that included diabetes support and education (DSE) [57]. Post hoc analysis of this study revealed that at one year, 11.5% of the participants in the ILI group achieved remission (partial or complete); however, remission rates subsequently decreased over time (9.2% at year two and 7.3% at year four). Nevertheless, the remission rates achieved through ILI were three to six times higher than those achieved in the DSE group. Lower baseline HbA1c, greater level of weight loss, shorter duration of T2D diagnosis, and lack of insulin use at baseline predicted higher remission rate in ILI participants [58].

Following the Look AHEAD study, other studies have evaluated a LCD for diabetes remission [59–61]. Most of these studies assessed remission over a short period of time in a small study sample. Bhatt et al. reported that six of the 12 individuals achieved partial remission at the end of the three-month intervention [61]. Ades et al. studied an intensive lifestyle program including calorie restriction and exercise, and reported that eight of the 10 individuals with recently diagnosed T2D achieved partial remission at six months, including one with complete remission [60]. The study ended at six months, therefore long term sustainability was not assessed. Another study assessing a one-year diabetes remission retrospectively among those undergoing 12 weeks of the intensive weight loss program "Why Wait" had a much lower remission rate of 4.5%, with 2.3% of them achieving partial remission, while another 2.3% had complete remission [59]. This study suggests that long-term maintenance of remission is a challenge. Moreover, diabetes remission was more likely reported in those who had a shorter diabetes duration, lower baseline HbA1c, and were taking fewer hypoglycemic medications [59,61].

An initial 2011 diabetes reversal study by Taylor and colleagues showed that a very low-calorie diet of 600 Kcal/day not only normalized glucose, HbA1c, and hepatic insulin sensitivity levels within a week, but also led to decreased hepatic and pancreatic triacylglycerol content and normalization of the insulin response within eight weeks [62]. At 12 weeks post-intervention, many of the improvements were maintained, but over a quarter of the patients had an early recurrence of diabetes. Further, average weight regain during the 12 weeks post-intervention was 20% [62]. As a follow-up to the 2011 study, the same group performed a larger and longer study with eight weeks of a very low-calorie meal replacement (624–700 kcal/day) followed by two weeks of solid food replacement and a weight maintenance program of up to six months [63]. In this study, those who achieved a fasting blood glucose of <7 mmol/L (<126 mg/dL) were categorized as responders, while others were categorized as non-responders. At six months, 40% of participants who initially responded to the intervention were still in T2D remission which was defined by achieving a fasting plasma glucose of <7mmol/L; the majority of those who remitted (60%) had a shorter diabetes duration (<4 years) [63].

These short-term studies were the foundation for a community-based cluster-randomized clinical trial called DiRECT (Diabetes Remission Clinical Trial). DiRECT enrolled a sample of 306 relatively healthy participants with T2D (people on insulin or with a diabetes duration longer than six years were excluded) [64] (Figure 1). They were cluster randomized to either standard diabetes care or an intervention using low-calorie meal replacement diet (825–853 kcal/day) for three to five months, followed by stepwise food re-introduction and a long-term weight maintenance program. At one-year follow-up, 46% of patients met the study criteria of diabetes remission (HbA1c <6.5% without antiglycemic medications) [64] and at two years the remission rate was 36% [65]. The DiRECT study has extended their follow-up an additional three years to assess the long-term impact on remission.

Taken together, evidence suggests that a LCD is effective in reversing diabetes in the short term up to two years, and its effectiveness was predominantly demonstrated in those with shorter duration since diabetes diagnosis. It is important to note that a substantial level of calorie restriction is needed to generate a sufficient level of weight loss for reversing diabetes. Short-term intervention with moderate energy restriction and metformin for modest weight loss was not as effective in reversing diabetes as compared to standard diabetes care [66]. Lifestyle intervention with severe energy restriction may have some deleterious effect on the body composition and physiology, which poses a concern for long-term health [67]. Furthermore, long-term achievement of diabetes remission, adherence to the diet, and weight loss maintenance after the diet remain a challenge. Studies have also suggested that physiological and metabolic adaptation of the body in response to caloric restriction may shift energy balance and hormonal regulation of weight toward weight regain after weight loss [67,68]. Thus, it is crucial that future studies are directed towards assessing the long-term sustainability of diabetes remission led by LCD and feasibility of this diet on the physiological adaptation and body composition changes.

3.3. *Carbohydrate-Restricted Diets (LC)*

Before the discovery of insulin in 1921, low carbohydrate (LC) diets were the most frequently prescribed treatment for diabetes [69,70]. The paradigm shifted both with the development of exogenous insulin and later with the emergence of the low-fat diet paradigm. A diet low in fat, which by default is high in carbohydrate, became the standard recommendation in guidelines around the globe [71]. Rather than preventing elevations in glucose, the goal became maintenance of blood sugar control via the increased use of glycemic control medications, including insulin [72]. Over the last decade, clinical studies have begun to resurrect the pre-insulin LC dietary approach. In response to the new evidence on the efficacy of carbohydrate restriction, low-carbohydrate has recently been endorsed as an eating pattern by the ADA and the European Association for the Study of Diabetes (EASD) [5,73]. In addition, the Veterans Affairs/Department of Defense (VA/DOD) guidelines now recommend carbohydrate restriction as low as 14% of energy intake in its most recent guidelines for treatment of diabetes (VA) [74].

LC diets are based on macronutrient changes rather than a focus on calorie restriction [75]. Although the exact definition varies, a low-carbohydrate diet usually restricts total carbohydrates to less than 130 grams per day, while a very low-carbohydrate or ketogenic diet usually restricts total carbohydrates to as low as 20–30 grams per day. Protein consumption is generally unchanged from a standard ADA diet (around 20% of intake), with the remaining energy needs met by fat from either the diet or mobilized body fat stores. Carbohydrate sources are primarily non-starchy vegetables with some nuts, dairy, and limited fruit [75].

A total of 32 separate trials examining carbohydrate restriction as a treatment for T2D were found when our search was performed [76–108]. However, for reasons that may include varied levels of carbohydrate restriction and differing levels of support given, not all studies had results that would be consistent with diabetes reversal. A number of shorter-term trials have found a significant between-group advantage of a low-carbohydrate intervention for T2D [80,84,92,97]. Data from longer-term trials are limited, and in some follow-up studies, the between-group advantage seen initially was lost or reduced, although it often remains significantly improved from baseline. This raises the question of long-term sustainability using this approach. Due to heterogeneity in methodology and definition of carbohydrate restriction, the ability to fully examine T2D reversal based on the existing studies is limited. Based upon a recent systematic review of LC, it appears that the greatest improvements in glycemic control and greatest medication reductions have been associated with the lowest carbohydrate intake [109]. In consideration of these limitations, it appears important to assess the level of carbohydrate restriction, support or other methods given to encourage sustainability, and length of follow-up.

A study comparing an ad libitum very low-carbohydrate (<20 g total) diet to an energy-restricted low-glycemic diet in T2D found greater reduction in HbA1c, weight, and insulin levels in the low-carbohydrate arm [89]. Additionally, 95% of participants in the low-carbohydrate arm reduced or eliminated glycemic control medications, compared to 62% in the low glycemic index arm at 24 weeks. Instruction was given in a one-time session with a dietician and included take-home materials for reference. A slightly longer study (34 weeks) trial [85] found that a very low-carbohydrate ketogenic diet intervention (20–50 g net carbs per day) resulted in HbA1c below the threshold for diabetes in 55% of the patients, compared to 0% of patients in the low-fat arm. The education sessions were all online and included behavior modification strategies and mindful eating which was aimed to address binge eating. New lessons were emailed to the patients weekly for the first 16 weeks and then every two weeks for the remainder of the study.

A small (34 participants) one-year study of an ad libitum, very low-carbohydrate diet compared to a calorie-restricted moderate carbohydrate diet found a significant reduction in HbA1c between groups favoring the low-carbohydrate arm [86]. At one year, 78% of participants who began the trial with a HbA1c above 6.5% no longer met the cutoff for the diagnosis of diabetes, no longer required any non-metformin medication, and significantly reduced or eliminated metformin. Total kilocalorie intake was not significantly different between the two groups, even with moderate carbohydrate restriction. Despite equal energy intake, the low carbohydrate group lost significantly more weight and had improved glycemic control, which indicates a potential mechanistic role for carbohydrate restriction itself. The support given was 19 classes over the 12-month period, tapering in frequency over time.

Another one-year trial [76] found significant HbA1c reduction in the subset of patients with diabetes (n = 54) assigned to an ad libitum low-carbohydrate diet (<30 total grams per day), compared to an energy-restricted low-fat diet. These results remained significant after adjusting the model for weight loss, indicating an effect of the carbohydrate reduction itself. The support given was four weekly sessions during the first month, followed by monthly sessions for the remaining 11 months.

A metabolic ward study on 10 patients with T2D [96] found that 24-h glucose curves normalized within two weeks on a very low-carbohydrate diet (<21 g total per day). This was in addition to medication reduction and elimination including insulin and sulfonylureas After accounting for body water changes, the average weight loss during the two-week period was 1.65 kg (average of <2% total body weight which is similar to the results of bariatric surgery, where normoglycemia is seen prior to significant weight loss. Interestingly, despite the diet being ad libitum other than the carbohydrate limit, the average energy intake decreased by 1000 kcal per day. Assuming no further change in glycemic control, HbA1c would be 5.6% after eight weeks, which would represent a reduction of 23%

from baseline. The fact that HbA1c reductions were greater than in other, longer-term outpatient studies may indicate that support of dietary changes is the key to longer-term success.

In our published trial providing significant support through the use of a continuous care intervention (CCI), we examined using a low-carbohydrate diet aimed at inducing nutritional ketosis in patients with T2D (n = 262), compared with usual care T2D patients (n = 87) [98] (Figure 1). At one year, the HbA1c decreased by 1.3% in the CCI, with 60% of completers achieving a HbA1c below 6.5% without hypoglycemic medication (not including metformin). Overall, medications were significantly reduced, including complete elimination of sulfonylureas and reduction or elimination of insulin therapy in 94% of users. Most cardiovascular risk factors showed significant improvement [110]. The one-year retention rate was 83%, which indicates that a non-calorie-restricted, low-carbohydrate intervention can be sustained. Improvements were not observed in the usual care patients. The newly released two-year results of this trial [106] show sustained improvements in normoglycemia, with 54% of completers maintaining HbA1c below 6.5% without medication or only on metformin. The retention rate at two years was 74%, further supporting the sustainability of this dietary intervention for diabetes reversal. Weight loss of 10% was seen at 2-years despite no intentional caloric restriction instruction. Additionally, this trial involved participants with a much longer duration of diabetes (8.4 years on average) than other nutrition trial interventions [58,64,65] and did not exclude anyone taking exogenous insulin. As duration of T2D and insulin use have both been identified to be negative factors in predicting remission after bariatric surgery [111,112], the 2-year results of this trial may be even more significant.

It is interesting to note that most studies utilize ad libitum intake in the carbohydrate-restricted arm. Despite this, in studies that have tracked energy intake, spontaneous calorie restriction has occurred [113,114]. In many trials where energy intake has been prescribed or weight loss has been equal, an advantage has been seen in glycemic control, weight, or both in the low-carbohydrate arm [86,91,107]. A better understanding of the role that caloric intake, whether prescribed or spontaneous, plays in the overall success is important. In cases of spontaneous energy intake reduction, elucidating the specific mechanism behind this reduction would help in the overall personalization of this approach.

Multiple studies have evaluated side effects or potential complications of carbohydrate restriction. The diet has been found to be safe and well tolerated although long term hard outcome data is lacking and should be a focus of future research. A transient rise in uric acid early in very low-carbohydrate restriction without an associated increase in gout or kidney stones has been documented [84,98,100]. Blood urea nitrogen (BUN) has been found to increase and decrease in different studies without an associated change in kidney function [87,98,100,115,116]. Recently, bone mineral density has been found to be unchanged despite significant weight loss after two years of a ketogenic diet intervention in patients with T2D [108]. While most studies show an improvement or no change in LDL-C levels in patients with T2D on a low-carbohydrate diet, there have been two studies that have found an increase in LDL-C in participants with T2D [99,111]. In one of the studies that found an increase in calculated LDL-C, a non-significant reduction in measured ApoB lipoproteins and unchanged non-HDL cholesterol were seen. Monitoring LDL-C or a measured value of potentially atherogenic lipoproteins such as ApoB should be considered. Lastly, micronutrient deficiency has been seen with a carbohydrate restricted diet, supplementation and monitoring should be given consideration with this intervention [56].

Although the use of very low-carbohydrate diets for diabetes reversal shows promising results, the lack of longer-term follow-up studies remains a limitation. Follow up is limited to two years, and therefore longer-term studies are needed to determine the sustainability of the metabolic improvements. Determining the appropriate method of support may be a key to the overall success with disease reversal.

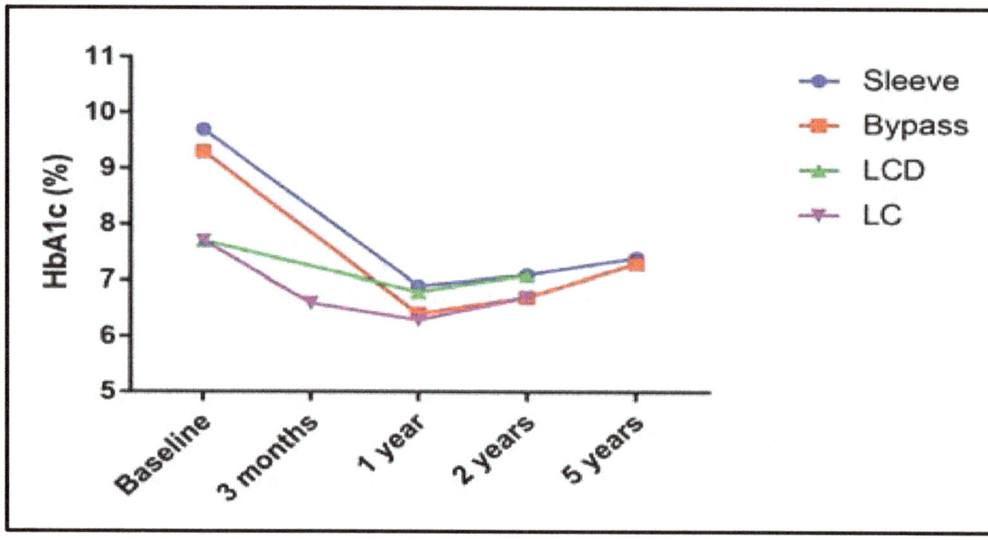

(A)

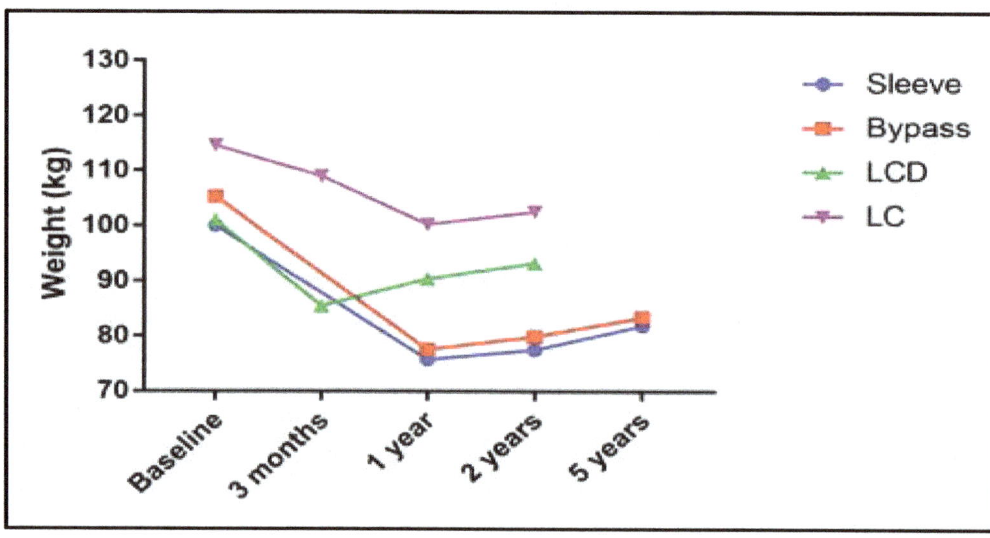

(B)

Figure 1. (**A**) Mean changes of hemoglobin A1c (HbA1c) from baseline to last published date for each study retrieved to represent the three methods of reversal; (**B**) mean changes of weight from baseline to last published date for each studies retrieved to represent the three methods of reversal. Note: We chose these three studies to represent the three methods of reversal based on publication date and relevance to diabetes reversal. Note that baseline characteristics differ. Surgery trial examined by sleeve gastrectomy and Roux-en-Y gastric bypass separately and were represented as sleeve and bypass in the graph. Surgery: STAMPEDE [34,35]. Low-calorie diets (LCD): DIRECT [65,66]; carbohydrate restriction (LC): IUH [99,107].

4. Summary

Additional evidence has become available in recent years suggesting that diabetes reversal is a possible alternative to consider in place of traditional diabetes treatment and management. In this paper, we provide a review of three methods that have been shown to successfully reverse type 2 diabetes. The current body of evidence suggests that bariatric surgery is the most effective method for overall efficacy and prolonged remission, even though concerns associated with surgical complications, treatment cost and complete lifestyle modification after surgery remain challenges for wide adoption of this approach. While both the LCD and LC dietary approaches are convincing for reversing diabetes in the short term (up to two years), long term maintenance of diabetes remission is still unproven. There are limited available data supporting long term maintenance of weight loss and its associated glycemic improvements in response to LCD; similarly, long-term adherence to a low carbohydrate diet will likely remain an obstacle without the development of proper patient education and optimal support for long-term behavioral change. Moreover, research in understanding the mechanism of diabetes reversibility in all three approaches and its overlapping mechanistic pathways are lacking; this is an area for future research emphasis.

There are similar identified negative predictors of remission for all three approaches. These factors include longer diabetes duration and increased severity, lower BMI, advanced age, poor glycemic control, and low C-peptide levels (indicating decreased endogenous insulin production) [117]. Further exploration into the heterogeneity of these factors will help personalize the approach, determine realistic goals for each patient, and should be considered during treatment discussions. Ongoing research into algorithm development will be helpful in this regard.

5. Conclusions

Overall, as a society we can no longer afford or tolerate the continued rising rates of diabetes. Despite many barriers within the healthcare system as a whole, providers are responsible on a daily basis for the lives of patients caught up in this unprecedented epidemic. The current standard of care may be suitable for some, but others would surely choose reversal if they understood there was a choice. The choice can only be offered if providers are not only aware that *reversal is possible* but have the education needed to review these options in a patient-centric discussion.

Author Contributions: Conceptualization, S.J.H. and S.J.A. Investigation, S.J.H., V.M.G., T.L.H., S.J.A. Writing—original draft, S.J.H., V.M.G., S.J.A. Writing—review and editing, S.J.H., V.M.G., T.L.H., S.J.A. All authors approved of the final manuscript.

Acknowledgments: We thank James McCarter and Stephen Phinney for their edits, which greatly improved the manuscript.

Abbreviations:

C	carbohydrate restriction
DSS-II	Diabetes Surgery Summit
RYGB	Roux-en-Y Gastric Bypass
SG	Sleeve Gastrectomy
CCK	cholecystokinin
PYY	peptide-tyrosine-tyrosine
GLP-1	glucagon-like peptide 1
LABS-2	Longitudinal Assessment of Bariatric Surgery 2
LCD	low-calorie diet
IMT	intensive medical intervention
DiRECT	Diabetes Remission Clinical Trial
ASD	European Association for the Study of Diabetes
VA/DOD	Veterans Affairs/Department of Defense

References

1. International Diabetes Federation. In *IDF Diabetes Atlas*, 8th ed.; International Diabetes Federation: Brussels, Belgium, 2017.
2. Centers for Disease Control and Prevention. National Diabetes Statistics Report, 2017. Available online: https://www.cdc.gov/diabetes/pdfs/data/statistics/national-diabetes-statistics-report.pd (accessed on 1 February 2019).

3. Home, P.; Riddle, M.; Cefalu, W.T.; Bailey, C.J.; Del Prato, S.; Leroith, D.; Schemthaner, G.; van Gaal, L.; Raz, I. Insulin therapy in people with Type 2 diabetes: Opportunities and challenges. *Diabetes Care* **2014**, *37*, 1499–1508. [CrossRef] [PubMed]
4. World Health Organization. Global Report on Diabetes. 2016. Available online: https://www.who.int/diabetes/publications/grd-2016/en/ (accessed on 1 February 2019).
5. Davies, M.J.; D'Alessio, D.A.; Fradkin, J.; Kernan, W.N.; Mathieu, C.; Mingrone, G.; Rossing, P.; Tsapas, A.; Wexler, D.J.; Buse, J.B. Management of hyperglycemia in Type 2 diabetes, 2018. A consensus report by the American Diabetes Association (ADA) and the European Association for the Study of Diabetes (EASD). *Diabetes Care* **2018**, *41*, 2669–2701. [CrossRef] [PubMed]
6. Ramos-Levi, A.M.; Cabrerizo, L.; Matia, P.; Sanchez-Pernaute, A.; Torres, A.J.; Rubio, M.A. Which criteria should be used to define type 2 diabetes remission after bariatric surgery. *BMC Surgery* **2013**, *13*, 8. [CrossRef] [PubMed]
7. Xiang, A.H.; Trigo, E.; Martinez, M.; Katkhouda, N.; Beale, E.; Wang, X.; Wu, J.; Chow, T.; Montgomery, C.; Nayak, K.S.; et al. Impact of gastric banding versus metformin on β-cell function in adults with impaired glucose tolerance or mild type 2 diabetes. *Diabetes Care* **2018**, *41*, 2544–2551. [CrossRef]
8. Diabetes Prevention Program Research Group. Long-term effects of metformin on diabetes prevention: Identification of subgroups that benefited most in the diabetes prevention program and diabetes prevention outcomes study. *Diabetes Care* **2019**, dc181970. [CrossRef]
9. Buse, J.B.; Caprio, S.; Cefalu, W.T.; Ceriello, A.; Del Prato, S.; Inzucchi, S.E.; McLaughlin, S.; Phillips, G.L., II; Robertson, R.P.; Rubino, F.; et al. How do we define cure of diabetes? *Diabetes Care* **2009**, *32*, 2133–2135. [CrossRef]
10. Karter, A.J.; Nundy, S.; Parker, M.M.; Moffet, H.H.; Huang, E.S. Incidence of remission in adults with Type 2 diabetes: The Diabetes & Aging Study. *Diabetes Care* **2014**, *37*, 3188–3195.
11. Steven, S.; Carey, P.E.; Small, P.K.; Taylor, R. Reversal of Type 2 diabetes after bariatric surgery is determined by the degree of achieved weight loss in both short- and long-duration diabetes. *Diabet Med.* **2015**, *32*, 47–53. [CrossRef] [PubMed]
12. Rubino, F.; Nathan, D.; Eckel, R.H.; Schauer, P.R.; Alberti, K.G.; Zimmet, P.Z.; Del Prato, S.; Ji, L.; Sadikot, S.M.; Herman, W.H.; et al. Delegates of the 2nd Diabetes Surgery Summit. Metabolic surgery in the treatment algorithm for type 2 diabetes: A joint statement by International Diabetes Organizations. *Diabetes Care* **2016**, *39*, 861–877. [CrossRef]
13. Anhe, F.F.; Varin, T.V.; Schertzer, J.D.; Marette, A. The Gut Microbiota as a Mediator of Metabolic Benefits after Bariatric Surgery. *Can. J. Diabetes* **2017**, *41*, 439–447. [CrossRef]
14. Medina, D.A.; Pedreros, J.P.; Turiel, D.; Quezada, N.; Pimentel, F.; Escalona, A.; Garrido, D. Distinct patterns in the gut microbiota after surgical or medical therapy in obese patients. *PeerJ* **2017**, *5*, e3443. [CrossRef]
15. Magouliotis, D.E.; Tasiopoulou, V.S.; Sioka, E.; Chatedaki, C.; Zacharoulis, D. Impact of Bariatric Surgery on Metabolic and Gut Microbiota Profile: A Systematic Review and Meta-analysis. *Obes. Surg.* **2017**, *27*, 1345–1357. [CrossRef]
16. Murphy, R.; Tsai, P.; Jullig, M.; Liu, A.; Plank, L.; Booth, M. Differential Changes in Gut Microbiota After Gastric Bypass and Sleeve Gastrectomy Bariatric Surgery Vary According to Diabetes Remission. *Obes. Surg.* **2017**, *27*, 917–925. [CrossRef] [PubMed]
17. Kaska, L.; Sledzinski, T.; Chomiczewska, A.; Dettlaff-Pokora, A.; Swierczynski, J. Improved glucose metabolism following bariatric surgery is associated with increased circulating bile acid concentrations and remodeling of the gut microbiome. *World J. Gastroenterol.* **2016**, *22*, 8698–8719. [CrossRef] [PubMed]
18. Penney, N.C.; Kinross, J.; Newton, R.C.; Purkayastha, S. The role of bile acids in reducing the metabolic complications of obesity after bariatric surgery: a systematic review. *Int. J. Obes. (Lond).* **2015**, *39*, 1565–1574. [CrossRef] [PubMed]
19. Sweeney, T.E.; Morton, J.M. The human gut microbiome: A review of the effect of obesity and surgically induced weight loss. *JAMA Surg.* **2013**, *148*, 563–569. [CrossRef]
20. Rubino, F.; Gagner, M. Potential of surgery for curing type 2 diabetes mellitus. *Ann. Surg.* **2002**, *236*, 554–559. [CrossRef]
21. Cohen, R.; Caravatto, P.P.; Correa, J.L.; Noujaim, P.; Petry, T.Z.; Salles, J.E.; Schiavon, C.A. Glycemic control after stomach-sparing duodenal-jejunal bypass surgery in diabetic patients with low body mass index. *Surg. Obes. Relat. Dis.* **2012**, *8*, 375–380. [CrossRef]

22. Federico, A.; Dallio, M.; Tolone, S.; Gravina, A.G.; Patrone, V.; Romano, M.; Tuccillo, C.; Mozzillo, A.L.; Amoroso, V.; Misso, G.; et al. Gastrointestinal Hormones, Intestinal Microbiota and Metabolic Homeostasis in Obese Patients: Effect of Bariatric Surgery. *In Vivo* **2016**, *30*, 321–330.
23. Peat, C.M.; Kleiman, S.C.; Bulik, C.M.; Carroll, I.M. The Intestinal Microbiome in Bariatric Surgery Patients. *Eur. Eat. Disord. Rev.* **2015**, *23*, 496–503. [CrossRef] [PubMed]
24. Sweeney, T.E.; Morton, J.M. Metabolic surgery: Action via hormonal milieu changes, changes in bile acids or gut microbiota? A summary of the literature. *Best Pract. Res. Clin. Gastroenterol.* **2014**, *28*, 727–740. [CrossRef]
25. Ma, I.T.; Madura, J.A. Gastrointestinal Complications after Bariatric Surgery. *Gastroenterol. Hepatol. (N Y).* **2015**, *11*, 526–535.
26. Rubino, F.; Schauer, P.R.; Kaplan, L.M.; Cummings, D.E. Metabolic surgery to treat type 2 diabetes: Clinical outcome and mechanisms of action. *Annu. Rev. Med.* **2010**, *61*, 393–411. [CrossRef] [PubMed]
27. Abraham, A.; Ikramuddin, S.; Jahansouz, C.; Arafat, F.; Hevelone, N.; Leslie, D. Trends in bariatric surgery: Procedure selection, revisional surgeries, and readmissions. *Obes. Surg.* **2016**, *26*, 1371–1377. [CrossRef] [PubMed]
28. Tack, J.; Deloose, E. Complications of bariatric surgery: Dumping syndrome, reflux and vitamin deficiencies. *Best Prac. Res. Clin. Gastroenterol.* **2014**, *28*, 741–749. [CrossRef] [PubMed]
29. Eisenbarg, D.; Azagury, D.E.; Ghiassi, S.; Grover, B.T.; Ki, J.J. ASMBS position statement on postprandial hyperinsulinemic hypoglycemia after bariatric surgery. *Surg. Obes. Relat. Dis.* **2017**, *13*, 371–378. [CrossRef]
30. Pories, W.J.; Mehaffey, J.H.; Staton, K.M. The surgical treatment of type two diabetes mellitus. *Surg Clin. N. Am.* **2011**, *91*, 821–836. [CrossRef]
31. Purnell, J.Q.; Selzer, F.; Wahed, A.S.; Pender, J.; Pories, W.; Pomp, A.; Dakin, G.; Mitchell, J.; Garcia, L.; Staten, M.A.; et al. Type 2 Diabetes Remission Rates After Laparoscopic Gastric Bypass and Gastric Banding: Results of the Longitudinal Assessment of Bariatric Surgery Study. *Diabetes Care* **2016**, *39*, 1101–1107. [CrossRef] [PubMed]
32. Salminen, P.; Helmio, M.; Ovaska, J.; Juuti, A.; Leivonen, M.; Peromaa-Haavista, P.; Hurme, S.; Soinio, M.; Nuutila, P.; Victorzon, M. Effect of laparoscopic sleeve gastrectomy vs. laparoscopic Roux-en-Y gastric bypass on weight loss at 5 years among patients with morbid obesity: The SLEEVEPASS randomized clinical trial. *JAMA* **2018**, *319*, 241–254. [CrossRef] [PubMed]
33. Schauer, P.R.; Kashyap, S.R.; Wolski, K.; Brethauer, S.A.; Kirwan, J.P.; Pothier, C.E.; Thomas, S.; Abood, B.; Nissen, S.E.; Bhatt, D.L. Bariatric surgery versus medical therapy in obese patients with diabetes. *N. Engl. J. Med.* **2012**, *366*, 1567–1576. [CrossRef]
34. Kashyap, S.R.; Bhatt, D.L.; Wolski, K.; Watanabe, R.M.; Abdul-Ghani, M.; Abood, B.; Pothier, C.E.; Brethauer, S.; Nissen, S.; Gupta, M.; et al. Metabolic effects of bariatric surgery in patients with moderate obesity and type 2 diabetes: Analysis of a randomized control trial comparing surgery with intensive medical treatment. *Diabetes Care* **2013**, *36*, 2175–2182. [CrossRef] [PubMed]
35. Schauer, P.R.; Bhatt, D.L.; Kirwan, J.P.; Wolski, K.; Aminian, A.; Brethauer, S.A.; Navaneethan, S.D.; Singh, R.P.; Pothier, C.E.; Nissen, S.E.; et al. Bariatric surgery versus intensive medical therapy for diabetes: 5-year outcomes. *N. Engl. J. Med.* **2017**, *376*, 641–651. [CrossRef] [PubMed]
36. Doble, B.; Wordsworth, S.; Rogers, C.A.; Welbourn, R.; Byrne, J.; Blazeby, J.M.; By-Band-Sleeve Trial Management Group. What are the real procedural costs of bariatric surgery? A systematic literature review of published cost analyses. *Obes. Surg.* **2017**, *27*, 2179–2192. [CrossRef] [PubMed]
37. Warren, J.A.; Ewing, J.A.; Hale, A.L.; Blackhurst, D.W.; Bour, E.S.; Scott, J.D. Cost-effectiveness of bariatric surgery: Increasing the economic viability of the most effective treatment for type II diabetes mellitus. *Am. Surgeon.* **2015**, *81*, 807–811.
38. Klein, S.; Ghosh, A.; Cremieux, P.Y.; Eapen, S.; McGavock, T.J. Economic impact of the clinical benefits of bariatric surgery in diabetes patients with BMI ≥ 35kg/m^2. *Obesity* **2011**, *19*, 581–587. [CrossRef] [PubMed]
39. Picot, J.; Jones, J.; Colquitt, J.L.; Gospodarevskaya, E.; Loveman, E.; Baxter, L.; Clegg, A.J. The clinical effectiveness and cost-effectiveness of bariatric (weight loss) surgery for obesity: A systematic review and economic evaluation. *Health Technol. Assess.* **2009**, *13*, 1–190. [CrossRef]
40. Schiavo, L.; Pilone, V.; Rossetti, G.; Barbarisi, A.; Cesaretti, M.; Iannelli, A. A 4-Week Preoperative Ketogenic Micronutrient-Enriched Diet Is Effective in Reducing Body Weight, Left Hepatic Lobe Volume, and Micronutrient Deficiencies in Patients Undergoing Bariatric Surgery: A Prospective Pilot Study. *Obes. Surg.* **2018**, *28*, 2215–2224. [CrossRef]

41. Leonetti, F.; Campanile, F.C.; Coccia, F.; Capoccia, D.; Alessandroni, L.; Puzziello, A.; Coluzzi, I.; Silecchia, G. Very low-carbohydrate ketogenic diet before bariatric surgery: Prospective evaluation of a sequential diet. *Obes. Surg.* **2015**, *25*, 64–71. [CrossRef]
42. Gumbs, A.A.; Pomp, A.; Gagner, M. Revisional bariatric surgery for inadequate weight loss. *Obes. Surg.* **2007**, *17*, 1137–1145. [CrossRef]
43. Velapati, S.R.; Shah, M.; Kuchkuntla, A.R.; Abu-Dayyeh, B.; Grothe, K.; Hurt, R.T.; Mundi, M.S. Weight Regain After Bariatric Surgery: Prevalence, Etiology, and Treatment. *Curr. Nutr. Rep.* **2018**, *7*, 329–334. [CrossRef] [PubMed]
44. Shoar, S.; Nguyen, T.; Ona, M.A.; Reddy, M.; Anand, S.; Alkuwari, M.J.; Saber, A.A. Roux-end-Y gastric bypass reversal: A systematic review. *Surg. Obes. Relat. Dis.* **2016**, *12*, 1366–1372. [CrossRef]
45. Bojsen-Moller, K.N. Mechanisms of improved glycemic control after Roux-en-Y gastric bypass. *Dan. Med. J.* **2015**, *62*, B5057. [PubMed]
46. Pories, W.J.; Swanson, M.S.; MacDonald, K.G.; Long, S.B.; Morris, P.G.; Brown, B.M.; Barakat, H.A.; de Ramon, R.A.; Israel, G.; Dolezal, J.M. Who would have thought it? An operation proves to be the most effective therapy for adult-onset diabetes mellitus. *Ann. Surg.* **1995**, *222*, 339–350. [CrossRef]
47. Sjostrom, L.; Lindroos, A.K.; Peltonen, M.; Torgerson, J.; Bouchard, C.; Carlsson, B.; Dahlgren, S.; Larsson, B.; Narbro, K.; Sjostrom, D.; et al. Lifestyle, diabetes and cardiovascular risk factors 10 years after bariatric surgery. *N. Engl. J. Med.* **2004**, *351*, 2683–2693. [CrossRef] [PubMed]
48. Bistrian, B.R.; Blackburn, G.L.; Flatt, J.P.; Sizer, J.; Scrimshaw, N.S.; Sherman, M. Nitrogen metabolism and insulin requirements in obese diabetic adults on a protein-sparing modified fast. *Diabetes* **1976**, *25*, 494–504. [CrossRef] [PubMed]
49. Bauman, W.A.; Schwartz, E.; Rose, H.G.; Eisenstein, H.N.; Johnson, D.W. Early and long term effects of acute caloric deprivation in obese diabetic patients. *Am. J. Med.* **1988**, *85*, 38–46. [CrossRef]
50. Hughes, T.A.; Gwynne, J.T.; Switzer, B.R.; Herbst, C.; White, G. Effects of caloric restriction and weight loss on glycemic control, insulin release and resistance, and atherosclerotic risk in obese patients with type II diabetes mellitus. *Am. J. Med.* **1984**, *77*, 7–17. [CrossRef]
51. Hammer, S.; Snel, M.; Lamb, H.J.; Jazet, I.M.; van der Meer, R.W.; Pijl, H.; Meinders, E.A.; Romijn, J.A.; de Roos, A.; Smit, J.W. Prolonged caloric restriction in obese patients with type 2 diabetes mellitus decreases myocardial triglyceride content and improves myocardial function. *J. Am. Coll. Cardiol.* **2008**, *52*, 1006–1012. [CrossRef]
52. Snel, M.; Jonker, J.T.; Hammer, S.; Kerpershoek, G.; Lamb, H.J.; Meinders, A.E.; Pijl, H.; de Roos, A.; Romijn, J.A.; Smit, J.W.A. Long-term beneficial effect of a 16-week very low calorie diet on pericardial fat in obese type 2 diabetes mellitus patients. *Obesity* **2012**, *20*, 1572–1576. [CrossRef]
53. Paisey, R.B.; Harvey, P.; Rice, S.; Belka, I.; Bower, L.; Dunn, M.; Taylor, P.; Paisey, R.M. An intensive weight loss programme in established type 2 diabetes and controls: Effect on weight and atherosclerosis risk factors at 1 year. *Diabet. Med.* **1998**, *15*, 73–79. [CrossRef]
54. Wing, R.R.; Blair, E.; Marcus, M.; Epstein, L.H.; Harvey, J. Year-long weight loss treatment for obese patients with type II diabetes: Does including an intermittent very-low-calorie diet improve outcome? *Am. J. Med.* **1994**, *97*, 354–362. [CrossRef]
55. Damms-Machado, A.; Weser, G.; Bischoff, SC. Micronutrient deficiency in obese subjects undergoing low calorie diet. *Nutr. J.* **2012**, 11. [CrossRef] [PubMed]
56. Gardner, C.D.; Kim, S.; Bersamin, A.; Dopler-Nelson, M.; Otten, J.; Oelrich, B.; Cherin, R. Micronutrient quality of weight-loss diets that focus on macronutrients: Results from the A to Z study. *Am. J. Clin. Nutr.* **2010**, *92*, 304–312. [CrossRef] [PubMed]
57. Ryan, D.H.; Espeland, M.A.; Foster, G.D.; Haffner, S.M.; Hubbard, V.S.; Johnson, K.C.; Kahn, S.E.; Knowler, W.C.; Yanovski, S.Z.; Look AHEAD Research Group. Look AHEAD (Action for Health in Diabetes): Design and methods for a clinical trial of weight loss for the prevention of cardiovascular disease in type 2 diabetes. *Control Clin Trials.* **2003**, *24*, 610–628. [PubMed]
58. Gregg, E.W.; Chen, H.; Wagenknecht, L.E.; Clark, J.M.; Delahanty, L.M.; Bantle, J.; Pownall, H.J.; Johnson, K.C.; Safford, M.M.; Kitabchi, A.E.; et al. Association of an intensive lifestyle intervention with remission of type 2 diabetes. *JAMA.* **2012**, *308*, 2489–2496. [CrossRef] [PubMed]
59. Mottalib, A.; Sakr, M.; Shehabeldin, M.; Hamdy, O. Diabetes remission after nonsurgical intensive lifestyle intervention in obese patients with Type 2 diabetes. *J. Diabetes Res.* **2015**, 468704. [CrossRef]

60. Ades, P.A.; Savage, P.D.; Marney, A.M.; Harvey, J.; Evans, K.A. Remission of recently diagnosed type 2 diabetes mellitus with weight loss and exercise. *J. Cardiopulm. Rehabil. Prev.* **2015**, *35*, 193–197. [CrossRef] [PubMed]
61. Bhatt, A.A.; Choudhari, P.K.; Mahajan, R.R.; Sayyad, M.G.; Pratyush, D.D.; Hasan, I.; Javherani, R.S.; Bothale, M.M.; Purandare, V.B.; Unnikrishnan, A.G. Effect of a low-calorie diet on restoration of normoglycemia in obese subjects with Type 2 diabetes. *Indian J. Endocrinol. Metab.* **2017**, *21*, 776–780. [PubMed]
62. Lim, E.L.; Hollingsworth, K.G.; Aribisala, B.S.; Chen, M.J.; Mathers, J.C.; Taylor, R. Reversal of type 2 diabetes: Normalisation of beta cell function in association with decreased pancreas and liver triacylglycerol. *Diabetol* **2011**, *54*, 2506–2514. [CrossRef]
63. Steven, S.; Hollingsworth, K.G.; Al-Mrabeh, A.; Avery, L.; Aribisala, B.; Caslake, M.; Taylor, R. Very low-calorie diet and 6 months of weight stability in type 2 diabetes: Pathophysiological changes in responders and nonresponders. *Diabetes Care* **2016**, *39*, 808–815. [CrossRef]
64. Lean, M.J.; Leslie, W.S.; Barnes, A.C.; Brosnahan, N.; Thom, G.; McCombie, L.; Peters, C.; Zhyzhneuskaya, S.; Al-Mrabeh, A.; Hollingsworth, K.G.; et al. Primary care-led weight management for remission of type 2 diabetes (DiRECT): An open-label, cluster-randomised trial. *Lancet.* **2018**, *391*, 541–551. [CrossRef]
65. Lean, M.E.J.; Leslie, W.S.; Barnes, A.C.; Brosnahan, N.; Thom, G.; McCombie, L.; Peters, C.; Zhyzhneuskaya, S.; Al-Mrabeh, A.; Hollingsworth, K.G.; et al. Durability of a primary care-led weight-management intervention for remission of type 2 diabetes: 2-year results of the DiRECT open-label, cluster-randomised trial. *Lancet Diabetes Endocrinol.* 2019. [CrossRef]
66. McInnes, N.; Smith, A.; Otto, R.; Vandermey, J.; Punthakee, Z.; Sherifali, D.; Balasubramaniam, K.; Hall, S.; Gerstein, HC. Piloting a remission strategy in type 2 diabetes: Results of a randomized controlled trial. *J. Clin. Endocrinol. Metab.* **2017**, *102*, 1596–1605. [CrossRef]
67. Fothergill, E.; Guo, J.; Howard, L.; Kerns, J.C.; Knuth, N.D.; Brychta, R.; Chen, K.Y.; Skarulis, M.C.; Walter, M.; Walter, P.J.; et al. Persistent metabolic adaptation 6 years after "The Biggest Loser" competition. *Obesity* **2016**, *24*, 1612–1619. [CrossRef] [PubMed]
68. Greenway, F.L. Physiological adaptations to weight loss and factors favouring weight regain. *Int. J. Obes.* **2015**, *39*, 1188–1196. [CrossRef]
69. Campbell, W.R. Dietetic treatment in diabetes mellitus. *Can. Med. Assoc. J.* **1923**, *13*, 487–492. [PubMed]
70. Westman, E.C.; Yancy, W.S.; Humphreys, M. Dietary treatment of diabetes mellitus in the pre-insulin era (1914–1922). *Perspect. Biol. Med.* **2006**, *49*, 77–83. [CrossRef]
71. Arky, R.; Wylie-Rosett, J.; El-Beheri, B. Examination of current dietary recommendations for individuals with diabetes mellitus. *Diabetes Care* **1982**, *5*, 59–63. [CrossRef]
72. Anderson, J.W.; Geil, P.B. New perspectives in nutrition management of diabetes mellitus. *Am. J. Med.* **1988**, *85*, 159–165. [CrossRef]
73. American Diabetes Association. Summary of Revisions: Standards of Medical Care in Diabetes-2019. *Diabetes Care* **2019**, *42*, S4–S6.
74. Department of Veteran Affairs and Department of Defense. VA/DoD Clinical Practice Guideline for the Management of Type 2 Diabetes Mellitus in Primary Care. Version 5.0. Available online: https://www.healthquality.va.gov/guidelines/cd/diabetes/ (accessed on 20 January 2019).
75. Westman, E.C.; Feinman, R.D.; Mavropoulos, J.C.; Vernon, M.C.; Volek, J.S.; Wortman, J.A.; Yancy, W.S.; Phinney, S.D. Low carbohydrate nutrition and metabolism. *Am. J. Clin. Nutr.* **2007**, *86*, 276–284. [CrossRef] [PubMed]
76. Stern, L.; Iqbal, N.; Seshadri, P.; Chicano, K.L.; Daily, D.A.; McGrory, J.; Williams, M.; Gracely, E.J.; Samaha, F.F. The effects of low-carbohydrate versus conventional weight loss diets in severely obese adults: One-year follow-up of a randomized trial. *Ann. Intern. Med.* **2004**, *140*, 778–785. [CrossRef]
77. Miyashita, Y.; Koide, N.; Ohtsuka, M.; Ozaki, H.; Itoh, Y.; Oyama, T.; Uetake, T.; Ariga, K.; Shirai, K. Beneficial effect of low carbohydrate in low calorie diets on visceral fat reduction in type 2 diabetic patients with obesity. *Diabetes Res. Clin. Pract.* **2004**, *65*, 235–241. [CrossRef] [PubMed]
78. Jönsson, T.; Granfeldt, Y.; Ahren, B.; Branell, U.C.; Pålsson, G.; Hansson, A.; Söderström, M.; Lindeberg, S. Beneficial effects of a Paleolithic diet on cardiovascular risk factors in type 2 diabetes: A randomized cross-over pilot study. *Cardiovasc. Diabetol.* **2009**, *8*, 3. [CrossRef] [PubMed]

79. Davis, N.J.; Tomuta, N.; Schechter, C.; Isasi, C.R.; Segal-Isaacson, C.J.; Stein, D.; Zonszein, J.; Wylie-Rosett, J. Comparative study of the effects of a 1-year dietary intervention of a low- carbohydrate diet versus a low-fat diet on weight and glycemic control in type 2 diabetes. *Diabetes Care* **2009**, *32*, 1147–1152. [CrossRef]
80. Daly, M.E.; Paisey, R.; Paisey, R.; Millward, B.A.; Eccles, C.; Williams, K.; Hammersley, S.; MacLeod, K.M.; Gale, T.J. Short-term effects of severe dietary carbohydrate-restriction advice in type 2 diabetes: A randomized controlled trial. *Diabet. Med.* **2006**, *23*, 15–20. [CrossRef]
81. Dyson, P.A.; Beatty, S.; Matthews, D.R. A low-carbohydrate diet is more effective in reducing body weight than healthy eating in both diabetic and non-diabetic subjects. *Diabet. Med.* **2007**, *24*, 1430–1435. [CrossRef]
82. Wolever, T.M.; Gibbs, A.L.; Mehling, C.; Chiasson, J.L.; Connelly, P.W.; Josse, R.G.; Leiter, L.A.; Maheux, P.; Rabasa-Lhoret, R.; Rodger, N.W.; et al. The Canadian trial of carbohydrates in diabetes (CCD), a 1-yr controlled of low-glycemic index dietary carbohydrate in type 2 diabetes: No effect on glycated hemoglobin but reduction in C-reactive protein. *Am. J. Clin. Nutr.* **2008**, *87*, 114–125. [CrossRef] [PubMed]
83. Iqbal, N.; Vetter, M.L.; Moore, R.H.; Chittams, J.L.; Dalton-Bakes, C.V.; Dowd, M.; Williams-Smith, C.; Cardillo, S.; Wadden, T.A. Effects of a low-intensity intervention that prescribed a low-carbohydrate vs. a low-fat diet in obese, diabetic participants. *Obesity (Silver Spring)* **2010**, *18*, 1733–1738. [CrossRef] [PubMed]
84. Goday, A.; Bellido, D.; Sajoux, I.; Crujeiras, A.B.; Burguera, B.; García-Luna, P.P.; Casanueva, F.F. Short-term safety, tolerability and efficacy of a very low-calorie ketogenic diet interventional weight loss program versus hypocaloric diet in patients with type 2 diabetes mellitus. *Nutr. Diabetes.* **2016**, *6*, e230. [CrossRef]
85. Saslow, L.R.; Mason, A.E.; Kim, S.; Goldman, V.; Ploutz-Snyder, R.; Bayandorian, H.; Daubenmier, J.; Hecht, F.M.; Moskowitz, J.T. An online intervention comparing a very low-carbohydrate ketogenic diet and lifestyle recommendations versus a plate method diet in overweight individuals with type 2 diabetes: A randomized controlled trial. *J. Med. Int. Res.* **2017**, *19*, e36. [CrossRef] [PubMed]
86. Saslow, L.R.; Daubenmier, J.J.; Moskowitz, J.T.; Kim, S.; Murphy, E.J.; Phinney, S.D.; Ploutz-Snyder, R.; Goldman, V.; Cox, R.M.; Mason, A.E.; et al. Twelve-month outcomes of a randomized trial of a moderate-carbohydrate versus very low-carbohydrate diet in overweight adults with type 2 diabetes mellitus or prediabetes. *Nutr. Diabetes.* **2017**, *7*, 304. [CrossRef]
87. Yamada, Y.; Uchida, J.; Izumi, H.; Tsukamoto, Y.; Inoue, G.; Watanabe, Y.; Irie, J.; Yamada, S. A non-calorie-restricted low-carbohydrate diet is effective as an alternative therapy for patients with type 2 diabetes. *Int. Med.* **2014**, *53*, 13–19. [CrossRef]
88. Guldbrand, H.; Dizdar, B.; Bunjaku, B.; Lindström, T.; Bachrach-Lindström, M.; Fredrikson, M.; Östgren, C.J.; Nystrom, F.H. In type 2 diabetes, randomisation to advice to follow a low-carbohydrate diet transiently improves glycaemic control compared with advice to follow a low-fat diet producing a similar weight loss. *Diabetologi.* **2012**, *55*, 2118–2127. [CrossRef]
89. Westman, E.C.; Yancy, W.S.; Mavropoulos, J.C.; Marquart, M.; McDuffie, J.R. The effect of a low-carbohydrate, ketogenic diet versus a low-glycemic index diet on glycemic control in type 2 diabetes mellitus. *Nutr. Metab.* **2008**, *19*, 36. [CrossRef]
90. Haimoto, H.; Iwata, M.; Wakai, K.; Umegaki, H. Long-term effects of a diet loosely restricting carbohydrates on HbA1c levels, BMI and tapering of sulfonylureas in type 2 diabetes: A 2-year follow-up study. *Diabetes Res. Clin. Pract.* **2008**, *79*, 350–356. [CrossRef] [PubMed]
91. Tay, J.; Thompson, C.H.; Luscombe-Marsh, N.D.; Wycherley, T.P.; Noakes, M.; Buckley, J.D.; Wittert, G.A.; Yancy, W.S., Jr.; Brinkworth, G.D. Effects of an energy-restricted low-carbohydrate, high unsaturated fat/low saturated fat diet versus a high-carbohydrate, low-fat diet in type 2 diabetes: A 2-year randomized clinical trial. *Diabetes Obes. Metab.* **2018**, *20*, 858–871. [CrossRef] [PubMed]
92. Wang, L.L.; Wang, Q.; Hong, Y.; Ojo, O.; Jiang, Q.; Hou, Y.Y.; Huang, Y.-H.; Wang, X.H. The effect of low-carbohydrate diet on glycemic control in patients with type 2 diabetes mellitus. *Nutrients* **2018**, *10*, 661. [CrossRef] [PubMed]
93. Larsen, R.N.; Mann, N.J.; Maclean, E.; Shaw, J.E. The effect of high-protein, low-carbohydrate diets in the treatment of type 2 diabetes: A 12 month randomised controlled trial. *Diabetologia* **2011**, *54*, 731–740. [CrossRef] [PubMed]
94. Sato, J.; Kanazawa, A.; Makita, S.; Hatae, C.; Komiya, K.; Shimizu, T.; Ikeda, F.; Tamura, Y.; Ogihara, T.; Mita, T.; et al. A randomized controlled trial of 130g/day low-carbohydrate diet in type 2 diabetes with poor glycemic control. *Clin. Nutr.* **2017**, *36*, 992–1000. [CrossRef]

95. Sanada, M.; Kabe, C.; Hata, H.; Uchida, J.; Inoue, G.; Tsukamoto, Y.; Yamada, Y.; Irie, J.; Tabata, S.; Tabata, M.; et al. Efficacy of a moderately low carbohydrate diet in a 36-month observational study of Japanese patients with Type 2 diabetes. *Nutrients* **2018**, *10*, 528. [CrossRef] [PubMed]

96. Boden, G.; Sargrad, K.; Homko, C.; Mozzoli, M.; Stein, T.P. Effect of a low carbohydrate diet on appetite, blood glucose levels, and insulin resistance in obese patients with type 2 diabetes. *Ann. Intern. Med.* **2005**, *142*, 403–411. [CrossRef] [PubMed]

97. Gannon, M.C.; Nuttall, F.Q. Effect of a high-protein, low-carbohydrate diet on blood glucose control in people with type 2 diabetes. *Diabetes* **2004**, *53*, 2375–2382. [CrossRef] [PubMed]

98. Hallberg, S.J.; McKenzie, A.L.; Williams, P.T.; Bhanpuri, N.H.; Peters, A.L.; Campbell, W.W.; Hazbun, T.L.; Volk, B.M.; McCarter, J.P.; Phinney, S.D.; et al. Effectiveness and safety of a novel care model for the management of type 2 diabetes at 1 year: An open-label, non-randomized, controlled study. *Diabetes Ther.* **2018**, *9*, 583–612. [CrossRef] [PubMed]

99. Krebs, J.D.; Bell, D.; Hall, R.; Parry-Strong, A.; Docherty, P.D.; Clarke, K.; Chase, J.G. Improvements in glucose metabolism and insulin sensitivity with a low-carbohydrate diet in obese patients with type 2 diabetes. *J. Am. Coll. Nutr.* **2013**, *32*, 11–17. [CrossRef] [PubMed]

100. Hussain, T.A.; Matthew, T.C.; Dashti, A.A.; Asfar, S.; Al-Zaid, N.; Dashti, H.M. Effect of low-calorie versus low-carbohydrate ketogenic diet in type 2 diabetes. *Nutrition* **2012**, *28*, 1016–1021. [CrossRef]

101. Sasakabe, T.; Haimoto, H.; Umegaki, H.; Wakai, K. Effects of a moderate low-carbohydrate diet on preferential abdominal fat loss and cardiovascular risk factors in patients with type 2 diabetes. *Diabetes Metab. Syndr. Obes.* **2011**, *4*, 167–174. [CrossRef] [PubMed]

102. Nielsen, J.V.; Joensson, E.A. Low carbohydrate diet in type 2 diabetes: Stable improvement of bodyweight and glycemic control during 44 months follow-up. *Nutr. Metab.* **2008**, *5*, 14. [CrossRef] [PubMed]

103. Dashti, H.M.; Mathew, T.C.; Khadada, M.; Al-Mousawi, M.; Talib, H.; Asfar, S.K.; Behbahani, A.I.; Al-Zaid, N.S. Beneficial effects of ketogenic diet in obese diabetic subjects. *Mol. Cell Biochem.* **2007**, *302*, 249–256. [CrossRef] [PubMed]

104. Yancy, W.S.; Foy, M.; Chalecki, A.M.; Vernon, A.C.; Westman, E.C. A low carbohydrate, ketogenic diet to treat type 2 diabetes. *Nutr. Metab.* **2005**, *2*, 34. [CrossRef] [PubMed]

105. Dashti, H.M.; Mathew, T.C.; Hussein, T.; Asfar, S.K.; Behbahani, A.; Khoursheed, M.A.; Al-Sayer, H.M.; Bo-Abbas, Y.Y.; Al-Zaid, N.S. Long-term effects of a ketogenic diet in obese patients. *Exp. Clin. Cardiol.* **2004**, *9*, 200–205.

106. Shai, I.; Schwarzfuchs, D.; Henkin, Y.; Shahar, D.R.; Witkow, S.; Greenberg, I.; Golan, R.; Fraser, D.; Bolotin, A.; Vardi, H.; et al. Weight loss with a low-carbohydrate, Mediterranean, or low-fat diet. *N. Engl. J. Med.* **2008**, *359*, 229–241. [CrossRef] [PubMed]

107. Elhayany, A.; Lustman, A.; Abel, R.; Attal-Singer, J.; Vinker, S. A low carbohydrate Mediterranean diet improves cardiovascular risk factors and diabetes control among overweight patients with type 2 diabetes mellitus: A 1-year prospective randomized intervention study. *Diabetes Obes. Metab.* **2010**, *12*, 204–209. [CrossRef]

108. Athinarayanan, S.J.; Adams, R.N.; Hallberg, S.J.; McKenzie, A.L.; Bhanpuri, N.H.; Campbell, W.W.; Volek, J.S.; Phinney, S.D.; McCarter, J.P. Long-term effects of a novel continuous remote care intervention including nutritional ketosis for the management of type 2 diabetes: A 2-year non-randomized clinical trial. *bioRxiv* **2018**, *476275*. [CrossRef]

109. Snorgaard, O.; Poulsen, G.M.; Andersen, H.K.; Astrup, A. Systematic review and meta-analysis of dietary carbohydrate restriction in patients with type 2 diabetes. *BMJ Open Diabetes Res. Care.* **2017**, *5*, e000354. [CrossRef] [PubMed]

110. Bhanpuri, N.H.; Hallberg, S.J.; Williams, P.T.; McKenzie, A.L.; Ballard, K.D.; Campbell, W.W.; McCarter, J.P.; Phinney, S.D.; Volek, J.S. Cardiovascular disease risk factor responses to a type 2 diabetes care model including nutritional ketosis induced by sustained carbohydrate restriction at one year: An open label, non-randomized, controlled study. *Cardiovasc. Diabetol.* **2018**, *17*, 56. [CrossRef]

111. Wang, G.F.; Yan, Y.X.; Yin, D.; Hui, Y.; Zhang, J.P.; Han, G.J.; Ma, N.; Wu, Y.; Xu, J.Z.; Yang, T. Predictive factors of Type 2 diabetes mellitus remission following bariatric surgery: A Meta-analysis. *Obes. Surg.* **2015**, *25*, 199–208. [CrossRef]

112. Yan, W.; Bai, R.; Li, Y.; Xu, J.; Zhong, Z.; Xing, Y.; Yan, M.; Lin, Y.; Song, M. Analysis of predictors of type 2 diabetes mellitus remission after roux-en-Y gastric bypass in 101 Chinese patients. *Obes. Surg.* **2019**. [CrossRef]
113. Brehm, B.J.; Seeley, R.J.; Daniels, S.R.; D'Alessio, D.A. A Randomized Trial Comparing a Very Low Carbohydrate Diet and a Calorie-Restricted Low Fat Diet on Body Weight and Cardiovascular Risk Factors in Healthy Women. *J. Clin. Endocrinol. Metab.* **2003**, *88*, 1617–1623. [CrossRef]
114. Nordmann, A.J.; Nordmann, A.; Briel, M.; Keller, U.; Yancy, W.S.; Brehm, B.J.; Bucher, H.C. Effects of a low-carbohydrate vs. low-fat diets on weight loss and cardiovascular risk factors. *Arch. Intern. Med.* **2006**, *166*, 285–293. [CrossRef] [PubMed]
115. Westman, E.C.; Yancy, W.S.; Edman, J.S.; Tomlin, K.F.; Perkins, CE. Effect of 6-month adherence to a very low carbohydrate diet program. *Am. J. Med.* **2002**, *113*, 30–36. [CrossRef]
116. Nuttall, F.Q.; Gannon, M.C. The metabolic response to a high-protein, low-carbohydrate diet in men with type 2 diabetes mellitus. *Metabolism* **2006**, *55*, 243–251. [CrossRef] [PubMed]
117. Min, T.; Barry, J.D.; Stephens, J.W. Predicting the Resolution of Type 2 Diabetes after Bariatric Surgical Procedures: A Concise Review. *J. Diabetes Metab.* **2015**, *6*, 617.

12

The Effects of a Low GI Diet on Cardiometabolic and Inflammatory Parameters in Patients with Type 2 and Gestational Diabetes

Omorogieva Ojo [1,*], Osarhumwese Osaretin Ojo [2], Xiao-Hua Wang [3] and Amanda Rodrigues Amorim Adegboye [4]

1 Faculty of Education and Health, Department of Adult Nursing and Paramedic Science, University of Greenwich, London SE9 2UG, UK
2 South London and Maudsley NHS Foundation Trust, University Hospital, Lewisham High Street, London SE13 6LH, UK
3 The School of Nursing, Soochow University, Suzhou 215006, China
4 Faculty of Education and Health, Department of Psychology, Social Work & Counselling, University of Greenwich, London SE9 2UG, UK
* Correspondence: o.ojo@greenwich.ac.uk

Abstract: The prevalence of diabetes is increasing globally, and its effect on patients and the healthcare system can be significant. Gestational diabetes mellitus (GDM) and type 2 diabetes are well established risk factors for cardiovascular disease, and strategies for managing these conditions include dietary interventions, such as the use of a low glycemic index (GI) diet. Aims: This review aimed to evaluate the effects of a low GI diet on the cardio-metabolic and inflammatory parameters in patients with type 2 diabetes and women with GDM and assess whether the effects are different in these conditions. Methods: This review was based on the preferred reporting items for systematic reviews and meta-analyses (PRISMA) guidelines. Three databases (EMBASE, Pubmed, and PsycINFO) were searched from inception to 20 February 2019 using search terms that included synonyms and Medical Subject Headings (MeSH) in line with the population, intervention, comparator, outcomes, and studies (PICOS) framework. Studies were evaluated for the quality and risk of bias. Results: 10 randomised controlled studies were included in the systematic review, while 9 were selected for the meta-analysis. Two distinct areas were identified: the effect of a low GI diet on lipid profile and the effect of a low GI diet on inflammatory parameters. The results of the meta-analysis showed that there were no significant differences ($p > 0.05$) between the low GI and higher GI diets with respect to total cholesterol, HDL, and LDL cholesterol in patients with type 2 diabetes. However, there was a significant difference ($p = 0.027$) with respect to triglyceride which increased by a mean of 0.06 mmol/L (0.01, 0.11) in patients with type 2 diabetes on higher GI diet. With respect to the women with GDM, the findings from the systematic review were not consistent in terms of the effect of a low GI diet on the lipid profile. The results of the meta-analysis did not show significant differences ($p > 0.05$) between low GI and higher GI diets with respect to adiponectin and C-reactive proteins in patients with type 2 diabetes, but a significant difference ($p < 0.001$) was observed between the two groups in relation to interleukin–6. Conclusion: This systematic review and meta-analysis have demonstrated that there were no significant differences ($p > 0.05$) between the low GI and higher GI diets in relation to total cholesterol—HDL and LDL cholesterol—in patients with type 2 diabetes. However, a significant difference ($p < 0.05$) was observed between the two groups with respect to triglyceride in patients with type 2 diabetes. The results of the effect of a low GI diet on the lipid profile in patients with GDM were not consistent. With respect to the inflammatory parameters, the low GI diet significantly decreased interleukin–6 in patients with type 2 diabetes compared to the higher GI diet. More studies are needed in this area of research.

Keywords: type 2 diabetes; gestational diabetes; glycemic index; randomised controlled trial; lipid profile; inflammatory parameters

---

1. Introduction

Globally, there is an increasing prevalence of diabetes, with over 420 million people living with the condition. This number has significant implications for health care provisions due to the impact of diabetes and its complications on those who have the condition [1,2]. Type 2 diabetes is usually characterised by insulin deficiency due to beta cell dysfunction and often involves insulin resistance [3]. On the other hand, hyperglycaemia first detected at any time during pregnancy is classified either as diabetes in pregnancy or Gestational Diabetes Mellitus (GDM), and are usually diagnosed based on the fasting and/or 2 h plasma glucose following a 75 g oral glucose load [4].

Both type 2 diabetes and GDM have implications for carbohydrate, protein and fat metabolism and may predispose individuals to acute and long-term complications [5]. About half of the women diagnosed with GDM proceed to develop type 2 diabetes within 5 to 10 years after giving birth [6]. Due to changing lifestyles, type 2 diabetes is increasingly diagnosed in children [7]. In 2013, over 3.2 million adults were diagnosed with diabetes in England and Wales, with prevalence rates of 6% and 6.7% in England and Wales, respectively [7]. In addition, about 90% of adults who are currently diagnosed with diabetes have type 2 diabetes, with the burden of the disease disproportionally affecting ethnic minorities, particularly Africans, African-Caribbeans, and South Asians [7].

GDM presents adverse risks to the mother and child during the pre- and post–natal period [4]. It was estimated that 21.3 million live births had some form of raised blood glucose or hyperglycaemia in 2017, and about 85.1% of these were due to GDM [6]. This represented about one in every seven births affected by GDM [6]. In England and Wales, of the estimated 700,000 women who give birth every year, about 5% have either pre-existing diabetes or GDM [8]. About 87.5% of these women who have diabetes during pregnancy have GDM [8]. Therefore, management strategies, including dietary interventions such as the use of a low glycemic index (GI) diet, have been recommended instead of a higher GI diet, in order to manage hyperglycaemia and mitigate related complications [8]. In our previous review on the effect of a low GI diet in patients with type 2 diabetes, Ojo et al. [9] found that a low GI diet was more effective in controlling glycated haemoglobin and fasting blood glucose compared with a higher GI diet in these patients. Therefore, this current review builds on the earlier systematic review and meta-analysis [9] by assessing the impact of a low GI diet on lipid profile and inflammatory markers.

Why is it important to do this review? GDM is closely associated with type 2 diabetes, as they share many key pathophysiological characteristics including progressive insulin resistance [3,10]. In addition, people who develop either type 2 diabetes or GDM have similar risk factors, such as ethnicity (South Asian or Afro–Caribbean), a high body mass index (BMI), family history, and advanced age [5,10].

Although low grade inflammation and insulin resistance are part of normal physiological adaptation of pregnancy, these processes are exacerbated in patients with GDM and obesity [11]. Elevated levels of inflammatory components, such as tumour necrosis factor alpha (TNF-α), have been shown to correlate with progressive insulin resistance in pregnancy and are associated with hyperinsulinaemia in obesity and in patients with type 2 diabetes [10]. The risks associated with GDM, including postpartum type 2 diabetes, increase with progressive hyperglycaemia [8,12]. Furthermore, both GDM and type 2 diabetes are well established risk factors for cardiovascular diseases [3,5,13].

This calls for scrutiny and a greater understanding of the role of low GI diets on inflammatory parameters and lipid profiles (cardiometabolic parameters) in these patients, as the biomarkers have implications for insulin resistance and cardiovascular mortality. We know this based on the knowledge that dietary interventions are useful approaches to managing type 2 diabetes and GDM.

Therefore, a study should involve an evaluation of the effect, and quality and quantity of the macro and micronutrients in the foods consumed. Of particular interest is the quality of carbohydrate in the diets of people with type 2 diabetes or GDM, often linked to its glycemic index (GI). Foods with low GI may improve glycemic control including the reduction in glycated haemoglobin (HbA1c) through improvement in peripheral insulin sensitivity [14–19]. However, the evidence regarding the effect of a low GI diet on lipid profiles is still conflicting.

Bouchie et al. [20] revealed that 5 weeks of a low GI diet was useful in improving plasma lipids in non-diabetic men who were moderately overweight. However, in normolipidemic well controlled patients with type 2 diabetes, Brand et al. [21] observed that low GI diets did not provide improvement in plasma lipids. Clar et al. [22], in their meta–analysis, noted that there is, presently, no compelling evidence that shows that low GI diets have significant beneficial effects on blood lipids. On the other hand, Schwingshacki and Hoffman [23] demonstrated that a low GI diet has beneficial effects with respect to pro–inflammatory markers, such as C–reactive protein (CRP) which may be useful in preventing obesity associated diseases. This study involved both patients who had type 2 diabetes and participants who were non–diabetic. The systematic reviews by Goff et al. [13], Clar et al. [22], and Fleming and Godwin [24] were based on assessing the effect of low GI diets on lipid profiles on either general participants or those with cardiovascular diseases. No previous review has assessed the effect of a low GI diet on both lipids and the inflammatory profile of patients with type 2 diabetes and/or GDM. Therefore, the current review evaluates the impact of a low GI diet on the cardio-metabolic and inflammatory parameters in patients with type 2 diabetes and GDM. This is based on the understanding that the control of cardio-metabolic parameters is a useful approach in managing patients with type 2 diabetes and women with GDM [4,25].

Objectives:

This is a systematic review and meta-analysis which:

- Evaluates the effect of a low GI diet on cardio-metabolic and inflammatory parameters in patients with type 2 diabetes and women with GDM.

2. Methods

This systematic review and meta-analysis was written according to the preferred reporting items for systematic reviews and meta-analyses (PRISMA) guidelines [26]. The eligibility criteria for paper inclusion according to type of study, participants, intervention, and outcomes are described below.

Types of Studies:

Randomised controlled studies were the only studies included in this review (Tables 1 and 2).

Type of Participants:

Patients with type 2 diabetes or pregnant women with gestational diabetes were the participants of interest in all the studies selected (Table 2).

Type of Interventions:

Diets with low GI were compared with diets with higher GI in patients with type 2 diabetes and in women with GDM. The classification of diets as having either low GI or higher GI was based on the lower GI values of the intervention diets (low GI diet).

2.1. Outcomes of Interest

The primary measures of interest were:

- Cardio-metabolic parameters: total cholesterol (TC) mmol/L, low density lipoprotein (LDL) cholesterol mmol/L, high density lipoprotein (HDL) cholesterol mmol/L, and triglycerides (TG) mmol/L.

The secondary outcome measures were:

- Inflammatory parameters: C–reactive protein (CRP) mg/L, Adiponectin mg/L, and Interleukin–6 (IL-6) mg/L.

2.2. Search Terms and Search Strategy

The process of searching for articles for this review relied on the Population, Intervention, Comparator, Outcome, and Study design (PICOS) approach [27] and involved electronic databases (EMBASE, Pubmed, and PsycINFO) from inception to 20 February 2019. A number of articles were identified through this process by using search terms, including Medical Subject Headings (MeSH) and synonyms. Boolean operators (AND/OR) were used to combine words and search terms (Table 1). The reference lists of included articles were manually searched for relevant papers.

2.3. Inclusion and Exclusion Criteria

The criteria for selecting studies are outlined in Table 2. No time or language restriction was applied. Only primary research studies that were randomised controlled trials were selected for this review. In addition, studies involving patients with type 2 diabetes or GDM and the use of low GI diets across the world were included. Those studies not meeting the criteria set out in Table 2 and the text were excluded from this review. In this regard, studies that had animals, patients with type 1 diabetes, children with diabetes, or healthy adults without diabetes were excluded from the current review (Table 2). In addition, observational studies and those involving dietary supplements were excluded. Therefore, a total of 9 studies were included in the meta-analysis (Figure 1).

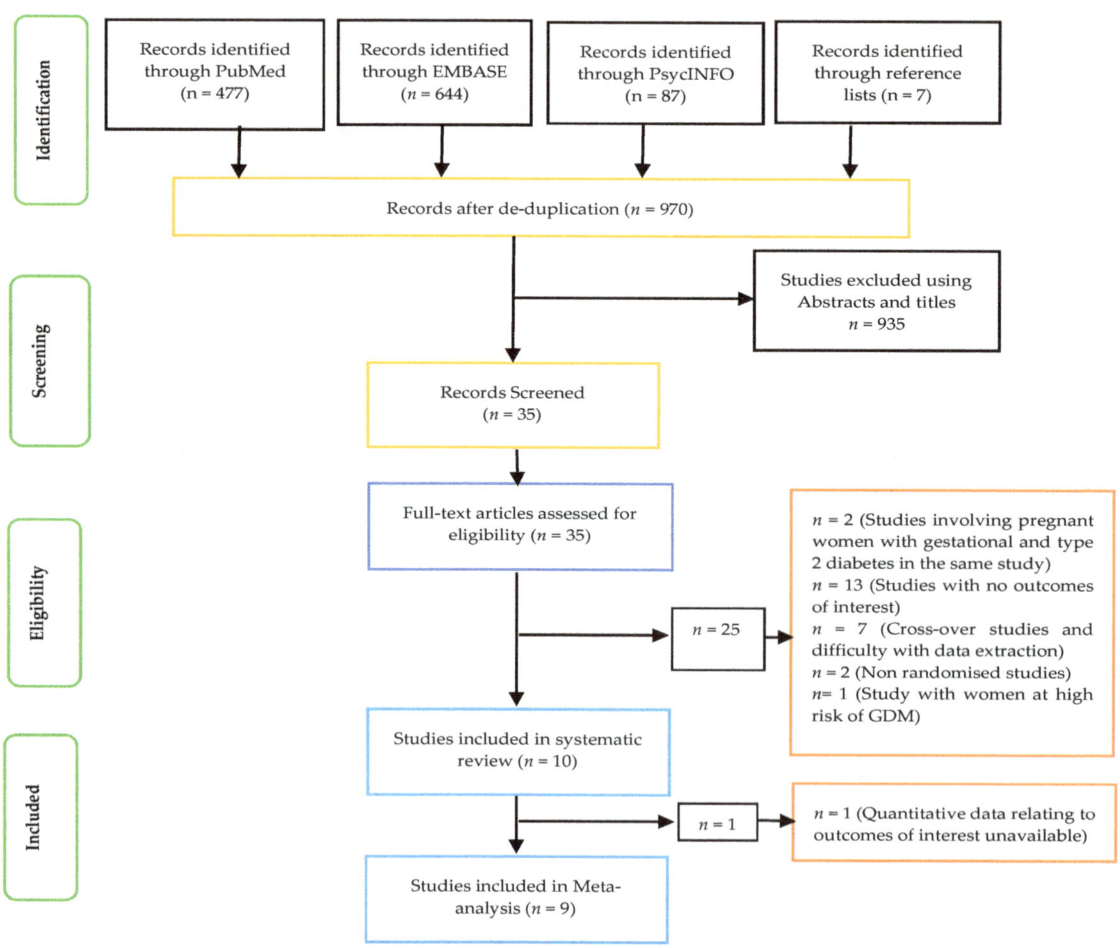

Figure 1. Prisma flow chart showing the studies included.

Table 1. Search Strategy and Search Terms.

Population	Intervention	Comparator	Study Designs	Combining Search Terms
Patients with Diabetes	**Low Glycemic Index (GI) Diet**	**Higher GI Diet**	**Randomised Controlled Trial**	
Type 2 diabetes OR diabetes OR Patients with diabetes OR diabetes mellitus OR Gestational diabetes OR gestational diabetes mellitus (GDM) OR gestational diabetes mellitus OR diabetes mellitus, gestational OR diabetes in pregnancy	GI diet OR glycemic index OR Glycemic Index Numbers OR glycemic load OR Glycemic Indices OR Glycemic Index Number		#1 Controlled clinical trial OR Randomised controlled trial OR placebo OR randomized OR groups OR drug therapy OR randomly OR trial #2 "Animals" NOT "Humans" #3 #1 NOT #2	Column 1 AND Column 2 AND Column 3

Table 2. Inclusion and Exclusion Criteria Based on PICOS Framework.

	Inclusion Criteria	Exclusion Criteria
Population	Patients with gestational diabetes or patients with type 2 diabetes	Studies involving participants with type 1 diabetes and animal studies. Studies that include children that have diabetes or adults that are healthy. Pre-existing diabetes in patients who are pregnant
Intervention	Low GI diet	Studies involving dietary supplements
Comparator	higher GI diet	Studies involving additional supplements
Outcomes	Primary outcome measures of interest: Cardio-metabolic: total cholesterol, low density lipoprotein (LDL) cholesterol, high density lipoprotein (HDL) cholesterol, triglycerides. Secondary outcome measures of interest: Inflammatory parameters: C–reactive protein, Adiponectin and Interleukin–6	Qualitative outcomes
Types of Study: Quantitative	Randomised controlled trials	Observational studies Letters Comments Reviews Editorials

2.4. *Quality Assessment and Risk of Bias of Included Studies*

The Critical Appraisal Skills Programme (CASP) checklist for randomised controlled trials [28] was used to evaluate the studies. In addition, the Cochrane risk of bias tool [29,30] was used to assess the methodological quality of the included studies. A grade (or score) was allocated to each trial on the basis of selection bias, performance bias, detection bias, attrition bias, and reporting bias. This process involved reviewing details about the similarity at baseline of the groups being compared, the blindness of the outcome measurement and participants, the randomisation method, dropout rates, selective reporting, and compliance with the intervention. On the basis of this information, studies were categorised into three groups: (a) low risk of bias, (b) unclear risk of bias, and (c) high risk of bias.

2.5. *Data Extraction and Management*

Statistical Analysis

Treatment effects were summarized as the weighted mean difference (WMD) with standard deviation by using the absolute change values from baseline to post-intervention for control and intervention groups. The meta-analysis was performed in stata (version 15.0, Stata Corp, College Station, TX, USA). Fixed-effects models were applied to estimate the overall weighted mean difference.

All results were presented with a 95% confidence interval (CI) and displayed on a forest plot and table, and the null hypothesis of no effect was rejected at $p \leq 0.05$. In addition to the forest plots, I^2 statistics were assessed to quantify the degree of heterogeneity. Values <25% were considered to be low, 25%–50% moderate, and >50% high. *Q* statistics was also used to assess heterogeneity. The null hypothesis of homogeneity was rejected if $p < 0.1$, given the low power of the test [29].

2.6. *Data Inclusion Decisions*

Gomes et al. [31] expressed their results as the median and interquartile ranges, which were converted to means and standard deviations [29]. In addition, for the meta-analysis, the units of measurements for the lipid parameters were converted to mmol/L, while for the inflammatory markers, they were converted to mg/L. The Grant et al. [32] study was not included in the meta-analysis, as the information provided showed that there were no significant differences ($p > 0.05$) between the low GI and the higher GI groups in terms of lipids and inflammatory markers. However, these results were not expressed in quantitative terms.

3. Results

Ten studies were selected for the systematic review (Table 3), and nine studies were included in the meta-analysis (Table 4). In addition, while four of the studies were conducted in Canada, two were carried out in China and one study each was carried out in Brazil, Greece, Malaysia, and the USA.The total number of subjects in the eight studies included in the meta-analysis in patients with type 2 diabetes involved 394 participants in the low GI group and 388 participants in the higher GI group. There were 41 subjects in the low GI group compared with 42 participants in the higher GI group in the only study on women with GDM.

Based on the systematic review (Tables 3 and 4) and meta-analysis, two distinct areas have been identified: the effect of a low GI diet on lipid profiles and the effect of a low GI diet on inflammatory parameters.

Table 3. The summary of studies selected for the review.

Citation	Country	Type of Diabetes	Length of Study	Study Type	Age (Years)	Sample Size	Interventions/Glycemic Index (GI) Values	Results/Conclusion
Gomes et al. [31]	Brazil	Type 2 diabetes	1 month	Parallel Design	42.4 ± 5.1	$n = 20$	Low GI diet v. higher GI diet (Mean ± SD) Baseline Higher GI: 66 ± 4 Low GI: 63 ± 6 Post-intervention Higher GI: 72 ± 3 Low GI: 54 ± 4	Serum non esterified fatty acid level increased in the higher GI group compared to the low GI group after intervention ($p = 0.032$). Low GI diet prevented the inflammatory responses induced by higher GI diet.
Grant et al. [32]	Canada	GDM	From 28 weeks gestation until delivery	Parallel Design	Higher GI: 34 ± 1.1 Low GI: 34 ± 0.1	Low GI: $n = 23$ Higher GI: $n = 24$	Higher GI v. Low GI (Mean ± SD) Higher GI: 58 ± 0.5 Low GI: 49 ± 0.8	The difference between the low GI and higher GI groups in respect of lipids and CRP were not statistically significant ($p > 0.05$).
Ma et al. [33]	China	GDM	12–14 Weeks	Parallel Design	Higher GI: 30.0 ± 3.5 Low GI: 30.1 ± 3.8 $p = 0.901$	Higher GI: $n = 42$ Low GL: $n = 41$	Higher GI v. Low GI (Mean ± SD) Baseline Higher GI: 56.1 ± 2.4 Low GI: 56.0 ± 2.1 Post-intervention Higher GI: 53.8 ± 2.5 Low GI: 50.1 ± 2.2	The increases in TC, TG and the decrease in HDL cholesterol were significantly lower ($p < 0.05$) in the low GI group compared with the higher GI group.
Jenkins et al. [34]	Canada	Type 2 diabetes	6 months	Parallel Design	(Mean ± SD) High-cereal fibre diet = 61 ± 9 Low-GI diet = 60 ± 10	210	Low GI diet v. high-cereal fibre diet Mean (95% CI) Baseline Higher GI: 81.5 (80.4–82.7) Low GI: 80.8 (79.6–82.0) Post-intervention Higher GI: 83.5 (82.4–84.7) Low GI: 69.6 (67.7–71.4)	HDL cholesterol increased by 1.7 mg/dL in the low GI group and decreased by −0.2 mg/dL in the higher GI group ($p = 0.005$). Reductions of the CRP were similar in the low GI and higher GI groups.
Jenkins et al. [35]	Canada	Type 2 diabetes	3 months	Parallel Design	(Mean±SEM) High-wheat fibre diet: 61 ± 1.0 Low-GI legume diet: 58 ± 1.3	121	Low GI legume diet v. high-wheat fibre diet Mean (95% CI) Baseline Higher GI: 78 (77–80) Low GI: 80 (79–82) Post-intervention Higher GI: 82 (81–83) Low GI: 66 (64–67)	Low GI legume produced significant decreases in TC ($p < 0.001$) and TG ($p < 0.001$) with no significant change in HDL cholesterol ($p = 0.19$). The relative reduction in TC and HDL cholesterol were greater in the low GI legume diet group compared with the higher GI diet group. No other lipid treatment differences were significant.

Table 3. *Cont.*

Citation	Country	Type of Diabetes	Length of Study	Study Type	Age (Years)	Sample Size	Interventions/Glycemic Index (GI) Values	Results/Conclusion
Ma et al. [36]	USA	Type 2 diabetes	12 months	Parallel Design	(Mean ± SD) 53.53 ± 8.40	40	Low GI diet v. American Diabetes Association diet (ADA) (Mean ± SEM) Baseline ADA: 82.03 ± 1.31 Low GI: 79.35 ± 1.36 Post-intervention ADA: 80.36 ± 1.40 Low GI: 76.64 ± 1.46	There were no significant differences between low GI and higher GI groups with respect to TC, HDL and TG.
Wolever et al. [37]	Canada	Type 2 diabetes	12 months	Parallel Design	(Mean ± SEM) Higher GI diet: 60.4 ± 1.1 Low GI diet: 60.6 ± 1.0	162	Low GI diet v. higher GI diet (Mean ± SEM) Baseline Higher GI: 61.5 ± 0.4 Low GI: 60.3 ± 0.4 Post-intervention Higher GI: 63.2 ± 0.4 Low GI: 55.1 ± 0.4	There were no significant effects for TC. With the low GI diet, mean triacylglycerol was 12% higher, HDL was 4% lower, the higher GI values were intermediate. The CRP with the low GI diet was 29% less than the higher GI diet ($p < 0.05$).
Yusof et al. [38]	Malaysia	Type 2 diabetes	12 weeks	Parallel Design	Not data	104	Low GI diet v. conventional carbohydrate exchange (CCE) (Mean ± SD) Baseline Higher GI: 64 ± 6 Low GI: 63 ± 5 Post-intervention Higher GI: 64 ± 5 Low GI: 57 ± 6	TG increased at week 4, then decreased at week 12 in the Low GI group and this was reversed in the CCE group. Serum HDL cholesterol increased significantly in both groups over time, although no significant differences were found between the two groups.
Argiana et al. [39]	Greece	Type 2 diabetes	12 weeks	Parallel Design	Control: 63.0 ± 1.3 Low GI: 61.3 ± 1.4	n = 61	Low GI diet v. Higher GI diet	The differences between the low GI diet and control diet with respect to HDL cholesterol at the end of the study was statistically significant ($p = 0.007$). A significant decrease ($p = 0.02$) in CRP was found in participants in the low GI diet group and the differences between the low GI and the higher GI groups were significant ($p = 0.007$) after the study. Serum IL–6 and adiponectin did not differ significantly in both groups at week 0 and week 12.
Cai et al. [40]	China	Type 2 diabetes	12 months	Parallel Design	56.7 ± 3.5	n = 130	Low GI diet v. Higher GI diet	After intervention, the levels of CRP-reactive protein and IL–6 in the low GI diet were significantly lower than the control group ($p < 0.05$).

Abbreviations: CCE (conventional carbohydrate exchange); Higher GI (Higher glycemic index); Low GI (Low glycemic index); n (Number); TC: total cholesterol; TG: triglyceride; CRP: C-reactive protein; IL–6: interleukin 6; v. (Versus).

Table 4. Cardio–metabolic and inflammatory parameters of studies included.

Citation	Baseline Versus Post-Intervention	HDL Cholesterol	LDL Cholesterol	Total Cholesterol	Triglyceride	C–Reactive Protein	Adiponectin	Interleukin–6
Gomes et al. [31]	Baseline mg/dL Median (Minimum/Maximum) Post-intervention	Higher GI: 43 (30/59) Low GI: 38 (27.6/45.2) Higher GI: 40 (30/54) Low GI: 41 (24.5/47)	No Data	Higher GI: 210.1 (180/273.5) Low GI: 200.4 (123/248.1) Higher GI: 211 (172/284) Low GI: 214.1 (145/288.5)	Higher GI: 180.2 (88.7/287) Low GI: 195 (68/372) Higher GI: 175.3 (132/311.2) Low GI: 205.1 (63/384.1)	(mg/L) Higher GI: 2.6 (0.8/7.3) Low GI: 2.7 (0.5/5.5) Higher GI: 2.8 (0.6/6.13) Low GI: 2.5 (0.1/6.9) $p = 0.44$	ng/mL Higher GI: 30.9 (29.8/31.4 Low GI: 30.1 (29.4/31.3) Higher GI: 30.8 (30.2/31.6) Low GI: 30.5 (26.7/93) $p = 0.74$	No Data
Ma et al. [33]	Baseline mmol/L (Mean ± SD) Post-intervention	Higher GI: 1.96 ± 0.39 Low GI: 1.89 ± 0.33 Higher GI: 1.85 ± 0.36 Low GI: 1.87 ± 0.34	Higher GI: 2.13 ± 0.60 Low GI: 2.19 ± 0.58 Higher GI: 2.16 ± 0.81 Low GI: 2.20 ± 0.54	Higher GI: 5.74 ± 0.74 Low GL: 5.79 ± 1.01 Higher GI: 5.97 ± 0.89 Low GI: 5.96 ± 1.02	Higher GI: 2.20 ± 0.60 Low GI:2.67 ± 1.27 Higher GI: 3.14 ± 1.05 Low GI: 3.09 ± 1.14	No Data	No Data	No Data
Jenkins et al. [34]	Baseline mg/dL (Mean) Post-intervention	Higher GI: 43.1 Low GI: 41.9 Higher GI: 42.8 Low GI: 43.6	Higher GI: 101.1 Low GI: 96.9 Higher GI: 101.3 Low GI: 95.3	Higher GI: 168.4 Low GI: 164.3 Higher GI: 168.4 Low GI: 162.6	Higher GI: 122.0 Low GI: 128.1 Higher GI: 122.2 Low GI: 124.6	Higher GI: 4.59 Low GI: 4.62 Higher GI: 2.82 Low GI: 3.02	No Data	No Data
Jenkins et al. [35]	Baseline mg/dL (95% CI) Post-intervention	Higher GI: 47 (44, 50) Low GI: 43 (40, 46) Higher GI: 48 (45, 52) Low GI: 43 (40, 45)	Higher GI: 91 (81, 101) Low GI: 84 (77, 92) Higher GI: 90 (81, 99) Low GI: 81 (74, 89)	Higher GI: 163 (151, 174) Low GI: 158 (147, 168) Higher GI: 161 (150, 172) Low GI: 149 (139, 160)	Higher GI: 124 (104, 145) Low GI: 149 (125, 173) Higher GI: 115 (96, 133) Low GI: 128 (107, 148)	No Data	No Data	No Data
Ma et al. [36]	Baseline mg/dL (Mean ± SEM) Post-intervention	Higher GI: 42.95 ± 2.26 Low GI: 45.42 ± 2.38 Higher GI: 44.29 ± 2.30 Low GI: 47.53 ± 2.43	Higher GI: 88.95 ± 7.52 Low GI: 93.16 ± 8.07 Higher GI: 71.49 ± 7.81 Low GI: 94.50 ± 8.32	Higher GI: 168.10 ± 9.06 Low GI: 175.58 ± 9.53 Higher GI: 149.71 ± 9.35 Low GI: 173.63 ± 0.06 $p = 0.09$	* Higher GI: 5.05 (0.14) Low GI: 4.99 (0.15) Higher GI: 4.93 (0.15) Low GI: 4.90 (0.16)	No Data	No Data	No Data
Wolever et al. [37]	Baseline mmol/L (Mean ± SEM) Post-intervention	Higher GI: 1.14 ± 0.05 Low GI: 1.21 ± 0.03 Higher GI: 1.19 ± 0.03 Low GI: 1.16 ± 0.03	Higher GI: 2.82 ± 0.13 Low GI: 3.02 ± 0.13 Higher GI: 3.0 ± 0.08 Low GI: 2.92 ± 0.05	Higher GI: 4.86 ± 0.16 Low GI: 5.09 ± 0.13 Higher GI: 5.04 ± 0.08 Low GI: 5.04 ± 0.08	Higher GI: 2.07 ± 0.15 Low GI: 1.87 ± 0.10 Higher GI: 2.0 ± 0.07 Low GI: 2.17 ± 0.07	** Higher GI: 3.34 (2.56, 4.26) Low GI: 2.64 (1.89, 3.70) Higher GI: 2.75 (2.33, 3.24) Low GI: 1.95 (1.68, 2.27)	No Data	No Data
Yusof et al. [38]	Baseline mmol/L (Mean ± SEM) Post-intervention	Higher GI: 1.18 ± 0.34 Low GI: 1.08 ± 0.30 Higher GI: 1.21 ± 0.05 Low GI: 1.14 ± 0.04	Higher GI: 2.78 ± 0.67 Low GI: 2.78 ± 0.67 Higher GI: 2.93 ± 0.14 Low GI: 2.67 ± 0.11	Higher GI: 4.56 ± 0.80 Low GI: 4.54 ± 0.75 Higher GI: 4.80 ± 0.16 Low GI: 4.54 ± 0.12	Higher GI: 1.35 ± 0.53 Low GI: 1.5 ± 0.47 Higher GI: 1.46 ± 0.08 Low GI: 1.59 ± 0.10	No Data	No Data	No Data
Argiana et al. [39]	Baseline mg/dL (Mean ± SEM) Post-intervention	Higher GI: 46.4 ± 1.8 Low GI: 43.1 ± 1.3 Higher GI: 46.1 ± 1.7 Low GI: 43.3 ± 1.2	Higher GI: 104.9 ± 5.1 Low GI: 107.0 ± 5.5 Higher GI: 104.2 ± 5.2 Low GI: 97.2 ± 6.2	Higher GI: 176.6 ± 5.2 Low GI: 173.9 ± 6.4 Higher GI: 175.8 ± 5.2 Low GI: 167.0 ± 4.1	Higher GI: 126.5 ± 10.8 Low GI: 119.2 ± 11.6 Higher GI: 127.5 ± 10.3 Low GI: 122 ± 9.3	*** Higher GI: 2.1 ± 0.5 Low GI: 4.4 ± 1.2 Higher GI: 2.8 ± 0.6 Low GI: 3.0 ± 0.8	*** Higher GI: 7.4 ± 1.6 Low GI: 12.2 ± 3.4 Higher GI: 8.3 ± 2.1 Low GI: 12.5 ± 1.5	**** Higher GI: 1.3 ± 0.2 Low GI: 1.4 ± 0.3 Higher GI: 2.0 ± 0.5 Low GI: 1.3 ± 0.2
Cai et al. [40]	Baseline mg/L (Not stated whether Mean or SD) Post-intervention	No Data	No Data	No Data	No Data	Higher GI: 8.03 ± 0.72 Low GI: 8.04 ± 0.75 Higher GI: 5.01 ± 0.32 Low GI: 3.68 ± 0.29	No Data	**** Higher GI: 12.26 ± 1.57 Low GI: 12.29 ± 1.44 Higher GI: 9.01 ± 0.83 Low GI: 7.97 ± 0.86

Abbreviations: CCE (conventional carbohydrate exchange); Higher GI (Higher glycemic index); Low GI (Low glycemic indexn (Number); TC: total cholesterol; TG: triglyceride; CRP: C-reactive protein; IL–6: interleukin 6. * mmol/L (Natural Logarithm); ** mg/L (Mean, 95% CIs); *** µg/mL (Mean ± SEM); **** pg/mL (Mean ± SEM); v. (Versus).

3.1. *Evaluation of the Risk of Bias of the Studies Selected*

Most of the studies demonstrated either a low risk of bias or an unclear risk of bias in all the domains evaluated (selection bias, performance bias, detection bias, attrition bias, and reporting bias) (Figure 2). However, Jenkins et al. [34] showed high risk of bias in the area of selection bias (Figure 3).

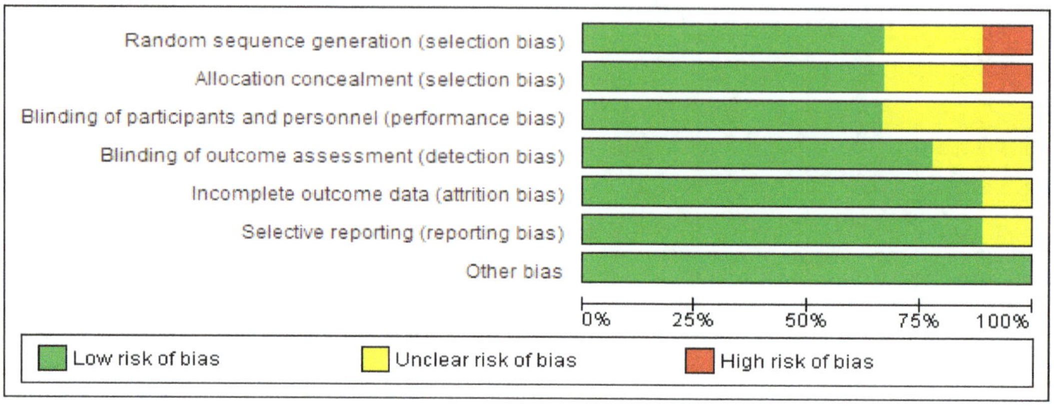

Figure 2. A summary risk of bias graph of included studies.

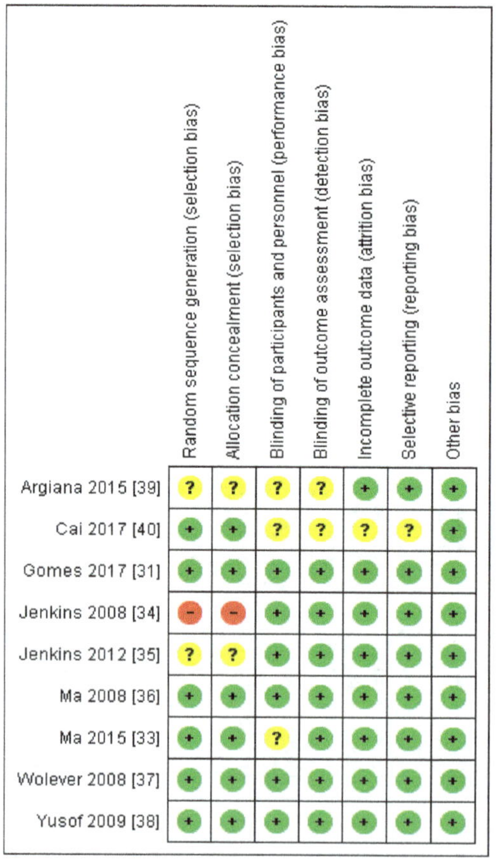

Figure 3. A risk of bias graph for each included study.

3.2. *The Effect of a Low GI Diet on Lipid Profile*

Grant et al. [32] found no significant differences ($p > 0.05$) between the low GI group compared to the higher GI group, with respect to the lipid profile in women with GDM (Table 3). In their study, Ma et al. [33] observed that the increases in total cholesterol (0.12 versus 0.23 mmol/L) and triglyceride

(0.41 versus 0.56 mmol/L), and the decrease in HDL cholesterol (−0.01 versus −0.11), were significantly lower ($p < 0.05$) than the higher GI group in women with GDM (Table 4).

In patients with type 2 diabetes, the results of the meta-analysis showed no significant differences ($p > 0.05$) between the low GI and higher GI groups with respect to HDL with a mean difference of 0.00 mmol/L (−0.02, 0.02) and LDL cholesterol with a mean difference of −0.14 mmol/L (−0.37, 0.09) (Figures 4 and 5, respectively).

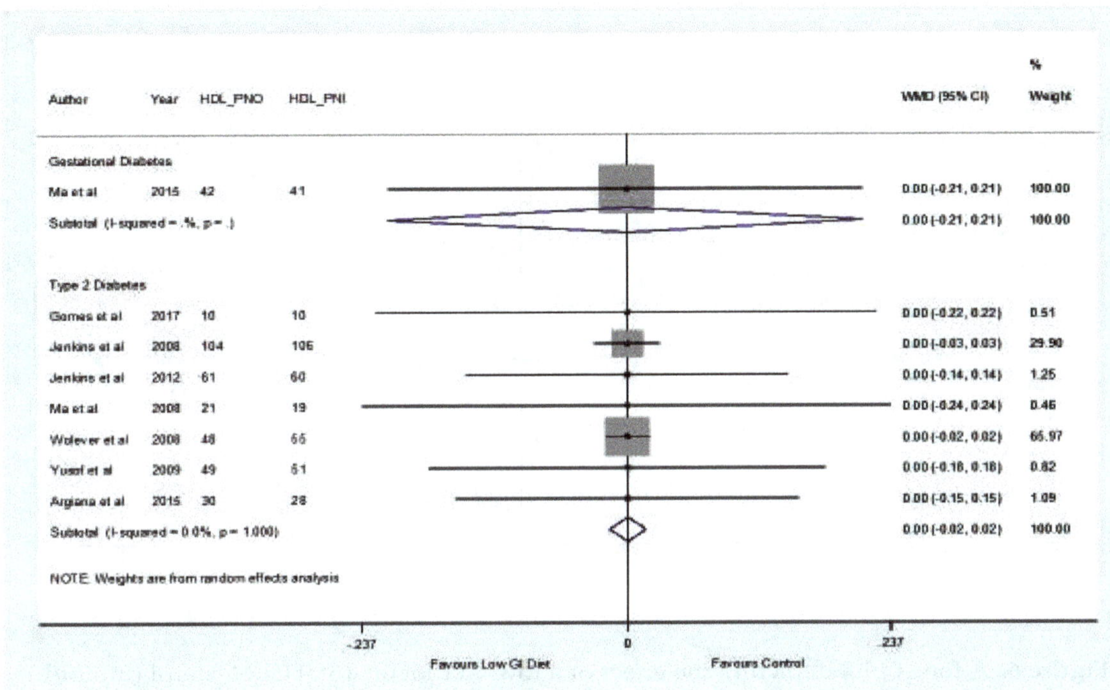

Figure 4. A forest plot showing the effects of a low GI diet on HDL cholesterol (mmol/L).

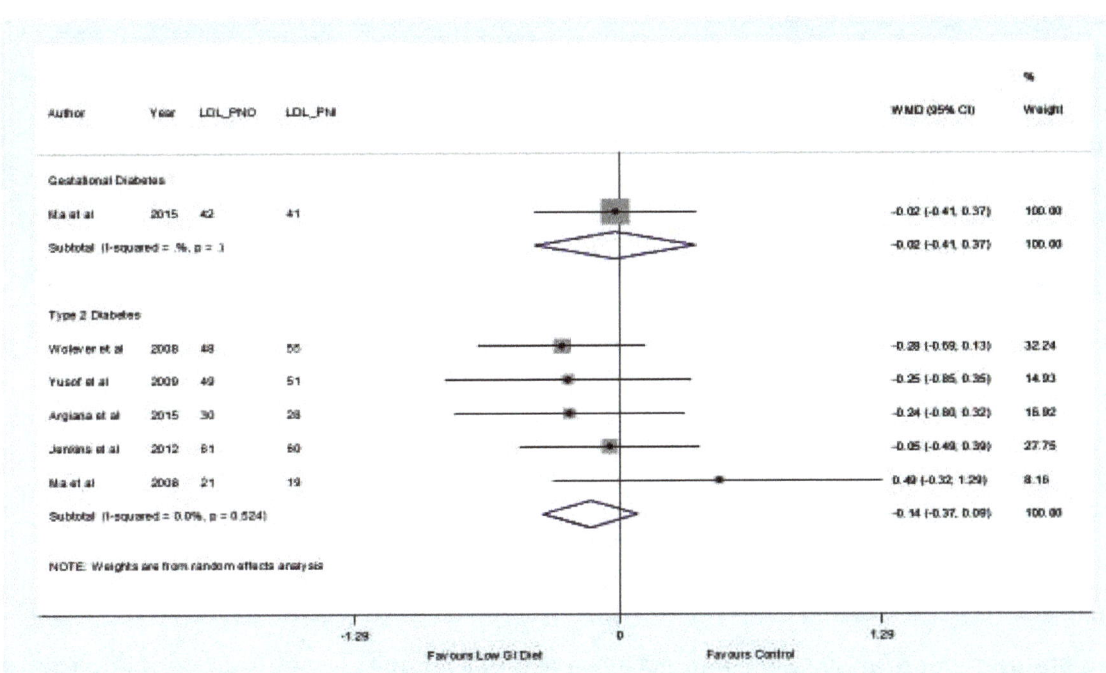

Figure 5. A forest plot showing the effect of a low GI diet on LDL cholesterol (mmol/L).

In addition, the findings from the meta-analysis found no significant difference ($p > 0.05$) between the two groups in relation to the total cholesterol which decreased by a mean of −0.08 mmol/L (−0.31, 0.16) (Figure 6) in the low GI group. The results showed that there was a significant difference ($p = 0.027$) with respect to triglycerides, which increased by a mean of 0.06 mmol/L (0.01, 0.11) in patients with type 2 diabetes in the higher GI group (Figure 7).

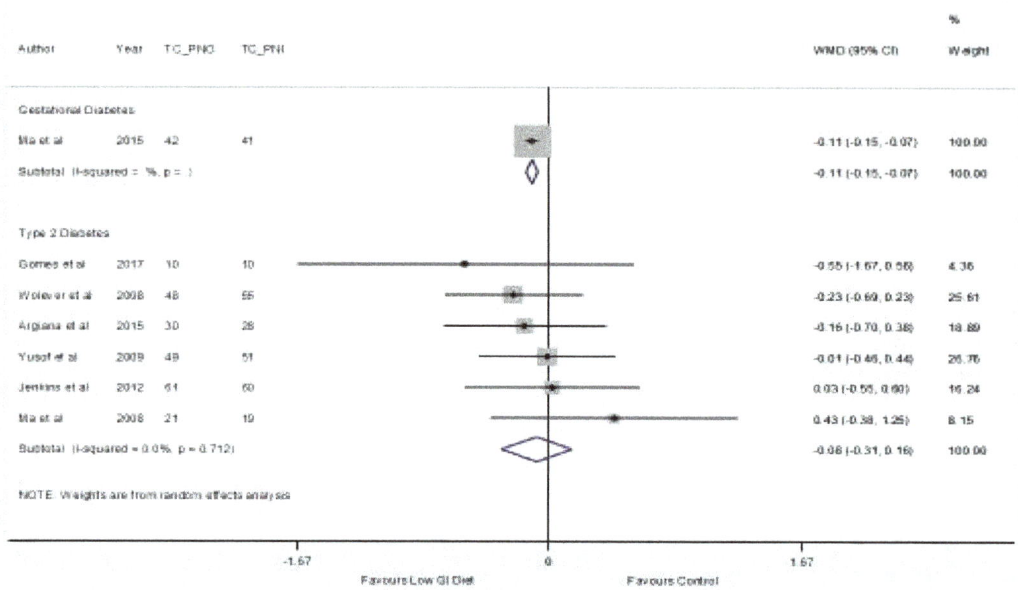

Figure 6. A forest plot depicting the effect of a low GI diet on Total Cholesterol (mmol/L).

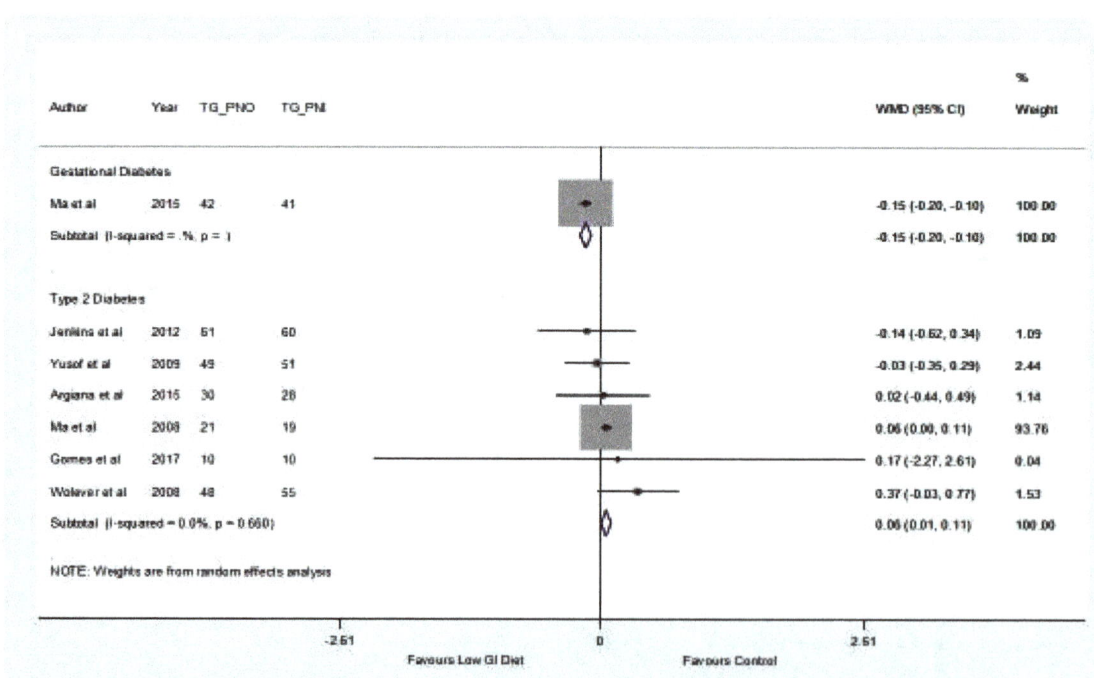

Figure 7. A forest plot depicting the effect of a low GI diet on Triglyceride (mmol/L).

3.3. *The Effect of a Low GI Diet on Inflammatory Parameters*

According to Grant et al. [32], there was no significant difference ($p > 0.05$) between the low GI and higher GI groups in relation to the C–reactive protein in women with GDM. In patients with type 2 diabetes, Gomes et al. [31] and Cai et al. [40] found that a low GI diet can reduce or prevent the inflammatory responses induced by a high GI diet. In addition, a low GI diet has been shown to reduce C–reactive protein levels significantly compared to a high GI diet [37,39].

With respect to serum interleukin–6 and adiponectin, Argiana et al. [39] did not find significant differences in both groups between week 0 and week 12 in patients with type 2 diabetes. The results of the meta-analysis did not show significant differences ($p > 0.05$) between low GI and higher GI diets with respect to adiponectin and C-reactive protein in patients with type 2 diabetes (Table 5). However, a significant difference ($p < 0.001$) was observed between the two groups in relation to interleukin–6 (Table 5), with the low GI diet decreasing interleukin–6 by a mean of −1.01 mg/L (−1.55, −0.48). A meta-analysis was not conducted for the patients with GDM with respect to inflammatory parameters due to the limited number of studies.

Table 5. Results of a meta-analysis of the effect of a low GI diet on inflammatory parameters.

Outcomes	Patients with Type 2 Diabetes			
	N Studies	Weighted Mean Difference (95% CI) mg/L	*p*-Value	I^2 %
Interleukin–6	2	−1.01 (−1.55, −0.48)	0.001	0.0
C–eactive Protein	5	−0.32 (−1.17, 0.53)	0.467	0.0
Adiponectin	2	0.01 (−0.00, 0.03)	0.072	0.0

4. Discussion

The results of the two studies [32,33] that evaluated the effects of low GI diets on lipid profiles in women with GDM were not consistent. While Grant et al. [32] did not find significant differences ($p > 0.05$) between the low GI and higher GI groups in relation to lipids, Ma et al. [33] found significant differences ($p < 0.05$) between the two groups with respect to total cholesterol, triglycerides, and HDL cholesterol. On the other hand, the results of the meta-analysis showed that there were no significant differences ($p > 0.05$) between the low GI diet and higher GI group with respect to total cholesterol, HDL, and LDL cholesterol in patients with type 2 diabetes (although the difference was statistically significant ($p < 0.05$) in relation to triglycerides, with higher GI diet increasing triglyceride levels). The differences observed between the effects of a low GI in patients with GDM compared to patients with type 2 diabetes in some of the metabolites may due to the limited number of studies in the current review and the differences in the pathophysiology of both conditions. In a previous meta-analysis, Fleming and Godwin [24] revealed that a low GI diet may help lower total cholesterol and LDL cholesterol. In addition, Goff et al. [13] found that low GI diets reduced total and LDL cholesterol and had no effect on HDL cholesterol and triglycerides. It is possible that the differences between the current review and the previous reviews in relation to some of the metabolites may be due to the participants included in the studies. While this review was based only on patients with GDM and type 2 diabetes, the earlier reviews were based on the general population [24] or included participants without diabetes [13].

The results of the effect of a low GI diet on inflammatory markers were variable in the studies selected in patients with GDM. However, the results of the meta-analysis showed that differences between low GI and higher GI groups were only significant ($p < 0.05$) in relation to interleukin–6, which decreased in the low GI group in patients with type 2 diabetes. These results are discussed below.

4.1. *The Effect of a Low GI Diet on Lipid Profile*

There appears to be controversy regarding the role of low GI diets in the prevention of cardiovascular diseases. The effect of GI on total cholesterol, LDL, and HDL cholesterol is not quite clear [39,41]. For example, in women with GDM, Grant et al. [32] reported no significant differences ($p > 0.05$) between the low GI and higher GI groups with respect to the lipids in women with GDM. However, Ma et al. [33] found that low GI diets improved blood lipids.

In patients with type 2 diabetes, Gomes et al. [31] found that a low GI diet reduced body fat. In the study by Jenkins et al. [34], it was observed that HDL cholesterol increased by 1.7 mg/dL in the low GI group and decreased by −0.2 mg/dL in the higher GI group ($p = 0.005$). In contrast, Wolever et al. [37] noted that HDL cholesterol was 4% lower in the low GI group, while the higher GI values were intermediate. Other studies [35,36,38] demonstrated no significant difference between the low GI and higher GI groups in relation to HDL cholesterol.

According to Jenkins et al. [35], low GI legumes produced significant decreases in total cholesterol level ($p < 0.001$) in patients with type 2 diabetes. The relative reduction in total cholesterol level was greater in the low GI legume diet group compared with the higher GI group [35]. However, Ma et al. [36] and Wolever et al. [37] did not find a significant difference between low GI and higher GI diets with respect to the total cholesterol in patients with type 2 diabetes.

Jenkins et al. [35] demonstrated that a low GI legume produced significant decreases in triglycerides ($p < 0.001$) in patients with type 2 diabetes. Decreases in triglycerides in the low GI group were also reported by Yusof et al. [38], although Wolever et al. [37] showed increased levels of triglycerides in the low GI group. On the other hand, Ma et al. [36] found no significant difference between low GI and higher GI with respect to triglycerides.

The mechanism by which dietary GI influences blood lipids has not been entirely elucidated [42]. This may explain the differences in the findings of the various studies. However, it has been suggested that high GI diets increase non esterified fatty acid concentrations after intervention compared to baseline, and increased levels of non-esterified fatty acids can cause beta cell dysfunction, insulin resistance, and reduced glucose uptake [31]. In other words, elevated levels of blood glucose, insulin, and free fatty acids following a high GI diet can induce insulin resistance, which could lead to increased triglyceride, a greater inflammatory response, and a decrease in HDL cholesterol [43,44].

Hyperinsulinaemia and insulin resistance are significantly correlated to dyslipidaemia and contribute to the changes in the plasma lipid profile [45]. Therefore, the potential effects of a low GI diet on cardiometabolic parameters may be caused by a reduction of hyperglycaemia, hyperinsulinaemia and levels of free fatty acids, which could lead to a reduced risk of insulin resistance, beta cell dysfunction, dyslipidaemia, and inflammatory response [45,46].

4.2. The Effect of a Low GI Diet on Inflammatory Parameters

Based on the findings of the meta-analysis in relation to the inflammatory parameters, low GI diets significantly decreased ($p < 0.05$) levels of interleukin-6 compared with the higher GI diets in patients with type 2 diabetes. Differences between the two groups were not statistically significant ($p > 0.05$) with respect to C-reactive proteins. The mechanism for this finding, with respect to interleukin-6, may due to hyperglycaemia in the higher GI group, which induces the release of inflammatory cytokines from monocytes [47]. Furthermore, the exposure of endothelial cells to varying levels of glucose concentration can increase the risk of oxidative stress and apoptosis and thus lead to the production of pro-inflammatory cytokines [39,48,49]. The results of this review confirm the findings of a previous study by Juanola-Falgaroma et al. [50], which found that subjects allocated a low GI diet showed significantly higher decreases in interleukin–6 after intervention.

This review has both clinical and public health implications in terms of our understanding of the role low GI diets in the management of cardiometabolic and inflammatory parameters in patients with diabetes.

5. Limitations

Although a total of nine studies were included in the meta-analysis, this number was limited by the two sub-groups of GDM and type 2 diabetes. More studies in each of the sub-groups would have further enhanced the wider application of the findings of this review. In addition, the lack of a consensus on what constitutes a low GI diet, and the variation in the GI levels of dietary interventions in the studies included, may have impacted the analysis of the findings of this review.

6. Conclusions

This systematic review and meta-analysis have demonstrated that there were no significant differences ($p > 0.05$) between low GI and higher GI diets in relation to total cholesterol, HDL, and LDL cholesterol in patients with type 2 diabetes. However, a significant difference ($p < 0.05$) was observed between the two groups with respect to triglycerides in patients with type 2 diabetes. The results of the effect of a low GI diet on the lipid profile in patients with GDM were not consistent. With respect to the inflammatory parameters, the low GI diet significantly decreased interleukin–6 in patients with type 2 diabetes than the higher GI diet. More studies are needed in this area of research.

Author Contributions: Conceptualization, O.O., O.O.O., X.-H.W., A.R.A.A.; methodology, O.O., O.O.O., X.-H.W., A.R.A.A.; validation, O.O., O.O.O., X.-H.W., A.R.A.A.; formal analysis, A.R.A.A. and O.O. and reviewed by O.O.O. and X.-H.W.; writing—original draft preparation, O.O.; writing—review and editing, O.O., O.O.O., X.-H.W., A.R.A.A.

References

1. International Diabetes Federation. Promoting Diabetes Care, Prevention and a Cure Worldwide. 2019. Available online: https://www.idf.org/ (accessed on 16 March 2019).
2. National Collaborating Centre for Chronic Conditions (NCCCC). *Type 2 Diabetes: National Clinical Guideline for Management in Primary and Secondary Care (Update)*; Royal College of Physicians: London, UK, 2008.
3. Poulakos, P.; Mintziori, G.; Tsirou, E.; Taousani, E.; Savvaki, D.; Harizopoulou, V.; Goulis, D.G. Comments on gestational diabetes mellitus: From pathophysiology to clinical practice. *Hormones (Athens, Greece)* **2015**, *14*, 335–344. [CrossRef] [PubMed]
4. World Health Organisation. Diagnostic Criteria and Classification of Hyperglycaemia First Detected in Pregnancy. 2013. Available online: http://apps.who.int/iris/bitstream/handle/10665/85975/WHO_NMH_MND_13.2_eng.pdf;jsessionid=09A82B923EF7A55CC6AB690976A1A1F3?sequence=1 (accessed on 16 March 2019).
5. Abell, S.K.; De Courten, B.; Boyle, J.A.; Teede, H.J. Inflammatory and Other Biomarkers: Role in Pathophysiology and Prediction of Gestational Diabetes Mellitus. *Int. J. Mol. Sci.* **2015**, *16*, 13442–13473. [CrossRef] [PubMed]
6. International Diabetes Federation. Care and Prevention Improving the Quality of Life of People with Diabetes and Those at Risk. 2019. Available online: https://www.idf.org/our-activities/care-prevention/gdm (accessed on 16 March 2019).
7. National Institute for Health and Care Excellence (NICE). Type 2 Diabetes in Adults: Management. 2015. Available online: nice.org.uk/guidance/ng28 (accessed on 1 March 2019).
8. National Institute for Health and Care Excellence (NICE). Diabetes in Pregnancy: Management from Preconception to the Postnatal Period. 2015. Available online: http://nice.org.uk/guidance/ng3 (accessed on 16 March 2018).
9. Ojo, O.; Ojo, O.O.; Adebowale, F.; Wang, X.-H. The Effect of Dietary Glycaemic Index on Glycaemia in Patients with Type 2 Diabetes: A Systematic Review and Meta-Analysis of Randomized Controlled Trials. *Nutrients* **2018**, *10*, 373. [CrossRef] [PubMed]
10. Hodson, K.; Robson, S.; Taylor, R. Gestational diabetes: Emerging concepts in pathophysiology. *Obstet. Med.* **2010**, *3*, 128–132. [CrossRef] [PubMed]
11. Daher, S. Gestational diabetes, inflammation and obesity: New insights into genetic markers and phenotype. *J. Reprod. Immunol.* **2012**, *94*, 6. [CrossRef]
12. American Diabetes Association. Life style management: Standards of Medical Care in Diabetes–2018. *Diabetes Care* **2018**, *41* (Suppl. 1), S38–S50. [CrossRef] [PubMed]
13. Goff, L.M.; Cowland, D.E.; Hooper, L.; Frost, G.S. Low glycaemic index diets and blood lipids: A systematic review and meta-analysis of randomised controlled trials. *Nutr. Metab. Cardiovasc. Dis.* **2013**, *23*, 1–10. [CrossRef]
14. Similä, M.E.; Valsta, L.M.; Kontto, J.P.; Albanes, D.; Virtamo, J. Low-, medium-and high-glycaemic index carbohydrates and risk of type 2 diabetes in men. *Br. J. Nutr.* **2011**, *105*, 1258–1264. [CrossRef]

15. Esfahani, A.; Wong, J.W.; Mirrahimi, A.; Villa, C.R.; Kendall, C.C. The application of the glycemic index and glycemic load in weight loss: A review of the clinical evidence. *IUBMB Life* **2011**, *63*, 7–13. [CrossRef]
16. Food and Agricultural Organisation (FAO). *Carbohydrates in Human Nutrition. Report of a Joint FAO/WHO Expert Consultation*; FAO (Food and Nutrition paper–66); FAO: Rome, Italy, 1998. Available online: http://www.fao.org/docrep/w8079e/w8079e00.htm (accessed on 16 January 2019).
17. Chiu, C.; Taylor, A. Dietary hyperglycemia, glycemic index and metabolic retinal diseases. *Prog. Retin. Eye Res.* **2011**, *30*, 18–53. [CrossRef]
18. Chang, K.T.; Lampe, J.W.; Schwarz, Y.; Breymeyer, K.L.; Noar, K.A.; Song, X.; Neuhouser, M.L. Low Glycemic Load Experimental Diet More Satiating Than High Glycemic Load Diet. *Nutr. Cancer* **2012**, *64*, 666–673. [CrossRef] [PubMed]
19. Russell, W.R.; Baka, A.; Björck, I.; Delzenne, N.; Gao, D.; Griffiths, H.R.; Weickert, M.O. Impact of Diet Composition on Blood Glucose Regulation. *Crit. Rev. Food Sci. Nutr.* **2016**, *56*, 541–590. [CrossRef] [PubMed]
20. Bouché, C.; Rizkalla, S.W.; Luo, J.; Vidal, H.; Veronese, A.; Pacher, N.; Fouquet, C.; Lang, V.; Slama, G. Five-week, low-glycemic index diet decreases total fat mass and improves plasma lipid profile in moderately overweight nondiabetic men. *Diabetes Care* **2002**, *25*, 822–828. [CrossRef] [PubMed]
21. Brand, J.C.; Colagiuri, S.; Crossman, S.; Allen, A.; Roberts, D.C.; Truswell, A.S. Low-glycemic index foods improve long-term glycemic control in NIDDM. *Diabetes Care* **1991**, *14*, 95–101. [CrossRef] [PubMed]
22. Clar, C.; Al-Khudairy, L.; Loveman, E.; Kelly, S.A.; Hartley, L.; Flowers, N.; Germanò, R.; Frost, G.; Rees, K. Low glycaemic index diets for the prevention of cardiovascular disease. *Cochrane Database Syst. Rev.* **2017**, *7*, CD004467. [CrossRef]
23. Schwingshackl, L.; Hoffmann, G. Long-term effects of low glycemic index/load vs. high glycemic index/load diets on parameters of obesity and obesity-associated risks: A systematic review and meta-analysis. *Nutr. Metab. Cardiovasc. Dis. NMCD* **2013**, *23*, 699–706. [CrossRef]
24. Fleming, P.; Godwin, M. Low-glycaemic index diets in the management of blood lipids: A systematic review and meta-analysis. *Fam. Pract.* **2013**, *30*, 485–491. [CrossRef]
25. Mendes, N.; Tavares Ribeiro, R.; Serrano, F. Beyond self-monitored plasma glucose and HbA1c: The role of non-traditional glycaemic markers in gestational diabetes mellitus. *J. Obstet. Gynaecol.* **2018**, *38*, 762–769. [CrossRef]
26. Moher, D.; Liberati, A.; Tetzlaff, J.; Altman, D.G. The PRISMA Group Preferred Reporting Items for Systematic Reviews and Meta-Analyses: The PRISMA Statement. *PLoS Med.* **2009**, *6*, e1000097. [CrossRef]
27. Methley, A.M.; Campbell, S.; Chew-Graham, C.; McNally, R.; Cheraghi-Sohi, S. PICO, PICOS and SPIDER: A comparison study of specificity and sensitivity in three search tools for qualitative systematic reviews. *BMC Health Serv. Res.* **2014**, *14*, 579. [CrossRef]
28. Critical Appraisal Skills Programme (CASP). Randomised Controlled Trial Checklist. 2017. Available online: https://casp-uk.net/wp-content/uploads/2018/01/CASP-Randomised-Controlled-Trial-Checklist-2018.pdf (accessed on 18 January 2019).
29. Higgins, J.P.T.; Green, S. *Cochrane Handbook for Systematic Reviews of Interventions*; Wiley-Blackwell: Hoboken, NJ, USA, 2009.
30. The Nordic Cochrane Centre. *Review Manager (RevMan) [Computer Program]*, Version 5.3.; The Nordic Cochrane Centre, The Cochrane Collaboration: Copenhagen, Denmark, 2014.
31. Gomes, J.G.; Fabrini, S.P.; Alfenas, R.G. Low glycemic index diet reduces body fat and attenuates inflammatory and metabolic responses in patients with Type 2 diabetes. *Arch. Endocrinol. Metab.* **2017**, *61*, 137–144. [CrossRef] [PubMed]
32. Grant, S.M.; Wolever, T.M.; O'Connor, D.L.; Nisenbaum, R.; Josse, R.G. Effect of a low glycaemic index diet on blood glucose in women with gestational hyperglycaemia. *Diabetes Res. Clin. Pract.* **2011**, *91*, 15–22. [CrossRef] [PubMed]
33. Ma, W.J.; Huang, Z.H.; Huang, B.X.; Qi, B.H.; Zhang, Y.J.; Xiao, B.X.; Li, Y.H.; Chen, L.; Zhu, H.L. Intensive low-glycaemic-load dietary intervention for the management of glycaemia and serum lipids among women with gestational diabetes: A randomized control trial. *Public Health Nutr.* **2015**, *18*, 1506–1513. [CrossRef] [PubMed]
34. Jenkins, D.A.; Kendall, C.C.; McKeown-Eyssen, G.; Josse, R.G.; Silverberg, J.; Booth, G.L.; Leiter, L.A. Effect of a low-glycemic index or a high-cereal fiber diet on Type 2 diabetes: A randomized trial. *JAMA* **2008**, *300*, 2742–2753. [CrossRef] [PubMed]

35. Jenkins, D.A.; Kendall, C.C.; Augustin, L.A.; Mitchell, S.; Sahye-Pudaruth, S.; Blanco Mejia, S.; Josse, R.G. Effect of legumes as part of a low glycemic index diet on glycemic control and cardiovascular risk factors in type 2 diabetes mellitus: A randomized controlled trial. *Arch. Intern. Med.* **2012**, *172*, 1653–1660. [CrossRef] [PubMed]
36. Ma, Y.; Olendzki, B.C.; Merriam, P.A.; Chiriboga, D.E.; Culver, A.L.; Li, W.; Pagoto, S.L. A randomized clinical trial comparing low-glycemic index versus ADA dietary education among individuals with type 2 diabetes. *Nutrition* **2008**, *24*, 45–56. [CrossRef]
37. Wolever, T.; Gibbs, A.; Mehling, C.; Chiasson, J.; Connelly, P.; Josse, R.; Ryan, E. The Canadian Trial of Carbohydrates in Diabetes (CCD), a 1-y controlled trial of low-glycemic-index dietary carbohydrate in type 2 diabetes: No effect on glycated hemoglobin but reduction in C-reactive protein. *Am. J. Clin. Nutr.* **2008**, *87*, 114–125. [CrossRef] [PubMed]
38. Yusof, B.M.; Talib, R.A.; Kamaruddin, N.A.; Karim, N.A.; Chinna, K.; Gilbertson, H. A low-GI diet is associated with a short-term improvement of glycaemic control in Asian patients with Type 2 diabetes. *Diabetes Obes. Metab.* **2009**, *11*, 387–396. [CrossRef]
39. Argiana, V.; Kanellos, P.T.; Makrilakis, K.; Eleftheriadou, I.; Tsitsinakis, G.; Kokkinos, A.; Perrea, D.; Tentolouris, N. The effect of consumption of low-glycemic-index and low-glycemic-load desserts on anthropometric parameters and inflammatory markers in patients with Type 2 diabetes mellitus. *Eur. J. Nutr.* **2015**, *54*, 1173–1180. [CrossRef]
40. Cai, X.; Wang, L.; Wang, X.; Liu, S. Effect of high dietary fiber low glycemic index diet on intestinal flora, blood glucose and inflammatory response in T2DM patients. *Biomed. Res.* **2017**, *28*, 9371–9375.
41. Pelkman, C.L. Effects of the glycemic index of foods on serum concentrations of high-density lipoprotein cholesterol and triglycerides. *Curr. Atheroscler. Rep.* **2001**, *3*, 456–461. [CrossRef] [PubMed]
42. Huffman, F.G.; Zarini, G.G.; Cooper, V. Dietary glycemic index and load in relation to cardiovascular disease risk factors in Cuban American population. *Int. J. Food Sci. Nutr.* **2010**, *61*, 690–701. [CrossRef] [PubMed]
43. Reaven, G.M. Pathophysiology of insulin resistance in human disease. *Physiol. Rev.* **1995**, *75*, 473–486. [CrossRef] [PubMed]
44. Ludwig, D.S. The glycemic index: Physiological mechanisms relating to obesity, diabetes, and cardiovascular disease. *JAMA* **2002**, *287*, 2414–2423. [CrossRef] [PubMed]
45. Radulian, G.; Rusu, E.; Dragomir, A.; Posea, M. Metabolic effects of low glycaemic index diets. *Nutr. J.* **2009**, *8*, 1–8. [CrossRef] [PubMed]
46. Aston, L.M. Glycaemic index and metabolic disease risk. *Proc. Nutr. Soc.* **2006**, *65*, 125–134. [CrossRef] [PubMed]
47. Devaraj, S.; Venugopal, S.K.; Singh, U.; Jialal, I. Hyperglycemia induces monocytic release of interleukin-6 via induction of protein kinase c-{alpha} and -{beta}. *Diabetes* **2005**, *54*, 85–91. [CrossRef]
48. Leiter, L.A.; Ceriello, A.; Davidson, J.A.; Hanefeld, M.; Monnier, L.; Owens, D.R.; Tajima, N.; Tuomilehto, J. Postprandial glucose regulation: New data and new implications. *Clin. Ther.* **2005**, *27* (Suppl. B), S42–S56. [CrossRef]
49. Risso, A.; Mercuri, F.; Quagliaro, L.; Damante, G.; Ceriello, A. Intermittent high glucose enhances apoptosis in human umbilical vein endothelial cells in culture. *Am. J. Physiol. Endocrinol. Metab.* **2001**, *281*, E924–E930. [CrossRef]
50. Juanola-Falgarona, M.; Salas-Salvado, J.; Ibarrola-Jurado, N.; Rabassa-Soler, A.; Diaz-Lopez, A.; Guasch-Ferré, M.; Hernández-Alonso, P.; Balanza, R.; Bullo, M. Effect of the glycemic index of the diet on weight loss, modulation of satiety, inflammation, and other metabolic risk factors: A randomized controlled trial. *Am. J. Clin. Nutr.* **2014**, *100*, 27–35. [CrossRef]

13

Zinc Intake and Status and Risk of Type 2 Diabetes Mellitus

José C. Fernández-Cao [1,2,*], Marisol Warthon-Medina [3,4], Victoria H. Moran [5], Victoria Arija [6], Carlos Doepking [1], Lluis Serra-Majem [7,8] and Nicola M. Lowe [4]

1 Department of Nutrition and Dietetics, Faculty of Heath Sciences, University of Atacama, Av. Copayapu 2862, Copiapó, 1530000 Atacama Region, Chile; carlos.doepking@uda.cl
2 Nutrition and Public Health, Universitat Rovira i Virgili, C/ Sant Llorenç 21, Reus, 43201 Tarragona, Spain
3 Food Databanks National Capability, Quadram Institute Bioscience, Norwich Research Park, Norwich, Norfolk NR4 7UA, UK; marisol@warthon-medina.com
4 International Institute of Nutritional Sciences and Food Safety Studies, University of Central Lancashire, Darwin Building c/o Psychology Scholl Office, Preston, Lancashire PR1 2HE, UK; NMLowe@uclan.ac.uk
5 Maternal and Infant Nutrition and Nurture Unit, University of Central Lancashire, Preston, Lancashire PR 1 2HE, UK; VLMoran@uclan.ac.uk
6 Research Group in Nutrition and Mental Health (NUTRISAM), Institut d'Investigació Sanitària Pere Virgili (IISPV), Rovira i Virgili University, Reus, 43201 Tarragona, Spain; victoria.arija@urv.cat
7 Research Institute of Biomedical and Health Sciences, University of Las Palmas de Gran Canaria and CHUIMI, Canarian Health Service, 35016 Las Palmas de Gran Canaria, Spain; lluis.serra@ulpgc.es
8 Consorcio CIBER, M.P. Fisiopatología de la Obesidad y Nutrición (CIBERObn), Instituto de Salud Carlos III (ISCIII), 28029 Madrid, Spain
* Correspondence: jose.fernandez.cao@uda.cl

Abstract: Zinc could have a protective role against type 2 diabetes mellitus (T2DM). This systematic review and meta-analysis aimed to evaluate the association between dietary, supplementary, and total zinc intake, as well as serum/plasma and whole blood zinc concentration, and risk of T2DM. Observational studies, conducted on cases of incident diabetes or T2DM patients and healthy subjects that reported a measure of association between zinc exposure and T2DM, were selected. Random effects meta-analyses were applied to obtain combined results. Stratified meta-analyses and meta-regressions were executed to assess sources of heterogeneity, as well as the impact of covariates on the findings. From 12,136 publications, 16 studies were selected. The odds ratio (OR) for T2DM comparing the highest versus lowest zinc intake from diet was 0.87 (95% CI: 0.78–0.98). Nevertheless, no association between supplementary or total zinc intake from both diet and supplementation, and T2DM was observed. A direct relationship was found between serum/plasma zinc levels and T2DM (OR = 1.64, 95% CI: 1.25–2.14). A moderately high dietary zinc intake, in relation to the Dietary Reference Intake, could reduce by 13% the risk of T2DM, and up to 41% in rural areas. Conversely, elevated serum/plasma zinc concentration was associated with an increased risk of T2DM by 64%, suggesting disturbances in zinc homeostasis.

Keywords: zinc intake; zinc status; trace elements; type 2 diabetes mellitus; systematic review; meta-analysis; epidemiology

1. Introduction

Diabetes mellitus is a major public health challenge worldwide, and is a key contributor to morbidity and mortality. In 2016, diabetes mellitus was listed as the seventh leading cause of death globally [1]. According to the International Diabetes Federation (IDF) Diabetes ATLAS, the global prevalence of diabetes among individuals aged 20–79 years in 2017 was 8.8% (95% confidence interval

(CI): 7.2–11.3), i.e., 424.9 million people, with a total healthcare expenditure estimated at just under USD 727 billion [2]. The number of people suffering from diabetes is expected to increase to 628.6 million in 2045, a prevalence of over 9.9% (95% CI: 7.5–12.7). Around 90% of cases of diabetes are type 2 diabetes (T2DM) [2]. This disease results from the body's ineffective use of insulin [1], and is the result of the interaction of multiple genetic and environmental factors [3].

The role of zinc in the etiology of T2DM has been widely reported in recent decades. Longitudinal large prospective cohort studies, such as the Nurses' Health Study (NHS) cohort [4] in the USA; the Australian Longitudinal Study on Women's Health cohort study [5]; the Malmö Diet and Cancer Study cohort [6] in Sweden; and the Japan Collaborative Cohort study [7], among others, have investigated the effect of dietary, supplementary, and/or total zinc intake on the risk of developing T2DM. The NHS cohort was the first to prospectively analyze these relationships, and it reported that the higher the total and/or dietary zinc intake, the lower the risk of T2DM over subsequent years [4]. Although a non-significant association was observed between supplementary zinc intake and risk of T2DM in the overall sample, an inverse relationship was seen in those participants with low dietary zinc intake [4]. There is currently no evidence that supports the use of zinc supplements in the prevention of T2DM [8]. Nevertheless, a recent clinical trial based on zinc supplementation has found a reduction in the progression to diabetes in prediabetic subjects [9]. Some subsequent prospective cohort studies, however, have failed to confirm some of the results reported in the NHS cohort [6,10–12]. A systematic review of prospective studies that aimed to examine the role of zinc intake and status on the risk of T2DM revealed inconsistencies between studies, and suggested the possible influence of confounding factors on these relationships [13].

Similarly, findings on the relationship between serum/plasma zinc concentration and T2DM are contradictory [14–16]. The prospective Kuopio Ischaemic Heart Disease Risk Factor (KIHD) cohort study of 2220 Finnish men followed over twenty years showed that higher serum zinc levels were associated with an increased risk of T2DM [14]. Conversely, a cross-sectional study of 128 Russian postmenopausal women found an inverse relationship between serum zinc and T2DM [17]. The relationship between whole blood zinc concentration and T2DM has been investigated by two studies carried out within the same population-based Nord-Trøndelag Health Study (HUNT3), but their results were inconclusive [18,19]. The study conducted on newly diagnosed T2DM patients found a positive association between whole blood zinc concentration and T2DM [18], while the study performed in previously diagnosed T2DM patients showed no association [19]. In our previous systematic review and meta-analysis, which aimed to compare whole blood zinc concentration between T2DM patients and non-diabetic subjects, we observed a lower whole blood zinc concentration in T2DM patients [20]. It should be noted that diabetic subjects had, at least, 10.2 ± 8.6 years of duration of diabetes. Therefore, the duration of diabetes may have an impact on this association, and it is important to clarify this relationship.

The mechanism whereby zinc could have an impact on the risk of T2DM has not been completely elucidated, however zinc is an essential trace element that is involved in the physiology of carbohydrate metabolism in many ways. Zinc participates in the adequate insulin synthesis, storage, crystallization, and secretion in the pancreatic β-cell, as well as action and translocation of insulin into the cells [21–24]. In addition, zinc seems to play a role in insulin sensitivity through the activation of the phosphoinositol-3-kinase/protein kinase B cascade [25]. Due to its insulin–mimetic action, zinc also stimulates glucose uptake in insulin-dependent tissues [26]. Moreover, zinc is implicated in the suppression of proinflammatory cytokines, such as interleukin-1β [27] and nuclear factor kβ [28], avoiding β-cells' death and protecting insulin. All of these functions of zinc could support its potential protective role against diabetes mellitus.

Much remains uncertain concerning the effect of zinc on the risk of developing T2DM. Therefore, the purpose of this comprehensive systematic review and meta-analysis of observational studies was to evaluate the association between dietary, supplementary, and total zinc intake, as well as serum/plasma zinc and whole blood concentration and risk of T2DM in the adult population. A secondary objective was to examine potential confounding factors that may impact on these relationships.

2. Materials and Methods

The protocol for this systematic review and meta-analysis of observational studies was registered in PROSPERO (2015: CRD42015020178) and can be accessed here: (http://www.crd.york.ac.uk/PROSPERO/display_record.php?ID=CRD42015020178). The study was conducted in accordance with the Meta-Analyses of Observational Studies in Epidemiology (MOOSE) criteria statement [29]. The MOOSE checklist is shown in Supplementary Materials Table S1.

2.1. Search Strategy

This systematic review and meta-analysis were carried out by six investigators within the framework of the EURopean micronutrient RECommendations Aligned (EURRECA) Network of Excellence, one aim of which was to undertake a series of systematic search for studies assessing the effect of zinc on different health outcomes. A comprehensive search was developed in MEDLINE (Ovid), Embase (Ovid), and The Cochrane Library (CENTRAL) up to January 2019, using search terms for ("study designs in humans") AND (Zinc) AND (intake OR status). Additional articles were identified through manual searching and citation tracking (Figure 1).

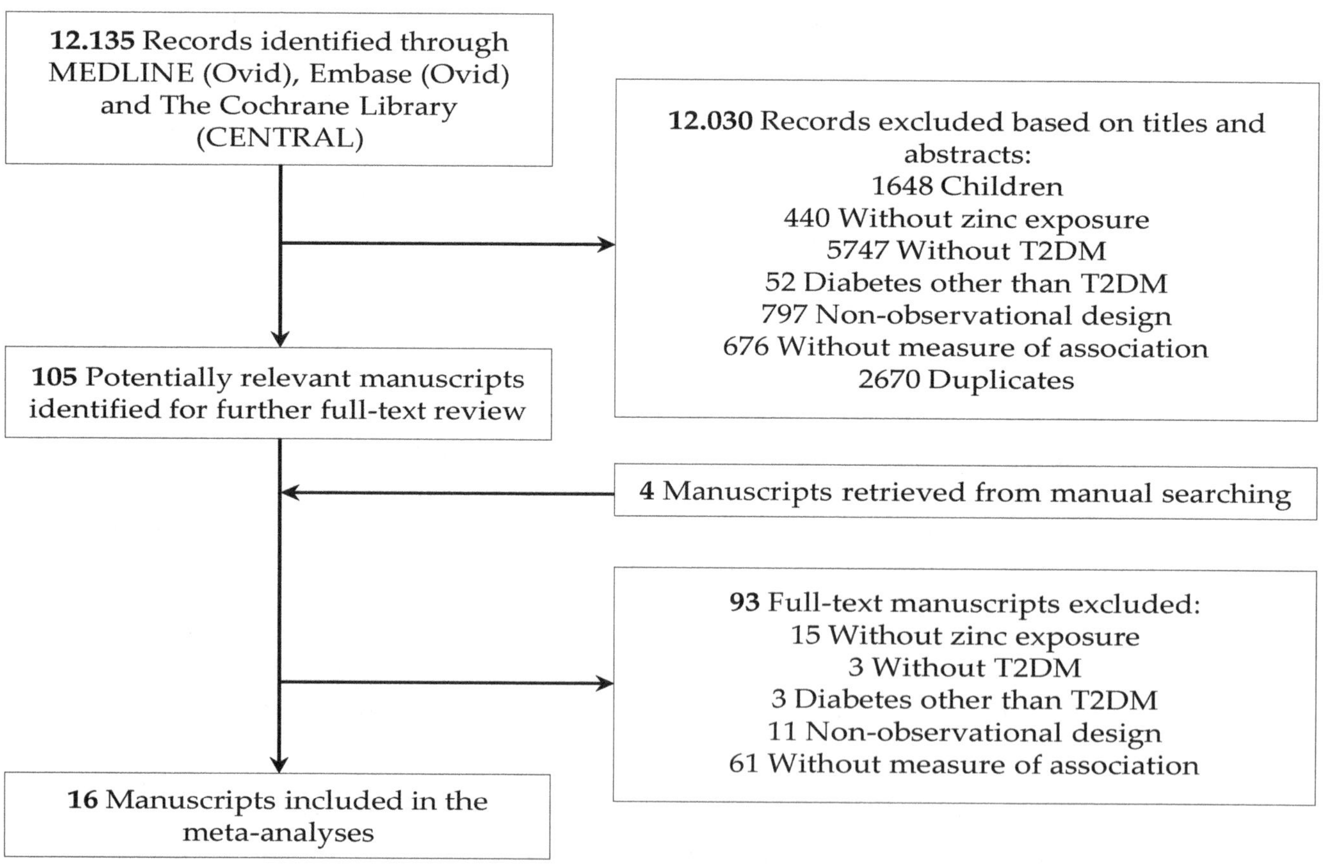

Figure 1. Flowchart of the selection process.

2.2. Study Eligibility Criteria

Studies were selected according to the following inclusion criteria: (1) studies of observational design, including prospective cohort, case-control, and cross-sectional; (2) studies conducted on human adults, with type 2 diabetes mellitus (T2DM) or cases of incident diabetes and healthy control individuals or controls of non-incident diabetes; (3) publications reported in English, Spanish or other

European languages; (4) studies that reported a measure of association, such as relative risk (RR), odds ratio (OD) or hazard ratio (HR), between dietary, supplementary, and/or total zinc intake and/or serum/plasma and/or whole blood zinc concentration and T2DM, through a multivariable adjusted analysis that compared the highest quantile of zinc exposure versus the lowest. Studies that compared user versus non-user of zinc supplements in relation to T2DM were also selected. Other kinds of observational study designs, such as case reports, case series or ecological studies; reviews; and experimental or quasi-experimental studies, as well as those with participants diagnosed with diabetes mellitus other than T2DM, were excluded.

2.3. Study Selection

Titles and abstracts of studies identified through the literature search were independently screened for eligibility. Subsequently, the full text of relevant studies was retrieved and examined further against the inclusion and exclusion criteria. Reasons for excluding studies were recorded. The selection process was independently completed by members of the research team (JCFC, MWM, VHM, CD, and NL). A 10% sample was cross-checked by another investigator (MWM) to ensure consistency between reviewers, and any discrepancy or disagreement was resolved by discussion until consensus was reached among the reviewers.

2.4. Data Extraction and Study Quality Assessment

One reviewer (JCFC) carried out the data extraction process using a data-extraction spreadsheet. Two other reviewers (VHM and NL) independently screened the accuracy of the extracted data. In order to avoid the inclusion of duplicate data in the meta-analyses, some strategies were applied: first, the name of the project was recorded for all studies that met the inclusion criteria, as well as the geographic location where the studies had been conducted; second, the lists of authors were compared among them. Complementary data from the same project was included for a qualitative summary.

From each manuscript selected for inclusion, the following data were extracted into an excel spreadsheet: study identification (first author's name, year of publication, and name of the project), study characteristics (study design, period of follow-up, measure of association, adjustment variables, quality score, country, geographic regions, geographic area, sample base, matched design, sample size for each group and total, zinc assessment method, zinc quantiles adjusted for energy, ascertainment of T2DM, percentage of T2DM subjects, effect size, and 95% confidence interval (CI) for the most adjusted model), and study population (age, gender, ethnicity, area of residence—dietary, supplementary and total zinc intake, as well as serum, plasma, and whole blood zinc concentration—BMI, fasting glucose levels, stage of diabetes). To incorporate relevant data in forms other than the mean and standard deviation, such as median and the interquartile range, estimation methods proposed by Wan et al., [24] were applied, which are valid for both normal and skewed data. When covariates of interest were expressed as a range, the midpoint of the range was assumed. If any of the data were missing, the authors were contacted for additional data.

The quality of studies selected was evaluated by one research investigator (JCFC) using the Strengthening the Reporting of Observational Studies in Epidemiology (STROBE) Statement [25]. The STROBE checklist is shown in Supplementary Materials Table S2. The quality score was used to assess its possible influence on results.

2.5. Statistical Analysis

Meta-analyses comparing the highest versus the lowest quantile of exposure to zinc intake and/or status were performed when at least two studies with a common exposure in relation to T2DM were available. For all meta-analyses, effect size and 95% CIs were log-transformed. Estimated standard errors were calculated from log 95% CIs by subtracting the lower bound of the CI from the upper bound and subsequently dividing by two times 1.96. The method of a random-effects model and the generic inverse variance method were used to calculate the pooled effect sizes, reported as OR and 95% CI. Relative risks and hazard ratios were deemed equivalent to ORs [30]. The most adjusted model of the multivariable analysis in the selected studies was used to estimate the effect size in all meta-analyses. Forest plots were created to visualize individual and global estimates. As the studies included in the meta-analysis on supplementary zinc intake and T2DM reported exposure either in quantiles or as dichotomous variable (user versus no user), a stratified meta-analysis was performed based on these criteria.

Univariate and multivariate meta-regressions with Knapp–Hartung modification [31] were conducted to examine the potential impact of certain covariates on effect size. To display relevant results of a single continuous covariate in univariate meta-regressions, bubble plots were created. This graph represents the fitted regression line together with circles representing the estimates from each study, sized according to the precision of each estimate (the inverse of its within-study variance). Multivariate meta-regressions models were executed adding the covariate with the strongest association in univariate analysis first and then adding the next one in turn. Covariates showing collinearity were removed from the final multivariate model. Finally, a meta-regression equation was generated using the intercept (a), as well as the regression coefficient (b) of a specific covariate, to know how the effect size (OR for T2DM) changes with a unit increase in the exploratory covariate ($\mathrm{Ln}\ (\mathrm{OR}_{\mathrm{T2DM}}) = (\mathrm{a}) + \mathrm{b} \times$ (covariate)).

Heterogeneity was assessed by the Cochran Q-statistic and the I^2 statistic to quantify the percentage of variation attributable to between-study heterogeneity [32]. I^2 values of 25%, 50%, and 75% were considered as low, medium, and high heterogeneity, respectively [33,34]. Potential sources of heterogeneity were explored through stratified analyses and univariate meta-regressions, even if an initial heterogeneity was non-significant [35], using different variables. Thus, categorical variables were: study design, study design and area of residence, measures of association, quality score, geographic regions, location, sample base, matched design, sample size, zinc intake assessment method, zinc serum/plasma assessment method, ascertainment of T2DM, diagnostic pattern, percentage of T2DM, gender, ethnicity, area of residence, group with higher serum/plasma zinc levels, zinc quantiles adjusted for energy. In addition, continuous variables were also used, such as sample size for each group and total, period of follow-up (years), quality score (%), percentage of T2DM subjects (%), age in cases and controls (years), age difference and ratio between cases and controls (years), serum/plasma zinc levels in cases and controls (μg/dL), serum/plasma zinc difference and ratio between cases and controls (μg/dL), BMI in cases and controls ($\mathrm{kg/m^2}$), BMI difference and ratio between cases and controls ($\mathrm{kg/m^2}$), fasting glucose levels in cases and controls (mmol/L), and fasting glucose difference and ratio between cases and controls (mmol/L). Multivariate meta-regressions were also utilized to examine further the covariates that had a significant influence on heterogeneity in univariate analysis. In addition, the proportion of between-study variance explained by one or more covariates was estimated through the adjusted R^2 ($R_A{}^2$). Likewise, the percentage of residual variation due to heterogeneity which remains unexplained by one or more covariates ($I_r{}^2$) was obtained.

To assess the power of each study on the overall pooled estimates, sensitivity analysis was performed using the leave-one-out method [36], where one study was excluded at a time, evaluating the impact of removing each of the studies on the summary results and the between-study heterogeneity. Furthermore, publication bias was investigated by visual inspection of funnel plots and quantitatively assessed using Egger's [37] and Begg's [38] tests. All analyses were performed with STATA statistical software, version 15.0. (STATA Corp., College Station, Texas, USA).

3. Results

The literature search strategy generated 12,136 publications, and 16 studies were finally selected for this systematic review and meta-analysis of observational studies [4–7,10–12,14–19,39–41]. There were no studies that were excluded for reasons of language. The details of the selection process and the reasons for exclusion are shown in the flowchart (Figure 1). The quality of selected publications, according to the Strengthening the Reporting of Observational Studies in Epidemiology (STROBE)

Statement [42], was high. The compliance percentages of the STROBE items were between 69 and 100%, 14 of the 16 selected studies above 80% [4–7,10–12,14–19,39,41]. The characteristics of the included studies for meta-analyses are summarized in Tables 1–3.

3.1. *Dietary Zinc Intake and T2DM*

Seven prospective cohort studies [4–7,10,11] and one cross-sectional study [39] were included in the meta-analysis of the association between dietary zinc intake and T2DM (Table 1). Five studies were carried out in the western countries (USA, the Nurses' Health Study (NHS) cohort [4], the Multi-Ethnic Study of Atherosclerosis (MESA) cohort [10], and the Coronary Artery Risk Development in Young Adults (CARDIA) cohort [11]; Australia, the Australian Longitudinal Study on Women's Health (ALSWH) cohort [5]; and Sweden, the Malmö Diet and Cancer Study (MDCS) cohort [6]), and two in the eastern countries (India [39], and Japan, the Japan Collaborative Cohort (JACC) [7]). This meta-analysis comprised 146,027 participants aged between 18 and 84 years, and of both genders, belonging to different ethnic groups (Hispanic, Caucasian, African American, Chinese or South Asian, among others), and areas of residence (rural or urban). During the follow-up of participants, between 4.8 years on average in the MESA cohort [10] and 24 years in the NHS cohort [4], 11,511 cases of T2DM were detected (7.8%). The percentage of T2DM cases was highly variable between the studies, from 2.5% in the JACC study [7] to 14.1% in the Swedish MDCS cohort [6].

Dietary zinc intake was collected using validated food frequency questionnaires (VFFQs) [4,5,7,10], validated diet history questionnaires (VDHQ) [6,11], or a 7-day dietary record [39]. The mean of dietary zinc intake ranged from 5.6 ± 1.6 mg/day in urban women from India [39] to 16.7 mg/day in urban subjects from the USA [11]. Ascertainment of T2DM was carried out through different criteria (fasting plasma glucose (FPG) and/or oral glucose tolerance test (OGTT), and/or self-reported, and/or using registries from different institutions, and/or use of antidiabetic drugs).

To evaluate the association between the dietary zinc intake and the T2DM, a meta-analysis was conducted (Figure 2). The pooled effect size for T2DM comparing the highest versus lowest dietary zinc intakes was 0.87 (95% CI: 0.78–0.98), with moderate to high heterogeneity ($I^2 = 64.5\%$, $p = 0.003$).

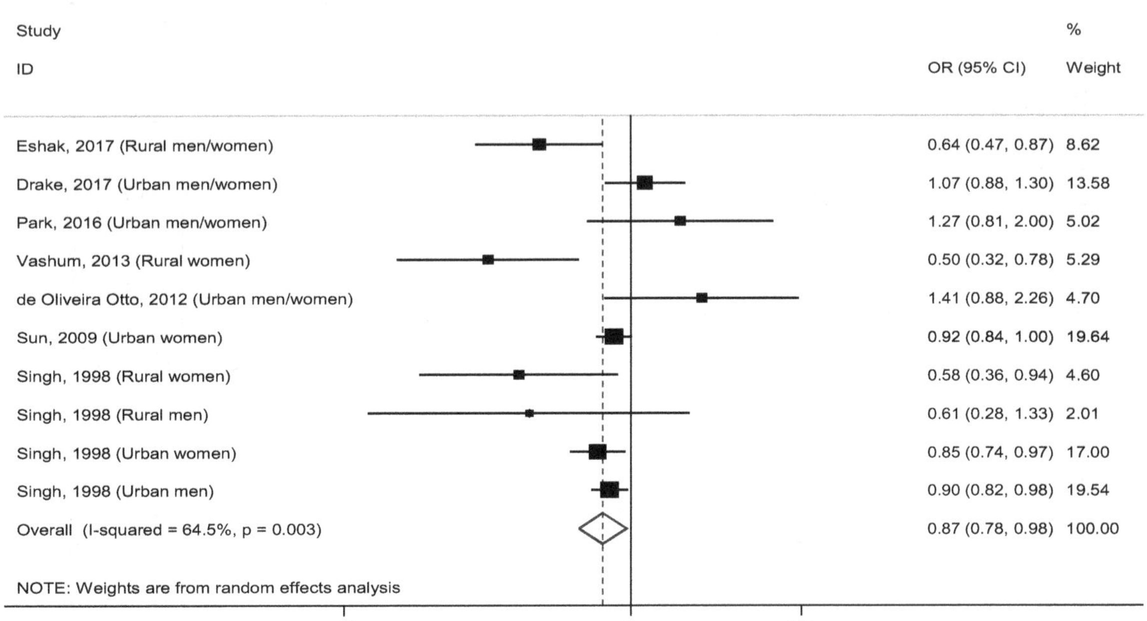

Figure 2. Forest plot of pooled effect size of the highest versus lowest dietary zinc intake for T2DM. Squares represent odds ratios (OR) for each study, and the size of the square is the study-specific statistical weight. Horizontal lines indicate the 95% CI of each study. Diamond represents the combined OR estimate with corresponding 95% CI.

Table 1. Characteristics of studies reporting the association between dietary zinc intake and risk of type 2 diabetes.

Author, Year (Study)	Location (Area)	Study Design	Follow-Up (Years)	Ethnicity	Gender	Age (Years) in Cases at Baseline (mean ± SD)	Age (Years) in Controls at Baseline (mean ± SD)	Sample Size (T2DM)	T2DM (%)	Ascertainment of T2DM	Zinc Assessment Method	Zinc Intake (mg/day) in Cases (mean ± SD)	Zinc Intake (mg/day) in Controls (mean ± SD)	Effect Size (95% CI)
Drake, 2017 (MDCS)	Sweden (urban)	Prospective cohort	Median: 19	White	Men/ Women	58.0 ± 7.0	57.8 ± 7.7	26,132 (3676)	14.1	FPG ≥ 7.0 mmol/L (twice), or registries	VDHQ	11.6 ± 3.6	11.1 ± 3.3	HR: 1.07 (0.88–1.30)
Eshak, 2017 (JACC)	Japan (rural, mostly)	Prospective cohort	5	Japanese	Men/ Women	Range: 40–65		16,160 (396)	2.5	Self-report	VFFQ	7.3 ± 0.8		OR: 0.64 (0.54–1.00)
Park, 2016 (CARDIA)	USA (urban)	Prospective cohort	23	African American, Caucasian	Men/ Women	Range: 18–30; 27.03 ± 3.61		3960 (418)	10.6	FPG ≥ 7.0 mmol/L, or 2-h 75-g OGTT ≥ 11.1 mmol/L, or HbA1c ≥ 6.5%, or drugs	VDHQ	16.7		HR: 1.27 (0.81–2.01)
Vashum, 2013 (ALSWH)	Australia (rural, mostly)	Prospective cohort	6	Australian	Women	Range: 45–50		8921 (333)	3.7	Self-report	VFFQ	10.7		OR: 0.50 (0.32–0.77)
de Oliveira Otto, 2012 (MESA)	USA (urban)	Prospective cohort	Mean: 4.8	White, Asian, African American, Hispanic	Men/ Women	Range: 45–84 61.8 ± 10.3		4982 (499)	10.0	FPG ≥ 6.99 mmol/L, or self-reported, or drugs	VFFQ	Median (standard error) 8.3 (4.4)		HR: 1.41 (0.88–2.27)
Sun, 2009 (NHS)	USA (urban)	Prospective cohort	24	White	Women	Range: 33–60		82,297 (6030)	7.3	Self-report	VFFQ	N/A	N/A	RR: 0.92 (0.84–1.00)
Singh, 1998	India (rural)	Cross-sectional study	N/A	South Asian	Men	25–64		894 (27)	3.0	FPG > 7.7 mmol/L, or 2-h 75-g OGTT > 11.1 mmol/L	7-day dietary record	8.8 ± 2.2		OR: 0.61 (0.35–1.66)
					Women			875 (24)	2.7			8.1 ± 2.1		OR: 0.58 (0.44–1.15)
	India (urban)				Men			904 (63)	7.0			7.0 ± 2.0		OR: 0.90 (0.82–0.98)
					Women			902 (45)	5.0			5.6 ± 1.6		OR: 0.85 (0.71–0.93)

Abbreviations: SD, Standard Deviation; T2DM, Type 2 Diabetes Mellitus; MDCS, Malmö Diet and Cancer Study; FPG, Fasting Plasma Glucose; VDHQ, Validated Diet History Questionnaire; HR, Hazard Ratio; CI, Confidence Interval; JACC, Japan Collaborative Cohort; VFFQ, Validated Food Frequency Questionnaire; OR, Odds Ratio; CARDIA, Coronary Artery Risk Development in Young Adults; OGTT, Oral Glucose Tolerance Test; HbA1c, Glycosylated Hemoglobin; ALSWH, Australian Longitudinal Study on Women's Health; MESA, Multi-Ethnic Study of Atherosclerosis; NHS, Nurses' Health Study; N/A, Not Applicable or Not Available; RR, Relative Risk.

Table 2. Characteristics of studies reporting the association between supplementary and total zinc intake and risk of type 2 diabetes.

Author, Year (Study)	Location (Area)	Study Design	Follow-Up (Years)	Ethnicity	Gender	Age (Years) in Cases at Baseline (mean ± SD)	Age (Years) in Controls at Baseline (mean ± SD)	Sample Size (T2DM)	T2DM (%)	Ascertainment of T2DM	Zinc Assessment Method	Zinc Intake (mg/day) in Cases (mean ± SD)	Zinc Intake (mg/day) in Controls (mean ± SD)	Effect Size (95% CI)
Supplementary zinc intake														
Drake, 2017 (MDCS)	Sweden (urban)	Prospective cohort	Median: 19	White	Men/ Women	58.0 ± 7.0	57.8 ± 7.7	26,132 (3676)	14.1	FPG ≥ 7.0 mmol/L (twice), or registries	VDHQ	12.3% user	17.7% user	HR: 0.83 (0.71–0.98)
Song, 2011 (NIH-AARP)	USA (urban)	Prospective cohort	10	White, mostly	Men/ Women	Range: 50–71		232,007 (14,130)	6.1	Self-report	Dietary survey	12.5% user	5.7% user	OR: 1.05 (0.98–1.13)
Sun, 2009 (NHS)	USA (urban)	Prospective cohort	24	White	Women with low dietary zinc intake	Range: 33–60		27,432 (2002)	7.3	Self-report	VFFQ	6.3% user in 1980–48.6% user in 2004		RR: 0.86 (0.74–0.99)
		Prospective cohort			Women with high dietary zinc intake			27,432 (2002)						RR: 1.05 (0.92–1.19)
Total zinc intake														
Drake, 2017 (MDCS)	Sweden (urban)	Prospective cohort	Median: 19	White	Men/ Women	58.0 ± 7.0	57.8 ± 7.7	26,132 (3676)	14.1	FPG ≥ 7.0 mmol/L (twice), or registries	VDHQ	12.9 ± 5.4	13.0 ± 6.2	HR: 1.05 (0.88–1.25)
Sun, 2009 (NHS)	USA (urban)	Prospective cohort	24	White	Women	Range: 33–60	N/A	82,297 (6030)	7.3	Self-report	VFFQ	Median range: 4.9–18.0	N/A	RR: 0.90 (0.82–0.99)

Abbreviations: SD, Standard Deviation; T2DM, Type 2 Diabetes Mellitus; MDCS, Malmö Diet and Cancer Study; FPG, Fasting Plasma Glucose; VDHQ, Validated Diet History Questionnaire; HR, Hazard Ratio; NIH-AARP, National Institutes of Health-American Association of Retired Persons Diet and Health Study; OR, Odds Ratio; NHS, Nurses' Health Study; N/A, Not Applicable or Not Available; VFFQ, Validated Food Frequency Questionnaire; RR, Relative Risk.

Table 3. Characteristics of studies reporting the association between serum/plasma and whole blood zinc concentration and risk of type 2 diabetes.

Author, Year	Location	Study Design	Follow-Up (Years)	Ethnicity	Gender	Age (Years) in Cases at Baseline (mean ± SD)	Age (Years) in Controls at Baseline (mean ± SD)	Sample Size (T2DM)	T2DM (%)	Ascertainment of T2DM	Zinc Assessment Method	Zinc Levels (μg/dL) in Diabetic Subjects (mean ± SD)	Zinc Levels (μg/dL) in Controls (mean ± SD)	Effect Size (95% CI)
Serum/plasma zinc concentration														
Yuan, 2018 (DFTJ)	China (urban)	Nested case-control	4.6	Chinese	Men/ Women	62.8 ± 7.2	62.9 ± 7.3	2078 (1039)	N/A	FPG ≥ 7.0 mmoL/L, or HbA1c ≥ 6.5%, or self-reported, or drugs	ICP-MS	169.6 ± 142.4	156.1 ± 126.5	OR: 1.09 (0.81–1.48)
Li, 2017	China (urban)	Cross-sectional	N/A	Chinese Han	Men/ Women	Range: 40–92, mean: 66.3	Range: 40–92, mean: 66.5	551 (122)	N/A	RPG ≥ 11.1 mmol/L and symptoms, 2-h OGTT ≥ 11.1 mmol/L, or FPG ≥ 7.0 mmol/L, or HbA1c ≥ 6.5%	ICP-MS	Median: 63.4	Median: 57.5	OR: 2.26 (1.29–3.98)
Zhang, 2017 (REACTION)	China (urban)	Cross-sectional	N/A	Chinese	Men/ Women	57.7 ± 7.4	55.2 ± 7.9	1837 (510)	N/A	Self-reported, or FPG > 7.0 mmol/L, or 2-h 75-g OGTT > 11.1 mmol/L	ICP-MS	109.0 ± 26.0	105.0 ± 25.0	OR: 1.79 (1.13–2.84)
Yary, 2016 (KIHD)	Finland (rural / urban)	Prospective cohort	20	N/A	Men	Range: 42–60		2220 (416)	18.7	Self-reported, or FPG ≥ 7.0 mmol/L or 2-h OGTT ≥ 11.1 mmol/L	AAS	95.0 ± 10.0	93.0 ± 12.0	HR: 1.39 (1.04–1.85)
Skalnaya, 2016	Russia (urban)	Cross-sectional	N/A	N/A	Women	55.8 ± 5.3	56.7 ± 6.1	128 (64)	N/A	HbA1c≥6.5%	ICP-MS	96.0 ± 0.2	105.0 ± 0.2	OR: 0.33 (0.14–0.76)
Shan, 2014	China (urban)	Cross-sectional	N/A	Chinese Han	Men/ Women	51.0 ± 10.8	42.5 ± 11.6	1578 (785)	N/A	WHO 1999 criteria	ICP-MS	115.0 ± 45.0	172.5 ± 73.0	OR: 0.09 (0.06–0.13)
Whole blood zinc concentration														
Simic, 2017 (HUNT3)	Norway (rural, mostly)	Cross-sectional	N/A	Caucasian, mostly	Men/ Women	65.4 ± 10.6	59.2 ± 12.2	876 (267)	N/A	Self-reported	ICP-MS	Median: 764.3 Range (10–90%): 643.6–893.3	Median: 751.2 Range (10–90%): 623.5–878.2	OR: 1.08 (0.59–1.97)
Hansen, 2017 (HUNT3)	Norway (rural, mostly)	Cross-sectional	N/A	Caucasian, mostly	Men/ Women	65.2 ± 10.3	61.4 ± 14.1	883 (128)	N/A	FPG ≥ 7.0 mmol/L and/or 2-h OGTT ≥ 11.1 mmol/L	ICP-MS	Median: 799.0 Range (10–90%): 675.0–881.0	Median: 754.0 Range (10–90%): 628.0–885.0	OR: 2.19 (1.05–4.59)

Abbreviations: SD, Standard Deviation; T2DM, Type 2 Diabetes Mellitus; DFTJ, Dongfeng–Tongji; FPG, Fasting Plasma Glucose; N/A, Not Applicable or Not Available; HbA1c, Glycosylated Hemoglobin; ICP-MS, Inductively Coupled Plasma Mass Spectrometry; OR, Odds Ratio; RPG, Random Plasma Glucose; OGTT, Oral Glucose Tolerance Test; REACTION, Risk Evaluation of cAncers in Chinese diabeTic Individuals: a lONgitudinal; KIHD, Kuopio IschaemicHeart Disease Risk Factor Study; AAS, Atomic Absorption Spectrophotometry; HR, Hazard Ratio; WHO, World Health Organization; HUNT, North-TrØndelag Health.

Through a stratified analysis based on the area of residence of participants, rural versus urban, (Figure 3) we observed a higher and significant effect size in rural areas (OR = 0.59, 95% CI: 0.48–0.73), and undetectable heterogeneity (I^2 = 0.0%, p = 0.843), meanwhile in urban areas the effect became non-significant (OR = 0.94, 95% CI: 0.86–1.02; I^2 = 43.9%, p = 0.113). Subsequently, we used the adjusted R^2 to examine how much of the heterogeneity was accounted for by the area of residence (Table 4), and we found that the heterogeneity was explained to a great extent (R_A^2 = 100.0%; I_r^2 = 17.8%). Interestingly, through a stratified analysis by the covariate "study design and area of residence", we observed that this protective effect of dietary zinc intake in rural areas was found in both cross-sectional and prospective studies (Figure 4). In this analysis, results were statistically significant, and heterogeneity was reduced (I^2 = 0.0%, $p > 0.050$) for all subgroups, except for prospective studies conducted in urban areas (OR = 1.04, 95% CI: 0.88–1.24; I^2 = 50.7%, p = 0.107).

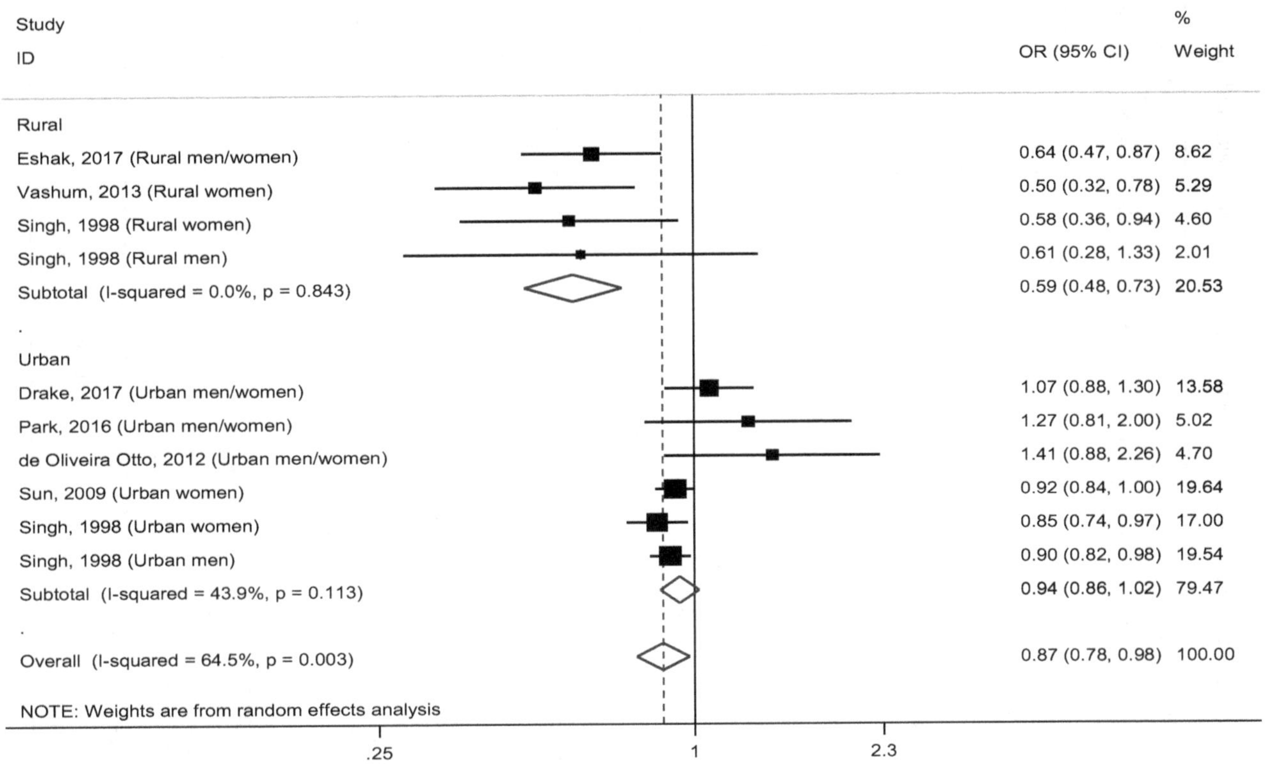

Figure 3. Forest plot of pooled effect size of the highest vs. lowest dietary zinc intake for T2DM according to area of residence (rural vs. urban). Squares represent ORs for each study, and the size of the square is the study-specific statistical weight. Horizontal lines indicate the 95% CI of each study. Diamond represents the combined OR estimate with corresponding 95% CI.

The corresponding adjusted R^2 for this covariate was 90.47%. However, the covariate that showed the greatest impact on the relationship studied was the percentage of T2DM, both as continuous and categorized variable. Thus, the stratified analysis (Figure 5) by this covariate categorized (<5/5–9.9/≥10) revealed a significant protective effect of dietary zinc intake in those studies with <5% of T2DM (OR = 0.59, 95% CI: 0.48–0.73; I^2 = 0.0%, p = 0.843), and those between 5–9.9% (OR = 0.90, 95% CI: 0.85–0.95; I^2 = 0.0%, p = 0.627), but not when it was higher than 10% (OR = 1.13, 95% CI: 0.96–1.34; I^2 = 0.0%, p = 0.499). It should be noted that the level of heterogeneity was reduced to 0.0% in all these subgroups. The importance of this covariate in the assessed relationship was supported by the large proportion of the between-study variance was explained (R_A^2 = 100.0%), as well as the undetectable percentage of the residual variation that was attributable to the between-study heterogeneity, after entering this covariate into a univariate meta-regression model (I_r^2 = 0.0%).

Table 4. Stratified meta-analyses and meta-regressions on the association between dietary zinc intake and risk of type 2 diabetes mellitus.

Subgroup	Studies (n)	Effect Size (95% CI)	Heterogeneity		Meta-Regressions					
			I^2 (%)	*p*-Value	Regression Coefficients (95% CI)	Standard Error	*p*-Value	Tau^2	I^2 Residual (%)	Adjusted R^2 (%)
Geographic area										
Western (1)	5	0.97 (0.77–1.22)	72.1%	0.006	−0.25 (−0.66; 0.17)	0.18	0.208	0.04	64.05%	6.68%
Eastern (2)	5	0.80 (0.70–0.92)	49.3%	0.096						
Geographic regions										
Oceania (1)	1	0.50 (0.32–0.78)	-	-	0.22 (0.04–0.39)	0.08	0.022	0.02	50.38%	67.68%
Asia (2)	5	0.80 (0.70–0.92)	49.3%	0.096						
America (3)	3	1.10 (0.82–1.47)	57.7%	0.094						
Europe (4)	1	1.07 (0.88–1.30)	-	-						
Area of residence										
Rural (1)	4	0.59 (0.48–0.73)	0.0%	0.843	0.45 (0.16; 0.73)	0.13	0.007	0.00	17.82%	100.0%
Urban (2)	6	0.94 (0.86–1.02)	43.9%	0.113						
Gender										
Men (1)	2	0.90 (0.82–0.98)	0.0%	0.331	0.14 (−0.17; 0.45)	0.13	0.330	0.06	67.67%	−30.54%
Women (2)	4	0.78 (0.65–0.95)	71.4%	0.015						
Men/Women (3)	4	1.02 (0.73–1.42)	74.1%	0.009						
Ethnicity										
White (1)	3	0.86 (0.66–1.12)	79.4%	0.008	0.10 (−0.06; 0.26)	0.07	0.194	0.06	68.30%	−17.63%
South Asian (2)	4	0.86 (0.77–0.95)	28.5%	0.241						
Japanese (3)	1	0.64 (0.47–0.87)	-	-						
Several ethnic groups (4)	2	1.34 (0.96–1.85)	0.0%	0.755						
Study design										
Prospective Cohort (1)	6	0.90 (0.73–1.12)	75.1%	0.001	−0.07 (−0.31; 0.16)	0.10	0.495	0.06	67.06%	−33.29%
Cross-sectional (2)	4	0.86 (0.77–0.95)	28.5%	0.241						
Study design and area of residence										
Prospective/Rural (1)	2	0.59 (0.46–0.76)	0.0%	0.367	0.18 (0.08; 0.29)	0.05	0.004	0.004	22.03%	90.47%
Cross-sectional/Rural (2)	2	0.58 (0.39–0.89)	0.0%	0.914						
Cross-sectional/Urban (3)	2	0.88 (0.82–0.95)	0.0%	0.489						
Prospective/Urban (4)	4	1.04 (0.88–1.24)	50.7%	0.107						
Measure of association										
Odds ratio (1)	5	0.75 (0.63–0.88)	63.2%	0.019	0.21 (0.05; 0.39)	0.07	0.016	0.02	49.76%	63.13%
Relative risk (2)	1	0.92 (0.84–1.00)	-	-						
Hazard ratio (3)	4	1.13 (0.96–1.34)	0.0%	0.499						

Table 4. *Cont.*

Subgroup	Studies (n)	Effect Size (95% CI)	Heterogeneity		Meta-Regressions					
			I^2 (%)	*p*-Value	Regression Coefficients (95% CI)	Standard Error	*p*-Value	Tau^2	I^2 Residual (%)	Adjusted R^2 (%)
Sample size										
<1000	4	0.86 (0.77–0.95)	28.5%	0.241	0.03 (−0.09; 0.14)	0.05	0.578	0.06	66.27%	−29.83%
1000–4999	2	1.34 (0.96–1.85)	0.0%	0.755						
5000–9999	2	0.59 (0.46–0.76)	0.0%	0.367						
≥10,000	2	0.97 (0.84–1.11)	47.9%	0.166						
Percentage of T2DM										
<5%	4	0.59 (0.48–0.73)	0.0%	0.843	0.31 (0.15; 0.46)	0.07	0.002	0.00	0.00%	100.0%
5–9.9%	3	0.90 (0.85–0.95)	0.0%	0.627						
≥10%	3	1.13 (0.96–1.34)	0.0%	0.499						
Zinc intake assessment method										
VFFQ (1)	4	0.80 (0.57–1.12)	80.3%	0.002	−0.01 (−0.28; 0.26)	0.12	0.906	0.07	68.24%	−40.61%
VDHQ (2)	2	1.10 (0.92–1.31)	0.0%	0.497						
7-day dietary record (3)	4	0.86 (0.77–0.95)	28.5%	0.241						
Zinc quantiles adjusted for energy										
Adjusted (1)	9	0.86 (0.76–0.96)	65.3%	0.003	0.42 (−0.40; 1.25)	0.36	0.271	0.04	65.34%	6.11%
Not adjusted (2)	1	1.27 (0.81–2.00)	-	-						
Ascertainment of T2DM										
FPG/OGTT (1)	4	0.86 (0.77–0.95)	28.5%	0.241	0.19 (−0.05; 0.43)	0.10	0.112	0.04	62.01%	11.25%
Self-reported (2)	3	0.70 (0.48–1.01)	82.6%	0.003						
Several criteria (3)	3	1.13 (0.96–1.34)	0.0%	0.499						
Diagnostic pattern										
One diagnostic pattern	7	0.81 (0.72–0.91)	61.7%	0.016	0.41 (0.06; 0.77)	0.15	0.027	0.02	53.12%	51.60%
Several diagnostic pattern	3	1.13 (0.96–1.34)	0.0%	0.499						
Study quality										
80–89	6	0.83 (0.71–0.97)	58.4%	0.035	−0.11 (−0.36; 0.58)	0.21	0.598	0.06	65.99%	−23.10%
≥90	4	0.92 (0.73–1.16)	74.0%	0.009						

Abbreviations: CI, Confidence Interval; VDHQ, Validated Diet History Questionnaire; VFFQ, Validated Food Frequency Questionnaire; T2DM, Type 2 Diabetes Mellitus; FPG, Fasting Plasma Glucose; OGTT, Oral Glucose Tolerance Test.

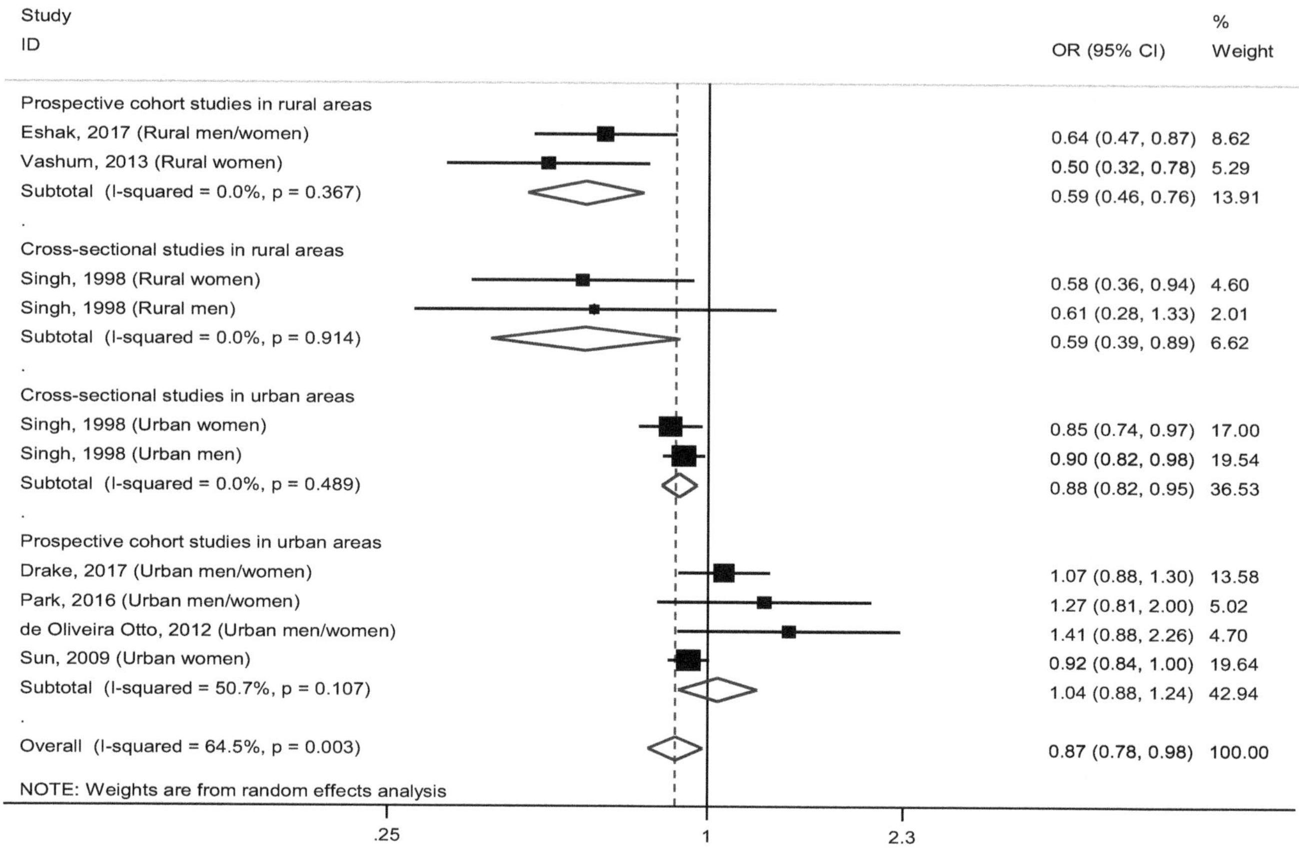

Figure 4. Forest plot of pooled effect size of the highest vs. lowest dietary zinc intake for T2DM according to study design and area of residence (prospective cohort studies in rural areas, cross-sectional studies in rural areas, cross-sectional studies in urban areas, and prospective cohort studies in urban areas). Squares represent ORs for each study, and the size of the square is the study-specific statistical weight. Horizontal lines indicate the 95% CI of each study. Diamond represents the combined OR estimate with corresponding 95% CI.

A multivariate meta-regression model adding the three covariates with a significantly higher impact on the association, showed that only a "percentage of T2DM" continued being significant (0.23, 95% CI: 0.02, 0.45, $p = 0.037$). Once the fourth covariate was introduced, none remained significant. When we analyzed the percentage of T2DM as a continuous variable, similar results were observed ($R_A^2 = 100.0\%$, $I_r^2 = 23.6\%$). A bubble plot was used to represent this covariate (Figure 6), and it was found that, as the percentage of T2DM increased, the protective effect of a moderately high dietary zinc intake was reduced in a relationship defined by the equation of the regression line: ($Ln(OR_{T2DM}) = (-0.4217314) + 0.0437897 \times$ (percentage of T2DM)).

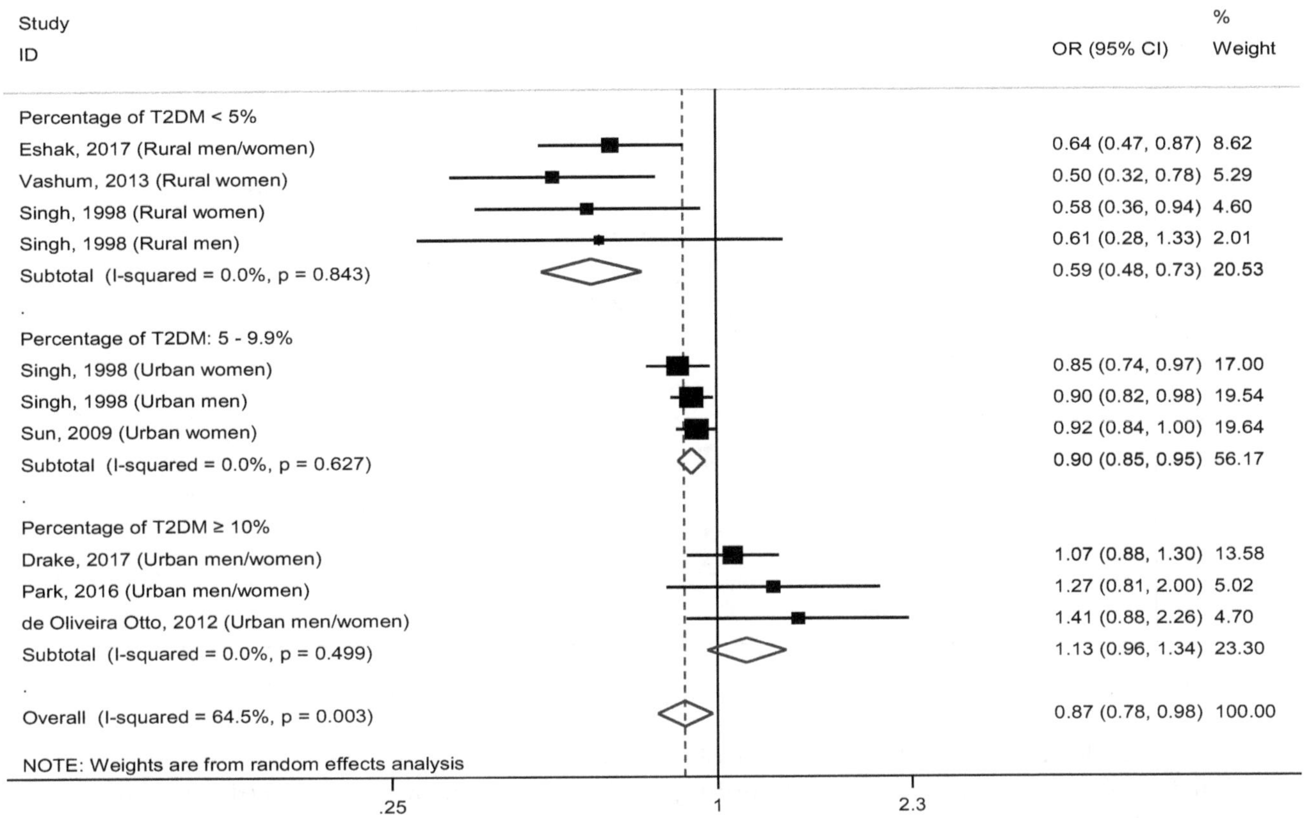

Figure 5. Forest plot of pooled effect size of the highest vs. lowest dietary zinc intake for T2DM according to the percentage of T2DM (<5%/5–9.9%/≥10%). Squares represent ORs for each study, and the size of the square is the study-specific statistical weight. Horizontal lines indicate the 95% CI of each study. Diamond represents the combined OR estimate with corresponding 95% CI.

The effect size ranged between (OR = 0.84, 95% CI: 0.75–0.96) after excluding the study carried out by Drake et al. [6], and (OR = 0.90, 95% CI: 0.81–0.99), after excluding the study conducted by Vashum et al. [5]. However, the combined overall effect size remained on the verge of statistical significance after removing the data obtained by Singh et al. [39] in urban Indian women (OR = 0.87, 95% CI: 0.76–1.00), or that of Eshak et al. [7] in Japanese subjects (OR = 0.90, 95% CI: 0.80–1.01). Finally, for this meta-analysis, an overall symmetry of the funnel plots was observed by visual inspection (Supplementary Materials Figure S1). This was confirmed by the Egger's (p = 0.429) and Begg's (p = 0.721) tests, indicating the absence of publication bias.

3.2. Supplementary Zinc Intake and T2DM

Three studies of 313,003 individuals assessed the association between supplementary zinc intake and T2DM (NHS cohort [4], National Institutes of Health-American Association of Retired Persons (NIH-AARP) Diet and Health Study [12], MDCS cohort [6]) (Table 2). The follow-up period of these prospective cohort studies ranged between 10 [12] to 24 years [4]. Participants were white (mostly) women [4] or subjects of both genders [6,12], aged between 33 and 71 years, and from urban areas. In total, 17,806 patients with incident diabetes (between 6.1 and 14.1%) were identified according to different diagnostic criteria (self-reported [4,12], or through an FPG ≥ 7.0 mmol/L measured twice, and institutional registries [6]).

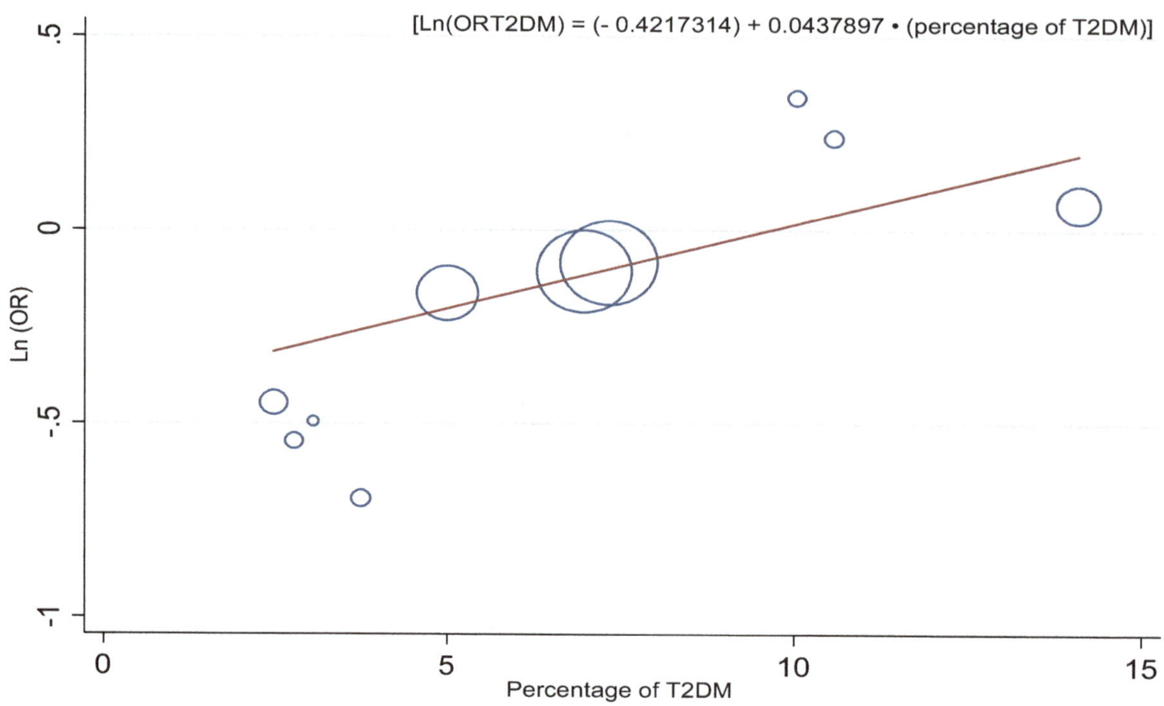

Figure 6. Bubble plot with a fitted meta-regression line of the relationship between the Ln(OR) and the percentage of T2DM. Circles are sized according to the precision of each estimate (the inverse of its within-study variance).

Supplementary zinc intake was determined using different food intake instruments, such as VFFQ [4], VDHQ [6], or dietary survey, including an FFQ and a short survey [12]. The percentage of patients with incident diabetes supplemented with zinc was around 12.5% [6,12], meanwhile in controls of non-incident diabetes, zinc supplementation ranged between 5.7% in the NIH-AARP Diet and Health Study [12], to 17.7%, in the MDCS cohort [6]. The NHS cohort reported a large increase in the proportion of women who were supplemented with zinc in 2004 (48.6%) compared with 1980 (6.3%) [4].

The association between supplementary zinc intake and the risk of T2DM was evaluated through a meta-analysis stratified by whether the analysis had been done comparing zinc supplement users versus non-users or comparing the highest versus lowest quantile of supplementary zinc intake, in order not to introduce bias in the analysis (Figure 7). Results revealed a non-significant association between zinc supplement users versus non-users and T2DM (OR = 0.94, 95% CI: 0.75–1.19; $I^2 = 85.4\%$, $p = 0.009$), and between higher supplementary zinc intake versus lower and T2DM (OR = 0.95, 95% CI: 0.78–1.16; $I^2 = 75.3\%$, $p = 0.044$), and an elevated heterogeneity in both cases.

Publication bias was unlikely in this meta-analysis, according to Egger's ($p = 0.186$), and Begg's ($p = 0.089$) tests (Figure S2).

3.3. *Total Zinc Intake and T2DM*

The final data set for the meta-analysis of total zinc intake and risk of T2DM included only two large prospective cohort studies [4,6] (Table 2). Nevertheless, both studies comprised 108,429 individuals, 9706 patients with incident diabetes and 98,723 controls of non-incident diabetes. Incidence of T2DM was 14.1% in the middle-aged Swedish cohort of urban men and women (MDCS) [6], and 7.3% in the American cohort of urban women (NHS) [4]. A VFFQ [4] and a VDHQ [6] were used to determine the total zinc intake, that ranged from 4.9 to 18.0 mg/day in the NHS cohort [4], and around 12.9 ± 5.4 mg/day in controls of non-incident diabetes and 13.0 ± 6.2 mg/day in patients with incident diabetes from the MDCS cohort [6].

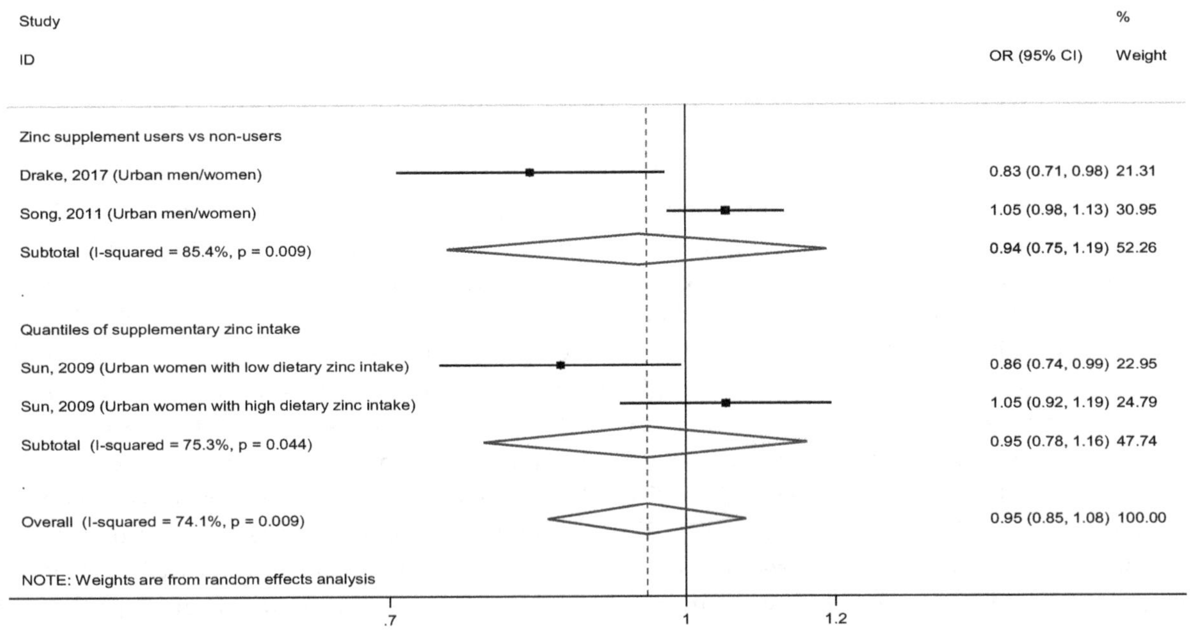

Figure 7. Forest plot of the pooled effect size of the highest versus lowest supplementary zinc intake for T2DM according to the analysis (zinc supplement users/non-users versus quantiles of supplementary zinc intake). Squares represent ORs for each study, and the size of the square is the study-specific statistical weight. Horizontal lines indicate the 95% CI of each study. Diamond represents the combined OR estimate with corresponding 95% CI.

After pooling data from both studies (Figure 8), we found that total zinc intake was not significantly associated with the incidence of T2DM (OR = 0.95, 95% CI: 0.82–1.11). There was moderate heterogeneity between the studies ($I^2 = 56.5\%$, $p = 0.129$). Moreover, no evidence of publication bias was found ($p = 1.000$) (Supplementary Materials Figure S3).

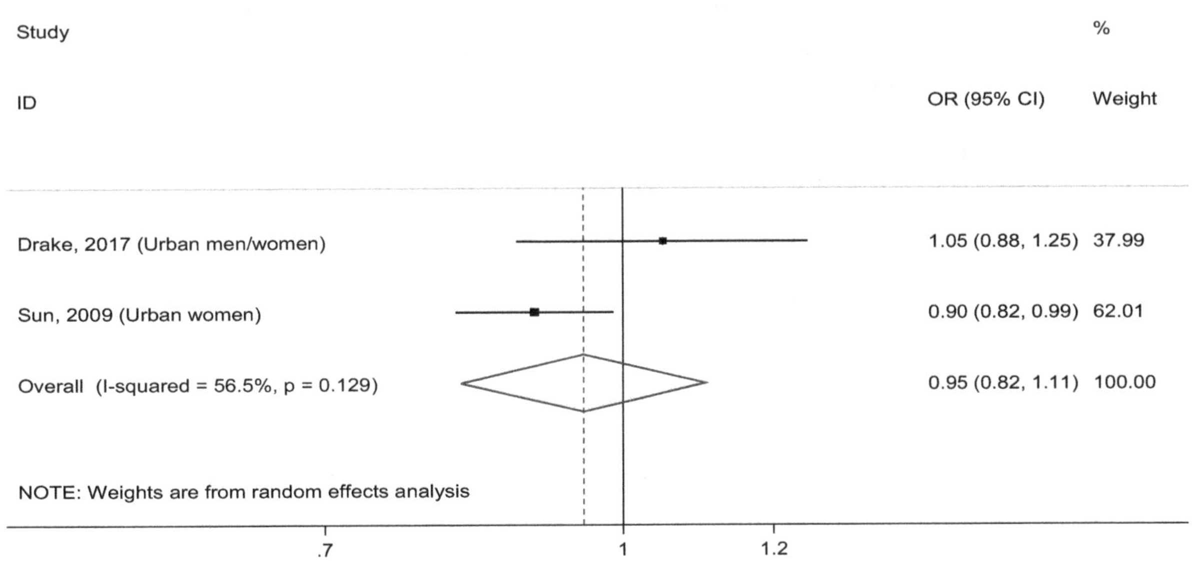

Figure 8. Forest plot of pooled effect size of the highest vs. lowest total zinc intake for T2DM. Squares represent ORs for each study, and the size of the square is the study-specific statistical weight. Horizontal lines indicate the 95% CI of each study. Diamond represents the combined OR estimate with corresponding 95% CI.

3.4. Whole Blood Zinc Concentration and T2DM

Only two cross-sectional studies carried out within the third survey of the population-based Nord-Trøndelag Health Study (HUNT3 Survey) were identified to assess the relationship between concentration of zinc in whole blood and T2DM [18,19]. The fact that both studies shared part of the same study sample prevented the execution of a meta-analysis to obtain a pooled result. Nevertheless, a qualitative summary was conducted to present the findings of these two studies (Table 3). Participants in both studies were men and women, mainly Caucasian, and aged around 61.5 ± 8.7 years old, who lived mainly in rural areas from Norway. The main difference between these two studies was the sampling strategy. Hansen et al. [18] selected 876 subjects at high risk for T2DM, but without previously known diabetes. In this study, 128 previously undiagnosed cases of T2DM, were detected by screening [18]. In contrast, Simic et al. [19] included 883 subjects, of which 267 had self-reported T2DM, i.e., they were patients in a more advanced stage of the disease. Curiously, while Hansen et al. [18] found a significant and positive association between a higher whole blood zinc concentration and the onset of T2DM (OR = 2.19, 95% CI: 1.05–4.59), Simic et al. [19] did not observe any significant relationship (OR = 1.08, 95% CI: 0.59–1.97). Differences in concentrations of zinc in whole blood between cases and controls, measured in both studies through inductively coupled plasma mass spectrometry (ICP-MS), were more evident in the study conducted by Hansen et al. [18] (median in cases: 799.0 µg/dL; median in controls: 754.0 µg/dL) compared to the one carried out by Simic et al. [19] (median in cases: 764.3 µg/dL; median in controls: 751.2 µg/dL). It is worth noting that the median whole blood zinc concentration in the control subjects in both studies was very similar, but not in those of the diabetic subjects.

3.5. Serum/Plasma Zinc Concentration and T2DM

Six observational studies (one prospective cohort study [14], one nested case-control study [15], and four cross-sectional studies [16,17,40,41]) were included in the meta-analysis of serum/plasma zinc concentration and T2DM (Table 3). Four studies were carried out on Chinese urban men and women between the ages of 40 and 90 years [15,16,40,41], one in Russian women with an average age of 56.3 ± 5.7 years [17], and one in Finnish men aged between 42 and 60 years [14]. The total number of cases of T2DM was 2936, among 8392 participants. The period of follow-up was between 4.6 years in the nested case control within the Dongfeng–Tongji (DFTJ) cohort [15], and 20 years in the KIHD study [14]. Serum/plasma zinc concentration was determined mainly by ICP-MS [15–17,40,41], meanwhile the KIHD used atomic absorption spectrophotometry (AAS) [14]. The levels of serum/plasma zinc in controls ranged from a median of 57.5 µg/dL to a mean of 172.5 ± 73.0 µg/dL; and in cases from a median of 63.4 µg/dL to a mean of 169.6 ± 142.4 µg/dL.

The combined effect size of T2DM for the highest versus lowest quantile of serum/plasma zinc concentration was 0.76 (95% CI: 0.29–2.01). However, a high level of heterogeneity was found ($I^2 = 97.1\%$, $p < 0.001$). Sensitivity analysis omitting one study at a time and calculating the heterogeneity for the remainder of the studies showed that the study conducted by Shan et al. [16] substantially influenced the overall heterogeneity, resulting in a reduction around 31% of this when it was excluded. In addition, the elimination of this study and the one carried out by Skalnaya et al. [17], decreased the level of heterogeneity by 44.5%, showing their impact on results (OR = 1.47, 95% CI: 1.11–1.95; $I^2 = 53.9\%$, $p = 0.090$). Nevertheless, the exclusion of any other study had a negligible effect on heterogeneity. When performing stratified analysis for "sample base" (Figure 9), a significant and positive association was found in the subgroup of "population or community-based studies" (OR = 1.64, 95% CI: 1.25–2.14), and a low heterogeneity ($I^2 > 22.5\%$, $p = 0.275$). On the other hand, "non-population or community-based studies" showed a very high level of heterogeneity ($I^2 > 98.0\%$, $p < 0.001$). Likewise, when it was stratified by the covariate "group with higher zinc levels", a relationship between serum/plasma zinc levels and T2DM (OR = 1.47, 95% CI: 1.11–1.95; $I^2 = 53.9\%$, $p = 0.090$) was observed in the subgroup of studies with higher zinc levels in the case group compared to controls (Table S3). Meanwhile, a significant negative relationship was found in the subgroup in which controls had higher serum/plasma concentration (OR = 0.16, 95% CI: 0.05–0.54), but with a high heterogeneity ($I^2 = 86.4\%$, $p = 0.007$). Finally, the difference in mean serum/plasma zinc concentration between cases and controls, as well its ratio, also explained, to a large extent, the heterogeneity observed ($R_A{}^2 = 85.2\%$, for mean difference; and $R_A{}^2 = 92.6\%$, for mean ratio), as expected.

Although the funnel plot showed some degree of asymmetry (Figure S3), we did not detect any risk of publication bias according to the Egger's ($p = 0.815$) or Begg's tests ($p = 0.707$).

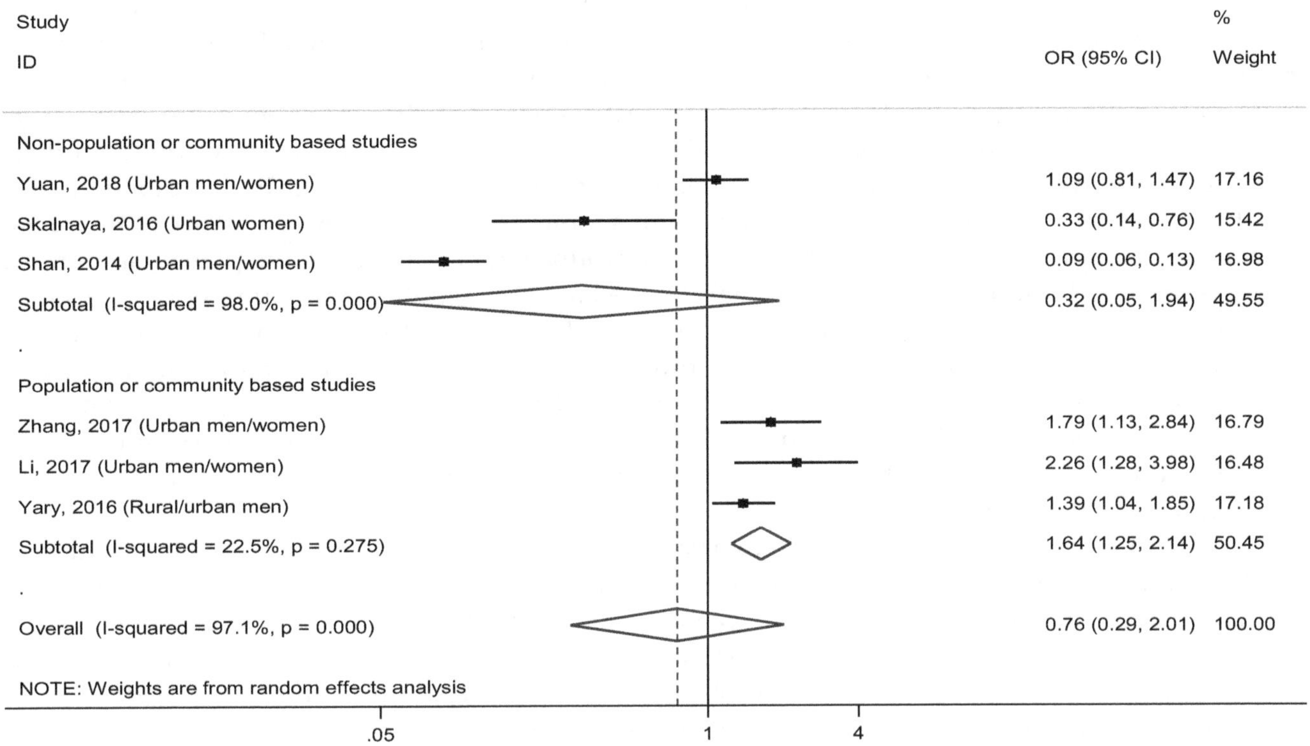

Figure 9. Forest plot of pooled effect size of the highest vs. lowest serum/plasma zinc concentration for T2DM according to the sample base (population/community-based studies vs. non-population/community-based studies). Squares represent ORs for each study, and the size of the square is the study-specific statistical weight. Horizontal lines indicate the 95% CI of each study. Diamond represents the combined OR estimate with corresponding 95% CI.

4. Discussion

This systematic review and meta-analysis of observational studies found an inverse association between dietary zinc intake and T2DM. This could suggest a potential beneficial role of zinc from diet to prevent the risk of this disease. In addition, the relationship seemed to be more evident in rural areas, and when the proportion of T2DM cases in the population was low or moderate. Conversely, a non-significant association between total or supplementary zinc intake and T2DM was observed, although data are limited. Whole blood zinc concentration could be directly related to T2DM only at an early phase of the diabetes disease, as suggested by results from the same cohort study. This hypothesis could not be examined for serum/plasma zinc concentration. Nevertheless, a positive relationship was found between this biomarker of zinc status and T2DM in population-based studies.

Our results suggest that a diet moderately elevated in zinc could help to prevent the development of T2DM. We tried to determine the cut-off point or range of dietary zinc intake with a protective effect against type 2 diabetes mellitus (T2DM); however, data were imprecise, heterogeneous, and not reported in all the studies. Despite these limitations in the data of the selected studies, it was notable that when the lowest quantiles (reference) did not reach the dietary reference intakes (DRI) according to the Institute Of Medicine (IOM) for adult men (11 mg/day) and women (8 mg/day) [43], those quantiles of dietary zinc intake that reached or moderately exceeded the DRI showed a protective effect, even in the intermediate quantiles [4,5]. Furthermore, when the highest quantiles of dietary zinc intake did not reach the DRI, no significant association was observed [10]. Interestingly, when the lowest quantiles of dietary zinc intake reached the DRI, the highest quantiles (>23.34 mg/day) did not show a protective effect on T2DM, and could even have a harmful impact on the risk of T2DM as observed in a model not fully adjusted [11]. These data seem to suggest that a dietary zinc intake within or slightly above the DRI could have a protective role on the risk of T2DM, but not when intake is very high. Consistent with our findings, several observational studies have shown a protective effect of a moderately high dietary zinc intake on cardiometabolic conditions, such as metabolic syndrome [44,45] and gestational hyperglycemia [46], and mortality by cardiovascular disease [47] and all causes [48]. Conversely, other studies have found no significant [10,49], or even direct associations [50,51] between dietary zinc intake and some of these cardiometabolic events. The first systematic review of prospective cohort studies on the association between zinc status, including dietary zinc intake, and risk of cardiovascular disease and T2DM [13] revealed a limited number of studies on this topic, as well as the inconsistence of their results. As the authors themselves suggested, the effect of confounding factors may have played an important role in the observed findings. In our meta-analysis we have evaluated a large number of confounding factors in order to identify and quantify those that could impact on the relationship between dietary zinc intake and T2DM. Gender is one of the confounding factors most reported in the above mentioned studies on the relationship between dietary zinc intake and metabolic syndrome [44,45], cardiovascular disease [13], and mortality [47]. Our results showed a similar significant inverse association between dietary zinc intake and T2DM in both men and women, suggesting that gender does not seem to have a relevant role in this relationship.

Interestingly, we observed that the covariate "area of residence" of participants (rural versus urban) had a key effect on our findings. While a strong inverse association was observed in studies conducted on participants living in rural areas, a null relationship was observed in those studies carried out on urban subjects (Figure 3). Interestingly, when we addressed these findings also taking into account the design of the studies, we observed a 41% reduction in the risk of T2DM in both cross-sectional and prospective studies conducted in rural areas (Figure 4). Conversely, the effect size was reduced to 12% in cross-sectional studies performed in urban areas, and in prospective cohort studies, the association was not significant. These observations support the hypothesis that living in urban areas may counteract the beneficial effect of an elevated dietary zinc intake on risk of T2DM. Accumulating evidence strongly suggests that the change from rural to urban environments may have a marked impact on lifestyle [52,53], resulting in the increase of certain risk factors, such as unhealthy diets, sedentary behavior, and smoking, among others, that account for a large contribution to global burden of major disease [54,55]. Thus, it has been revealed that T2DM risk factors are more common in urban than in rural areas [56]. The greater exposure to risk factors in urban environments could explain the small or null protective effect of the intake of zinc from diet against the risk of T2DM. Indeed, it is known that there is higher prevalence of T2DM in urban compared to rural areas [2,56]. According to the International Diabetes Federation (IDF) Diabetes ATLAS edition 2017, the global prevalence of diabetes in urban areas was 10.2%, i.e., 279.2 million people aged between 20–79 years, meanwhile in rural areas was notably lower, 6.9% (145.7 million) [2]. In addition, the number of people living with diabetes in urban areas is expected to increase to 472.6 million in 2045, due mainly to global urbanization [2].

It is interesting that the covariate which had the greatest impact on the association between dietary zinc intake and T2DM was the proportion of T2DM cases identified in each study, both as a continuous and categorized variable. When we conducted a meta-regression introducing the percentage of T2DM as a continuous variable, we found that for each percentage point that increased this covariate, the protective effect of a moderately high dietary zinc intake, relative to the DRI, against T2DM decreased 0.04 (95% CI: 0.01, 0.07, $p = 0.010$). Through a meta-regression equation represented in a bubble plot, we observed that when the proportion of T2DM subjects reached 10%, the protective effect from dietary zinc intake was nullified (Figure 6). Consistently, the three studies with a proportion of T2DM subjects of 10% or more, did not find a significant association between dietary zinc intake and T2DM [6,10,11]. In addition, stratified analysis based on the percentage of T2DM in each study (<5%, 5%–9.9%, and ≥10%) showed an undetectable heterogeneity in all the three subgroups ($I^2 = 0.0\%$, $p > 0.100$), which provides high reliability to the results. Furthermore, a significant inverse association was found between intake of zinc from diet and T2DM when the percentage of T2DM was lower than 10%, and with the highest effect size when that was less than 5% (Figure 5). It should be noted that the studies with less proportion of T2DM subjects (<5%) were those carried out in rural areas, while those with the highest percentage of diabetics (5%–9.9%, and ≥10%) were the studies conducted in urban areas. In addition, among studies of urban areas, those with a moderate proportion of T2DM (5%–9.9%) retained a significant association between dietary zinc intake and T2DM, although it was more attenuated than those in rural areas. Nevertheless, the studies with higher percentage of T2DM did not find any significant relationship (Figure 5). These results suggest that in rural areas, with less T2DM risk factors, and consequently, less T2DM prevalence, the association between dietary zinc intake and T2DM is significant and the effect size is strong; meanwhile, in urban areas, with a greater exposure to T2DM risk factors and a higher T2DM prevalence, the association is still significant but with a low effect size when T2DM prevalence is moderate, and not significant when the T2DM prevalence is high.

Only two studies have evaluated the effect of a high total zinc intake on the risk of T2DM [4,6], and the overall pooled estimates showed no significant association (Figure 8). The NHS cohort showed a moderate protective effect of total zinc intake, while the MDCS cohort did not find a relationship. Consistent with results from the meta-analysis of the dietary zinc intake, the NHS cohort [4] had a moderate proportion of T2DM (7.3%), meanwhile the MDCS cohort [6] presented the highest percentage of T2DM of all included studies in this systematic review (14.1%). This supports the hypothesis previously raised regarding the impact of the T2DM prevalence on the association between zinc intake and risk of T2DM.

Although, there is currently some evidence of the beneficial effect of zinc supplementation on glycemic control in T2DM patients [9,57], scarce studies support the use of zinc supplements in the prevention of this disease [8]. A recent clinical trial based on zinc supplementation has found a reduction in the progression to T2DM in prediabetic subjects, in addition to an improvement in blood glucose and insulin levels, insulin resistance, and β–cell function [9]. Observational studies that have assessed the association between supplementary zinc intake and risk of T2DM are also scarce [4,6,12]. The overall pooled estimates did not show any significant relationship, neither comparing zinc supplement users versus non-users, nor comparing the highest versus lowest quantile of supplementary zinc intake (Figure 7). Those studies that compared zinc supplement users versus non-users against the risk of T2DM, failed to differentiate between participants who obtained zinc from multivitamin/mineral supplements from those taking individual zinc supplements [6,12]. Thus, a synergistic effect or an interaction between minerals and vitamins supplemented, along with zinc, could have affected the relationship between supplementary zinc intake and the risk of T2DM. Interestingly, the NHS cohort reported a significant inverse association in participants with low dietary zinc intake, but not in those with high dietary zinc intake [4]. In addition, dietary zinc intake was more strongly associated with a lower risk of T2DM among those participants with low zinc intakes from supplements. This seems to suggest that only when the zinc intake is insufficient, zinc supplementation may have benefits. However, when dietary intake is adequate, additional zinc intake from supplementation may not confer further benefit.

To the best of our knowledge, only two cross-sectional studies, conducted within the same population-based HUNT3 study, have evaluated the association between whole blood zinc concentration and T2DM [18,19]. However, the results were dissimilar, likely due to characteristics of participants selected during the sampling. Interestingly, Hansen et al. [18] reported a significant and positive association between whole blood zinc concentration and T2DM, in previously undiagnosed diabetic patients and control subjects [18]. Meanwhile, Simic et al. [19], did not find a significant relationship in previously diagnosed T2DM patients and control subjects. These results seem to suggest that when T2DM is in the early stages, i.e., newly diagnosed, zinc levels are more elevated than non-diabetic subjects, and progressively they are reduced as the disease progresses, which is consistent with our previous systematic review and meta-analysis [20]. That meta-analysis which aimed to compare whole blood zinc concentration between T2DM patients and non-diabetic subjects, showed that duration of T2DM had a relevant influence on concentration of zinc in whole blood [20]. In addition, we found a lower whole blood zinc concentration in T2DM patients; however, this group had, at least, 10.2 ± 8.6 years of duration of diabetes, and differences between cases and controls in that study were not observed [58], in concordance with the study of Simic et al. [19], among previously diagnosed T2DM participants [19].

Since the use of whole blood zinc concentration may be not representative of the total zinc body burden [56], we also assessed the association between zinc and T2DM, through a more reliable biomarker of zinc status, the serum/plasma zinc concentration [59]. We wanted to contrast the hypothesis regarding the impact of the T2DM phases on serum/plasma zinc concentration; however, data were limited to carry out that analysis. Only six studies evaluated this relationship, and results were inconsistent [14–17,40,41], which was highlighted by high heterogeneity observed after the results were combined. Two of the included studies were responsible for 44.5% of the heterogeneity detected [16,17]. After both studies were excluded, the combined result was more reliable (OR = 1.47, 95% CI: 1.11–1.95; $I^2 = 53.9\%$, $p = 0.090$). Curiously, these two studies, together with the third that contributed more to the global heterogeneity, were conducted on non-population or community-based studies, i.e., hospital-based settings [16], retired employees of a motor company [15] and postmenopausal women on a voluntary basis [17], so the results could not be extrapolated to the general population. However, the other three studies were carried out on population [14] or community-based [40,41] studies. Stratified analysis according to the "sample base" (Figure 9) showed a high heterogeneity in the "non-population or community-based studies" group ($I^2 = 98.0\%$, $p < 0.001$), and a low heterogeneity in the "population or community-based studies" group ($I^2 = 22.5\%$, $p = 0.275$). The pooled estimates for this last subgroup revealed a direct and significant association between serum/plasma zinc concentration and T2DM (OR = 1.64, 95% CI: 1.25–2.14). This finding is not consistent with a previous meta-analysis that compared serum/plasma zinc levels between T2DM patients and healthy controls [60]. Results of this previous meta-analysis showed significantly lower serum/plasma zinc concentration in diabetic subjects compared to healthy controls, but with high heterogeneity. The high heterogeneity suggests that results were influenced by confounding factors, but its source was not analyzed in that meta-analysis. Finally, a recent cross-sectional study reported that urinary zinc levels were positively associated with T2DM [61]. These findings suggest this is a response mechanism against zinc excess in serum/plasma in diabetic patients, and it seems to be in concordance with the direct relationship between serum/plasma and T2DM that we observed in our meta-analysis.

Several limitations in the present systematic review and meta-analysis should be considered. First, the number of results and studies included in meta-analyses was small, and stratified analyses might have insufficient power to identify potential confounding factors, as well as to detect potential sources of heterogeneity. To correct this weakness, random effects meta-regressions were carried out. Furthermore, our findings were likely to be influenced by imprecise measurement of zinc intake. However, VFFQ and VDHQ were used to assess dietary, supplementary, and/or total zinc intake, in all but two studies. In addition, differences in diagnostic criteria for the ascertainment of T2DM over the years could have introduced misclassification bias and could affect results. Finally, meta-analyses were based on observational studies, which are prone to confounding and reverse causation. Nevertheless, for meta-analyses of dietary, supplementary and/or total zinc intake, all but one of the included studies were prospective cohort studies, which allows stronger inferences than cross-sectional studies [62].

Our study has also several strengths. Firstly, the comprehensive and robust search strategy within the framework of the EURRECA Network of Excellence was designed to avoid the loss of relevant studies. Moreover, there were no studies that were excluded for reasons of language, avoiding language bias. In addition, standard tests and visual inspection of funnel plots did not show any evidence for risk of publication bias in any meta-analysis. Furthermore, included studies were of high quality, according to the STROBE Statement [42]. The meta-analyses included 575,851 subjects, had a wide geographical spread, and a diverse ethnicity, giving more validity to the results. Finally, heterogeneity was low or moderate in most of the meta-analyses, which also contributes to the study validity.

The important role of zinc on carbohydrate metabolism via several mechanisms is well established, and this could explain the protective effect of dietary zinc intake on risk of T2DM observed in our meta-analysis. Zinc is involved in synthesis, storage, crystallization, and secretion, as well as the action of insulin and translocation of insulin into the cells [21–24]. In addition, zinc seems to play a role in insulin sensitivity through the activation of the phosphoinositol-3-kinase/protein kinase B cascade [25]. It has also a role insulin–mimetic, being involved in the regulation process of glucose homeostasis [26]. Moreover, zinc may participate in the suppression of proinflammatory cytokines, such as interleukin-1β [27] and nuclear factor kβ [28], avoiding β-cells' death and protecting insulin. The underlying mechanism whereby higher serum/plasma and/or whole blood zinc concentration could be related to T2DM is unclear. However, strong evidence supports disturbances in zinc homeostasis associated with T2DM, that could not be linked to zinc status [63,64]. In recent years, it has been proposed that the cellular zinc transport system may play a key role in the pathophysiology of T2DM [65,66]. Thus, differences between diabetic patients and healthy controls in gene expressions for most zinc transporters has been observed [63]. This zinc dyshomeostasis may be caused in the early stages of T2DM, as observed in a trend of increased serum zinc levels from healthy to prediabetic and diabetic postmenopausal women [67].

5. Conclusions

Findings from this systematic review and meta-analysis revealed a potential protective effect of a moderately high dietary zinc intake, related to the DRI, on the risk of T2DM. The relationship seems to be stronger and more evident in rural compared to urban areas. In addition, T2DM prevalence may be also a confounding factor for this association, being stronger when the prevalence is low, weak when it is moderate, and disappearing with a high prevalence. Conversely, no associations were observed between total or supplementary zinc intake and T2DM. However, more data are required to explore this relationship more fully.

In addition, an elevated serum/plasma zinc concentration is associated with an increased risk of T2DM in the general population. Meanwhile, high whole blood zinc concentration could be associated with T2DM, likely only at an early phase of the diabetes disease. Additional studies are required to confirm these results, and determine the role of serum/plasma and whole blood zinc concentration in the pathophysiology of T2DM.

Supplementary Materials:
Figure S1: Funnel plot of publication biases of studies included in the meta-analysis of the association between dietary zinc intake and T2DM. Each dot stands for an individual study. Figure S2: Funnel plot of publication biases of studies included in the meta-analysis of the association between supplementary zinc intake and T2DM. Each dot stands for an individual study. Figure S3: Funnel plot of publication biases of studies included in the meta-analysis of the association between serum/plasma zinc concentration and T2DM. Each dot stands for an individual study. Table S1: MOOSE Checklist for Meta-analyses of Observational Studies. Table S2: STROBE Statement Checklist. Table S3: Stratified meta-analyses and meta-regressions on the association between serum/plasma zinc concentration and risk of type 2 diabetes mellitus.

Author Contributions: Conceptualization, N.M.L. and V.H.M.; methodology, N.M.L., V.H.M., M.W.-M., and J.C.F.-C.; formal analysis, J.C.F.-C.; investigation, J.C.F.-C., M.W.-M., V.H.M., V.A., C.D., L.S.-M., and N.M.L.; writing—original draft preparation, J.C.F.-C.; writing—review and editing, J.C.F.-C., M.W.-M., V.H.M., V.A., C.D., L.S.-M., and N.M.L.; supervision, N.M.L.

Acknowledgments: JCFC thanks the support from the University Staff Training (FPU) grant by the Ministry of Education, Spain; and the mobility aid for university staff in training by the Ministry of Education, Spain. JCFC also thanks the support from the project ATA 1756 of the Ministry of Education of Chile.

References

1. World Health Organization Noncommunicable Diseases: Key Facts. Available online: http://www.who.int/news-room/fact-sheets/detail/noncommunicable-diseases (accessed on 7 February 2019).
2. International Diabetes Federation (IDF) IDF Diabetes Atlas 8th Edition. Available online: http://www.diabetesatlas.org/ (accessed on 7 February 2019).
3. Qi, L.; Hu, F.B.; Hu, G. Genes, environment, and interactions in prevention of type 2 diabetes: A focus on physical activity and lifestyle changes. *Curr. Mol. Med.* **2008**, *8*, 519–532. [CrossRef] [PubMed]
4. Sun, Q.; Van Dam, R.M.; Willett, W.C.; Hu, F.B. Prospective study of zinc intake and risk of type 2 diabetes in women. *Diabetes Care* **2009**, *32*, 629–634. [CrossRef]
5. Vashum, K.P.; McEvoy, M.; Shi, Z.; Milton, A.H.; Islam, M.R.; Sibbritt, D.; Patterson, A.; Byles, J.; Loxton, D.; Attia, J. Is dietary zinc protective for type 2 diabetes? Results from the Australian longitudinal study on women's health. *BMC Endocr. Disord.* **2013**, *13*, 40. [CrossRef] [PubMed]
6. Drake, I.; Hindy, G.; Ericson, U.; Orho-Melander, M. A prospective study of dietary and supplemental zinc intake and risk of type 2 diabetes depending on genetic variation in SLC30A8. *Genes Nutr.* **2017**, *12*, 30. [CrossRef] [PubMed]
7. Eshak, E.S.; Iso, H.; Maruyama, K.; Muraki, I.; Tamakoshi, A. Associations between dietary intakes of iron, copper and zinc with risk of type 2 diabetes mellitus: A large population-based prospective cohort study. *Clin. Nutr.* **2018**, *37*, 667–674. [CrossRef]
8. El Dib, R.; Gameiro, O.L.F.; Ogata, M.S.P.; Módolo, N.S.P.; Braz, L.G.; Jorge, E.C.; do Nascimento, P.; Beletate, V. Zinc supplementation for the prevention of type 2 diabetes mellitus in adults with insulin resistance. *Cochrane Database Syst. Rev.* **2015**, CD005525. [CrossRef]
9. Ranasinghe, P.; Wathurapatha, W.S.; Galappatthy, P.; Katulanda, P.; Jayawardena, R.; Constantine, G.R. Zinc supplementation in prediabetes: A randomized double-blind placebo-controlled clinical trial. *J. Diabetes* **2018**, *10*, 386–397. [CrossRef] [PubMed]
10. De Oliveira Otto, M.C.; Alonso, A.; Lee, D.-H.; Delclos, G.L.; Bertoni, A.G.; Jiang, R.; Lima, J.A.; Symanski, E.; Jacobs, D.R.; Nettleton, J.A. Dietary Intakes of Zinc and Heme Iron from Red Meat, but Not from Other Sources, Are Associated with Greater Risk of Metabolic Syndrome and Cardiovascular Disease. *J. Nutr.* **2012**, *142*, 526–533. [CrossRef]
11. Park, J.S.; Xun, P.; Li, J.; Morris, S.J.; Jacobs, D.R.; Liu, K.; He, K. Longitudinal association between toenail zinc levels and the incidence of diabetes among American young adults: The CARDIA Trace Element Study. *Sci. Rep.* **2016**, *6*, 23155. [CrossRef] [PubMed]
12. Song, Y.; Xu, Q.; Park, Y.; Hollenbeck, A.; Schatzkin, A.; Chen, H. Multivitamins, Individual Vitamin and Mineral Supplements, and Risk of Diabetes Among Older U.S. Adults. *Diabetes Care* **2011**, *34*, 108–114. [CrossRef]
13. Chu, A.; Foster, M.; Samman, S. Zinc status and risk of cardiovascular diseases and type 2 diabetes mellitus–A systematic review of prospective cohort studies. *Nutrients* **2016**, *8*, 707. [CrossRef]
14. Yary, T.; Virtanen, J.K.; Ruusunen, A.; Tuomainen, T.-P.; Voutilainen, S. Serum zinc and risk of type 2 diabetes incidence in men: The Kuopio Ischaemic Heart Disease Risk Factor Study. *J. Trace Elem. Med. Biol.* **2016**, *33*, 120–124. [CrossRef]
15. Yuan, Y.; Xiao, Y.; Yu, Y.; Liu, Y.; Feng, W.; Qiu, G.; Wang, H.; Liu, B.; Wang, J.; Zhou, L.; et al. Associations of multiple plasma metals with incident type 2 diabetes in Chinese adults: The Dongfeng-Tongji Cohort. *Environ. Pollut.* **2018**, *237*, 917–925. [CrossRef]
16. Shan, Z.; Bao, W.; Zhang, Y.; Rong, Y.; Wang, X.; Jin, Y.; Song, Y.; Yao, P.; Sun, C.; Hu, F.B.; et al. Interactions Between Zinc Transporter-8 Gene (SLC30A8) and Plasma Zinc Concentrations for Impaired Glucose Regulation and Type 2 Diabetes. *Diabetes* **2014**, *63*, 1796–1803. [CrossRef]
17. Skalnaya, M.G.; Skalny, A.V.; Yurasov, V.V.; Demidov, V.A.; Grabeklis, A.R.; Radysh, I.V.; Tinkov, A.A. Serum Trace Elements and Electrolytes Are Associated with Fasting Plasma Glucose and HbA1c in Postmenopausal Women with Type 2 Diabetes Mellitus. *Biol. Trace Elem. Res.* **2017**, *177*, 25–32. [CrossRef]
18. Hansen, A.F.; Simić, A.; Åsvold, B.O.; Romundstad, P.R.; Midthjell, K.; Syversen, T.; Flaten, T.P. Trace elements in early phase type 2 diabetes mellitus—A population-based study. The HUNT study in Norway. *J. Trace Elem. Med. Biol.* **2017**, *40*, 46–53. [CrossRef] [PubMed]

19. Simić, A.; Hansen, A.F.; Åsvold, B.O.; Romundstad, P.R.; Midthjell, K.; Syversen, T.; Flaten, T.P. Trace element status in patients with type 2 diabetes in Norway: The HUNT3 Survey. *J. Trace Elem. Med. Biol.* **2017**, *41*, 91–98. [CrossRef]
20. Fernández-Cao, J.C.; Warthon-Medina, M.; Hall Moran, V.; Arija, V.; Doepking, C.; Lowe, N.M. Dietary zinc intake and whole blood zinc concentration in subjects with type 2 diabetes versus healthy subjects: A systematic review, meta-analysis and meta-regression. *J. Trace Elem. Med. Biol.* **2018**. [CrossRef] [PubMed]
21. Coffman, F.D.; Dunn, M.F. Insulin-metal ion interactions: The binding of divalent cations to insulin hexamers and tetramers and the assembly of insulin hexamers. *Biochemistry* **1988**, *27*, 6179–6187. [CrossRef]
22. Keller, S.R. Role of the insulin-regulated aminopeptidase IRAP in insulin action and diabetes. *Biol. Pharm. Bull.* **2004**, *27*, 761–764. [CrossRef]
23. Meyer, J.A.; Spence, D.M. A perspective on the role of metals in diabetes: Past findings and possible future directions. *Metallomics* **2009**, *1*, 32–41. [CrossRef]
24. Moore, W.T.; Bowser, S.M.; Fausnacht, D.W.; Staley, L.L.; Suh, K.-S.; Liu, D. Beta Cell Function and the Nutritional State: Dietary Factors that Influence Insulin Secretion. *Curr. Diabetes Rep.* **2015**, *15*, 76. [CrossRef]
25. Tang, X.; Shay, N.F. Zinc has an insulin-like effect on glucose transport mediated by phosphoinositol-3-kinase and Akt in 3T3-L1 fibroblasts and adipocytes. *J. Nutr.* **2001**, *131*, 1414–1420. [CrossRef]
26. Chabosseau, P.; Rutter, G.A. Zinc and diabetes. *Arch. Biochem. Biophys.* **2016**, *611*, 79–85. [CrossRef]
27. Von Bülow, V.; Rink, L.; Haase, H. Zinc-mediated inhibition of cyclic nucleotide phosphodiesterase activity and expression suppresses TNF-alpha and IL-1 beta production in monocytes by elevation of guanosine 3′,5′-cyclic monophosphate. *J. Immunol.* **2005**, *175*, 4697–4705. [CrossRef]
28. Prasad, A.S.; Bao, B.; Beck, F.W.J.; Kucuk, O.; Sarkar, F.H. Antioxidant effect of zinc in humans. *Free Radic. Biol. Med.* **2004**, *37*, 1182–1190. [CrossRef]
29. Stroup, D.F.; Berlin, J.A.; Morton, S.C.; Olkin, I.; Williamson, G.D.; Rennie, D.; Moher, D.; Becker, B.J.; Sipe, T.A.; Thacker, S.B. Meta-analysis of observational studies in epidemiology: A proposal for reporting. Meta-analysis Of Observational Studies in Epidemiology (MOOSE) group. *JAMA* **2000**, *283*, 2008–2012. [CrossRef]
30. Greenland, S. Quantitative methods in the review of epidemiologic literature. *Epidemiol. Rev.* **1987**, *9*, 1–30. [CrossRef]
31. Knapp, G.; Hartung, J. Improved tests for a random effects meta-regression with a single covariate. *Stat. Med.* **2003**. [CrossRef]
32. Huedo-Medina, T.B.; Sánchez-Meca, J.; Marín-Martínez, F.; Botella, J. Assessing heterogeneity in meta-analysis: Q statistic or I^2 index? *Psychol. Methods* **2006**, *11*, 193–206. [CrossRef]
33. Higgins, J.P.T.; Thompson, S.G. Quantifying heterogeneity in a meta-analysis. *Stat. Med.* **2002**, *21*, 1539–1558. [CrossRef]
34. Higgins, J.P.T. Measuring inconsistency in meta-analyses. *BMJ* **2003**, *327*, 557–560. [CrossRef]
35. Thompson, S.G.; Higgins, J.P.T. How should meta-regression analyses be undertaken and interpreted? *Stat. Med.* **2002**, *21*, 1559–1573. [CrossRef]
36. Patsopoulos, N.A.; Evangelou, E.; Ioannidis, J.P.A. Sensitivity of between-study heterogeneity in meta-analysis: Proposed metrics and empirical evaluation. *Int. J. Epidemiol.* **2008**, *37*, 1148–1157. [CrossRef]
37. Egger, M.; Davey Smith, G.; Schneider, M.; Minder, C. Bias in meta-analysis detected by a simple, graphical test. *BMJ* **1997**, *315*, 629–634. [CrossRef]
38. Begg, C.B.; Mazumdar, M. Operating Characteristics of a Rank Correlation Test for Publication Bias. *Biometrics* **1994**, *50*, 1088. [CrossRef]
39. Singh, R.B.; Niaz, M.A.; Rastogi, S.S.; Bajaj, S.; Gaoli, Z.; Shoumin, Z. Current Zinc Intake and Risk of Diabetes and Coronary Artery Disease and Factors Associated with Insulin Resistance in Rural and Urban Populations of North India. *J. Am. Coll. Nutr.* **1998**, *17*, 564–570. [CrossRef]
40. Li, X.T.; Yu, P.F.; Gao, Y.; Guo, W.H.; Wang, J.; Liu, X.; Gu, A.H.; Ji, G.X.; Dong, Q.; Wang, B.S.; et al. Association between Plasma Metal Levels and Diabetes Risk: A Case-control Study in China. *Biomed. Environ. Sci.* **2017**, *30*, 482–491. [CrossRef]
41. Zhang, H.; Yan, C.; Yang, Z.; Zhang, W.; Niu, Y.; Li, X.; Qin, L.; Su, Q. Alterations of serum trace elements in patients with type 2 diabetes. *J. Trace Elem. Med. Biol.* **2017**, *40*, 91–96. [CrossRef]

42. Von Elm, E.; Altman, D.G.; Egger, M.; Pocock, S.J.; Gøtzsche, P.C.; Vandenbroucke, J.P. The Strengthening the Reporting of Observational Studies in Epidemiology (STROBE) statement: Guidelines for reporting of observational studies. *Der Internist* **2008**, *49*, 688–693. [CrossRef]
43. Panel on Micronutrients: Subcommittee on Upper Reference Levels of Nutrients; Subcommittee on Interpretation and Uses of Dietary Reference Intakes; Standing Committee on the Scientific Evaluation of Dietary Reference Intakes; Food and Nutrition Board, Institute of Medicine. *Dietary Reference Intakes for Vitamin A, Vitamin K, Arsenic, Boron, Chromium, Copper, Iodine, Iron, Manganese, Molybdenum, Nickel, Silicon, Vanadium, and Zinc*; National Academies Press: Washington, DC, USA, 2001.
44. Suarez-Ortegón, M.F.; Ordoñez-Betancourth, J.E.; Aguilar-de Plata, C. Dietary zinc intake is inversely associated to metabolic syndrome in male but not in female urban adolescents. *Am. J. Hum. Biol.* **2013**, *25*, 550–554. [CrossRef]
45. Al-Daghri, N.; Khan, N.; Alkharfy, K.; Al-Attas, O.; Alokail, M.; Alfawaz, H.; Alothman, A.; Vanhoutte, P. Selected Dietary Nutrients and the Prevalence of Metabolic Syndrome in Adult Males and Females in Saudi Arabia: A Pilot Study. *Nutrients* **2013**, *5*, 4587–4604. [CrossRef]
46. Bo, S.; Lezo, A.; Menato, G.; Gallo, M.-L.; Bardelli, C.; Signorile, A.; Berutti, C.; Massobrio, M.; Pagano, G.F. Gestational hyperglycemia, zinc, selenium, and antioxidant vitamins. *Nutrition* **2005**, *21*, 186–191. [CrossRef]
47. Eshak, E.S.; Iso, H.; Yamagishi, K.; Maruyama, K.; Umesawa, M.; Tamakoshi, A. Associations between copper and zinc intakes from diet and mortality from cardiovascular disease in a large population-based prospective cohort study. *J. Nutr. Biochem.* **2018**, *56*, 126–132. [CrossRef]
48. Bates, C.J.; Hamer, M.; Mishra, G.D. Redox-modulatory vitamins and minerals that prospectively predict mortality in older British people: The National Diet and Nutrition Survey of people aged 65 years and over. *Br. J. Nutr.* **2011**, *105*, 123–132. [CrossRef]
49. Shi, Z.; Yuan, B.; Qi, L.; Dai, Y.; Zuo, H.; Zhou, M. Zinc intake and the risk of hyperglycemia among Chinese adults: The prospective Jiangsu Nutrition Study (JIN). *J. Nutr. Health Aging* **2010**, *14*, 332–335. [CrossRef]
50. Milton, A.H.; Vashum, K.P.; McEvoy, M.; Hussain, S.; McElduff, P.; Byles, J.; Attia, J. Prospective Study of Dietary Zinc Intake and Risk of Cardiovascular Disease in Women. *Nutrients* **2018**, *10*, 38. [CrossRef]
51. Shi, Z.; Chu, A.; Zhen, S.; Taylor, A.W.; Dai, Y.; Riley, M.; Samman, S. Association between dietary zinc intake and mortality among Chinese adults: Findings from 10-year follow-up in the Jiangsu Nutrition Study. *Eur. J. Nutr.* **2018**, *57*, 2839–2846. [CrossRef]
52. McDade, T.W.; Adair, L.S. Defining the "urban" in urbanization and health: A factor analysis approach. *Soc. Sci. Med.* **2001**, *53*, 55–70. [CrossRef]
53. Pretorius, S.; Sliwa, K. Perspectives and perceptions on the consumption of a healthy diet in Soweto, an urban African community in South Africa. *SA Hear.* **2017**, *8*, 178–183. [CrossRef]
54. Lopez, A.D.; Mathers, C.D.; Ezzati, M.; Jamison, D.T.; Murray, C.J.L. Global and regional burden of disease and risk factors, 2001: Systematic analysis of population health data. *Lancet (London, England)* **2006**, *367*, 1747–1757. [CrossRef]
55. Ezzati, M.; Lopez, A.D.; Rodgers, A.; Vander Hoorn, S.; Murray, C.J.L. Comparative Risk Assessment Collaborating Group Selected major risk factors and global and regional burden of disease. *Lancet (London, England)* **2002**, *360*, 1347–1360. [CrossRef]
56. Al-Moosa, S.; Allin, S.; Jemiai, N.; Al-Lawati, J.; Mossialos, E. Diabetes and urbanization in the Omani population: An analysis of national survey data. *Popul. Health Metr.* **2006**, *4*, 5. [CrossRef]
57. Jayawardena, R.; Ranasinghe, P.; Galappatthy, P.; Malkanthi, R.; Constantine, G.; Katulanda, P. Effects of zinc supplementation on diabetes mellitus: A systematic review and meta-analysis. *Diabetol. Metab. Syndr.* **2012**, *4*, 13. [CrossRef]
58. Forte, G.; Bocca, B.; Peruzzu, A.; Tolu, F.; Asara, Y.; Farace, C.; Oggiano, R.; Madeddu, R. Blood metals concentration in type 1 and type 2 diabetics. *Biol. Trace Elem. Res.* **2013**, *156*, 79–90. [CrossRef]
59. Lowe, N.M.; Fekete, K.; Decsi, T. Methods of assessment of zinc status in humans: A systematic review. *Am. J. Clin. Nutr.* **2009**, *89*, 2040S–2051S. [CrossRef]
60. Sanjeevi, N.; Freeland-Graves, J.; Beretvas, S.N.; Sachdev, P.K. Trace element status in type 2 diabetes: A meta-analysis. *J. Clin. Diagn. Res.* **2018**, *12*, OE01–OE08. [CrossRef]
61. Liu, B.; Feng, W.; Wang, J.; Li, Y.; Han, X.; Hu, H.; Guo, H.; Zhang, X.; He, M. Association of urinary metals levels with type 2 diabetes risk in coke oven workers. *Environ. Pollut.* **2016**, *210*, 1–8. [CrossRef]

62. Carlson, M.D.A.; Morrison, R.S. Study design, precision, and validity in observational studies. *J. Palliat. Med.* **2009**, *12*, 77–82. [CrossRef]
63. Chu, A.; Foster, M.; Hancock, D.; Petocz, P.; Samman, S. Interrelationships among mediators of cellular zinc homeostasis in healthy and type 2 diabetes mellitus populations. *Mol. Nutr. Food Res.* **2017**, *61*. [CrossRef]
64. Ranasinghe, P.; Pigera, S.; Galappatthy, P.; Katulanda, P.; Constantine, G.R. Zinc and diabetes mellitus: Understanding molecular mechanisms and clinical implications. *Daru* **2015**, *23*, 44. [CrossRef]
65. Tamaki, M.; Fujitani, Y.; Hara, A.; Uchida, T.; Tamura, Y.; Takeno, K.; Kawaguchi, M.; Watanabe, T.; Ogihara, T.; Fukunaka, A.; et al. The diabetes-susceptible gene SLC30A8/ZnT8 regulates hepatic insulin clearance. *J. Clin. Investig.* **2013**, *123*, 4513–4524. [CrossRef]
66. Myers, S.A.; Nield, A.; Chew, G.-S.; Myers, M.A. The Zinc Transporter, Slc39a7 (Zip7) Is Implicated in Glycaemic Control in Skeletal Muscle Cells. *PLoS ONE* **2013**, *8*, e79316. [CrossRef]
67. Skalnaya, M.G.; Skalny, A.V.; Tinkov, A.A. Serum copper, zinc, and iron levels, and markers of carbohydrate metabolism in postmenopausal women with prediabetes and type 2 diabetes mellitus. *J. Trace Elem. Med. Biol.* **2017**, *43*, 46–51. [CrossRef]

14

A Multifunctional Bread Rich in Beta Glucans and Low in Starch Improves Metabolic Control in Type 2 Diabetes

Paolo Tessari [1,*] and Anna Lante [2]

1 Department of Medicine (DIMED), University of Padova, 35128 Padova PD, Italy
2 Department of Agronomy, Food, Natural Resources, Animals & Environment (DAFNAE), University of Padova, 35123 Padova PD, Italy; anna.lante@unipd.it
* Correspondence: paolo.tessari@unipd.it;

Abstract: Design: Functional foods may be useful for people with diabetes. The soluble fibers beta glucans can modify starch digestion and improve postprandial glucose response. We analyzed the metabolic effects of a specifically designed 'functional' bread, low in starch, rich in fibers (7 g/100 g), with a beta glucan/starch ratio of (7.6:100, g/g), in people with type 2 diabetes mellitus. Methods: Clinical and metabolic data from two groups of age-, sex- and glycated hemoglobin-matched diabetic subjects, taking either the functional bread or regular white bread, over a roughly six-month observation period, were retrieved. Results: Bread intake did not change during the trial. The functional bread reduced glycated hemoglobin by ~0.5% (absolute units) vs. pre-treatment values ($p = 0.028$), and by ~0.6% vs. the control group ($p = 0.027$). Post-prandial and mean plasma glucose was decreased in the treatment group too. Body weight, blood pressure and plasma lipids did not change. The acceptance of the functional bread was good in the majority of subjects, except for taste. Conclusions: A starch-restricted, fiber-rich functional bread, with an increased beta glucan/starch ratio, improved long term metabolic control, and may be indicated in the dietary treatment of type 2 diabetes.

Keywords: plasma glucose; beta glucan; starch; metabolic control; fibers

---

1. Introduction

Background and Aims

Type 2 diabetes mellitus (T2DM) is a disease with high prevalence and increasing incidence. The world population currently affected by T2DM is about 400 million, and it is expected to grow to more than 600 million by 2040 [1]. The increase of T2DM is largely due to changes of lifestyle [2], i.e., excess dietary intake combined to low physical activity. Therefore, diet represents a cornerstone for both prevention and therapy of T2DM, and a tool to maintain plasma glucose values close to normal.

Carbohydrates (CHO) are the key nutritional factors conditioning circulating glucose levels, particularly in the post-prandial state. In order to prevent excessive post-prandial glycemicexcursions, dietary CHO should be predominantly represented by starch (>90% of total CHO), with less than 10% by either mono- or di-saccharides [3]. Furthermore, since T2DM is associated with a constellation of conditions (obesity, dyslipidemia, hypertension) and risk factors (e.g., for cardiovascular disease) recognized in the concept of the 'metabolic syndrome' [4–6], food capable of addressing most, if not all these abnormalities, can be recommended. Thus, current understanding is that foods and diets for T2DM patients are considered, for the present, to be energy controlled, with a low glycemic index (GI), and with favorable effects on blood pressure and dyslipidemia. A reduction of cardiovascular (CV) risk and the prevention of long term diabetic complications are also expected to result from long-term use of such 'ideal' foods.

Post-prandial glucose increments in diabetes may be blunted by foods containing starch and/or simple CHO with a slow absorption rate, thus resulting in a low GI. Besides by the CHO type itself, CHO absorption may be modulated by a variety of additional factors, such as starch characteristics (i.e., resistance to digestion), fiber type and content, and by the presence of other compounds that can decrease carbohydrate intestinal digestion and absorption. Conversely, the guidelines for dietary treatment of hypertension, obesity and dyslipidemia include a reduction of sodium and energy intakes, and a control of intestinal lipid absorption. Thus, targeting some, if not all, these risk factors, by means of functional foods seems to be both recommended and promising in the dietary management of both diabetes and the metabolic syndrome, through health-beneficial properties conveyed by natural components and/or by added ingredients [7].

Functional foods rich in natural fibers, such as beta glucans, are among those most-widely studied and employed. Beta glucans are naturally-occurring soluble fibers of some cereals (oats and barley), composed of mixed-linkage (1,3)(1,4)-β-D-glucose units, mainly consisting of the linear polysaccharide (1→3), (1→4)-β-D-glucan. Beta glucans increase viscosity in the upper digestive tract, thus reducing postprandial glucose and insulin responses [8]. An optimal beta glucan/starch ratio has been proposed as a method to decrease starch digestion in functional breads [9].

Bread is a staple food and a fundamental source of CHO worldwide in everyday diet. Therefore, the design of a bread with targeted functional properties could retain a major impact on nutrition and on metabolic parameters.

In this study, we examined the metabolic effects of long-term (roughly six months) substitution of regular white bread with a functional bread, starch-restricted and rich in fiber (mostly beta glucans), in the everyday diet of persons with type 2 diabetes.

2. Methods

2.1. Study Design and Participants

In the context of a comprehensive analysis of clinical and biochemical parameters of people with type 2 diabetes mellitus, data from T2DM subjects of both sexes, collected at their regularly-scheduled outpatient visits at the Diabetes Center of the Padova University Hospital, Italy, were retrieved. This was an observational, controlled study with parallel groups, performed following recently published guidelines and format (http://www.consort-statement.org/). The subjects' inclusion criteria were: a diabetes duration longer than 2 years; an unsatisfactory diabetes control (HbA_1c values greater than 7%); age between 50 and 80 years; treatment with diet only, or diet plus oral hypoglycemic agents (OHA) and/or basal insulin; and a reported daily intake of at least 50 g CHO as either white bread, breadsticks or other bread substitutes. The patients were visited at 3–6 months intervals.

2.2. Interventions

The patients had routinely been recommended to consume foods considered to be beneficial to peoples with diabetes, such as low calorie items, with CHO predominantly represented by starch, with a high fiber content and/or a low glycemic index, and low amounts of fats of animal origin. Furthermore, the patients had been informed about the availability in supermarkets, of flour products enriched with fibers and/or other compounds that could be beneficial to control glucose levels. They were encouraged to prepare homemade bread using any of these flour products, as a substitute of their usually consumed white bread made of refined flour.

At subsequent examinations, the type of bread used by every subjects was recorded. Therefore, two groups of subjects could be selected over time: those who had shifted to the use of one of the functional bread types ('functional bread' group), and those who had been still using their regular white bread ('control' group). Among the former, the starting time of consumption of either the functional flour and/or bread, and its type, were retrieved and recorded. For the sake of homogeneity, we report here data of those subjects consuming only one type of these fiber-enriched products, i.e., a flour labelled Salus® (produced by Ruggeri srl, Padova, Italy), that was the most largely used. These subjects were included into the 'functional bread' group. The data of the case-control group, i.e., that of patients who were consuming their regular bread, were collected in a similar fashion. The matching criteria with the 'functional bread' group were age, sex, absolute HbA_1c values as well as absence of HbA_1c changes between the two selected time intervals (i.e., approximately ~6–7 months. apart), greater than $\pm 1\%$ (absolute value). For both groups, other inclusion criteria were: no variation in both hypoglycemic and other drug therapy, and no major intercurrent diseases over the chosen observation periods. A total of eleven subjects in each group were selected.

The target observations interval after the 'start' time point was set between 3 and 12 months. Each patient had been advised to maintain his/her usual dietary habits and nutrient intake, except for the type of bread used. The 24-h recall method was used to assess dietary intake of the day before each visit. The data of each patients were handled rigorously in anonymous fashion. Of the 20 subjects originally enrolled into the 'functional bread group', only eleven completed the intended observational time period. The causes for drop-out were: insufficient bread intake (less than 40 g of starch equivalents per day, possibly preventing the detection of a significant effect by substitution with the functional bread); intercurrent diseases and/or changes of therapy; major dietary changes and/or failure to observe the standard recommendations for people with T2DM.

As controls, two sets of data were used. First, each patient's own HbA_1c value(s) in the 3–12 month period antecedent either the start of consumption of the functional bread/flour, or a comparable period of use of the regular bread in the 'control' group, were recorded. These data are referred to as the 'previous' time points. Each patient was thus the control of him/herself. Second, data collected after use of either the 'functional bread' and of the 'control bread', as described above, recorded over the subsequent 3–12 months from the 'start' time point, were retrieved.

The subjects were either in the fasting state or had consumed their breakfast at home before coming to the Diabetes Centre. Breakfast composition was pretty reproducible in the same subject on the two/three visits, but different from patient to patient. In general, the patients consumed a medium-to-low-calorie Italian breakfast, consisting of milk, coffee (or tea), cereals (or bread slices), dressed with a thin layer of jam with a low sugar content, and/or one fruit, and/or one portion of yoghurt.

On the occasion of each visit, the patients' glucose value (either in the fasting state or 2-h post-breakfast, the latter labeled as 'post-prandial' value), were determined by a reflectometer. These directly determined values were averaged with those retrieved from the home glucose monitoring of each patients, in the two–three days preceding the visit. Thus, both the fasting and post-breakfast data were the mean of these values.

The local Ethics Committee of Padova University Hospital had approved, as part of broader clinical data investigations in diabetes, the retrieval in anonymous form, of clinical and biochemical data from medical records of the diabetic patients (Approval N. 14809, released on 11 March 2016).

2.3. Bread Preparation

The functional bread was prepared at home by every subject using the instructions of the producer(s). Typically, a Moulinex bread machine (model. OW 3101, Moulinex, Groupe Seb Italia Spa, Milan, Italy) was employed. The composition of the functional bread (Salus®) flour and that of the refined flour used for the preparation of the control white bread, are reported on Table 1. The botanical source of the Beta-glucans was oat, as reported by the producers on the label of flour Salus (see Reg. (CE) n. 1924/2006 and Reg. (CE) n. 1160/2011). The mix of ingredients to prepare the functional bread was contained in packs of 500 g containing about 20 g of β-glucan and 200 g of starch.

Table 1. Flour composition of the 'functional' and the 'control' (made with refined wheat white flour) breads.

Expressed per 100 g	Functional Bread	Control Bread
Edible part (%)	100	100
Water (g)	43	29
Protein (g)	12	8.6
Lipid (g)	1.2	0.4
Cholesterol (mg)	n.d.	0
Available carbohydrates (g)	31	66.9
Starch (g)	30.2	59.1
Soluble sugars (g)	0.8	1.9
Solubile fiber (g)	2.3	1.46
as beta-glucan	2.3	0
Insolubile fiber (g)	4.7	1.72
Total fiber (g)	7	3.2
Beta-glucan/starch	7.62	0
Energy (kJ)	827	1209
Energy (kcal)	197	289
Salt (mg)	885	1465
Sodium (mg)	354	586

The carbohydrates unit is expressed as g/100 g of the sum of glucose and starch. In this value, fiber is not included.

Bread baking was carried out using standard conditions for a white bread, as indicated by the manufacturer, as follows. Five hundred grams of the ingredient's mixture and 430 mL of water were added into the bread machine's pan. The bread maker took three hours to bake a loaf of bread. From about 450 g dough, 320–360 g cooked bread are obtained with a moisture percent ranging between 42%–43%. A bread loaf of 100 g contained about 2.3 g of β-glucans.

In order to determine consumer acceptability, a simple 5-point hedonic scale (questionnaire) for each sensorial attribute, was used, where 5 was the highest (i.e., extremely positive) score ('like very much') and 1 the lowest (i.e., extremely negative) ('dislike very much'). Participants were asked to rate odor, taste (salty and sweet), texture (soft and crisp) and general acceptance on the five-point Likert scale [10].

2.4. Outcome

The data of plasma glucose, HbA_1c, lipids, blood pressure, and weight were retrieved from each subject's medical records on the regularly scheduled visits. The methods of analyses were those standardized in the central analysis laboratory of the Padova University Hospital [11]. The post-prandial glucose values refer to measurements taken ~2 h after the meal (breakfast). The mean glucose concentrations resulting from the fasting and the post-prandial values was also calculated.

2.5. Sample Size and Statistical Analysis

By considering the primary end-point, i.e., a relative change of HbA_1c of 0.6% (as absolute units) between the treated vs. the control group, and assuming a population mean of HbA_1c of 8%, and an SD of 10% of the mean, a significant effect ($\alpha = 0.05$, $1 - \beta = 0.80$), would be attained by the sample size here studied.

All data were expressed as means ± standard error (SE). The two-way analysis of variance (ANOVA) for repeated measurements, followed by post-hoc test, was employed, to compare the data of the test group with those of the case-control group. The two tailed Student's t test for either paired or unpaired data was employed as appropriate. A p value < 0.05 was taken as statistically significant.

3. Results

The basal, pre-treatment clinical data of the patients are reported on Table 2. There was no statistical difference between the treatment and the control groups in any clinical or biochemical parameter. Although there were some differences between the two groups in drug consumption, no subject modified his/her current therapy (including both hypoglycemic agents and other drugs) during the test period, both in the test and in the control group. The subjects allocated to the 'functional bread' group had reported a daily intake of CHO (as bread, breadsticks, cereals or other bread substitutes) of approximately 70 ± 10 g. In the control group, the estimated intake of CHO (starch)-equivalents was similar. From medical records there were no evidence of changes in everyday diet in any of the selected subjects.

Table 2. Clinical characteristics of the type 2 diabetic subjects, included in either the functional bread or the control group. Data are expressed as means ± SE.

Parameter	Functional Bread Group	Control Bread Group
Number	11	11
Sex (M/F)	4/7	4/7
Age (years)	68.6 ± 1.9	68.0 ± 2.3
Body weight (kg)	72.9 ± 3.6	76.2 ± 4.0
BMI (kg/m^2)	27.8 ± 1.2	27.9 ± 1.3
Months between measurements	6.0 ± 0.5	6.9 ± 0.8
range	4–9	3–11
Therapy:		
Metformin	8	10
Sulphonylureas/Glinides	3	2
Insulin	1	2
Incretins	5	7
Statins	2	8
ACE-I/ARB	2	7
Beta-blockers/Antiadrenergics	4	1
Diuretics	2	4
Aspirin	2	1
Other	7	4

Abbreviations: BMI: Body Mass Index; ACE-I: angiotensin-conversion-enzyme inhibitors; ARB: angiotensin-receptor-blockers.

Following the time point defined as 'start', clinical and biochemical data were retrieved, after 6.0 ± 0.5 months in the 'treatment' group, and after 6.9 ± 0.8 months in the control group (p = NS between the two groups).

In the treatment group, the use of the functional bread resulted in (insignificantly) lower fasting glucose concentrations (by −20.4 ± 16.7 mg/dL, i.e., −1.15 ± 0.92 mmol/L, $p > 0.05$ by paired t test), but in significantly lower postprandial glucose concentrations (by −16.4 ± 6.3 mg/dL, i.e., −0.91 ± 0.35 mmol/L, $p = 0.045$ by paired t test). The resulting average glucose concentrations were reduced by −17.4 ± 8.0 mg/dL (i.e., by −0.97 ± 0.44 mmol/L, $p = 0.08$ by paired t test) (Table 3).

In contrast, in the control group, modest though insignificantly greater fasting (by +2.8 ± 9.9 mg/dL, i.e., +0.15 ± 0.55 mmol/L), post-prandial (by +29.0 ± 10.6 mg/dL, i.e., +1.6 ± 0.6 mmol/L) and mean (by +12.7 ± 6.6 mg/dL, i.e., +0.71 ± 0.34 mmol/L) plasma glucose concentrations were observed. As a result, a significant difference between the two groups was observed (by ANOVA, as interaction effect), as regards both the post-prandial ($p = 0.011$) and the mean ($p = 0.02$) glucose concentrations (Table 3).

Table 3. Hemoglobin A_1c (HbA_1c) (as percent, %), fasting plasma glucose (FPG), post-prandial plasma glucose (PPG) and mean plasma glucose (MPG), in the 'functional bread' and in the 'control' treatment groups, before ('start') and after ('end') the observation periods. Data are expressed as means ± SE.

	Functional Bread Group		Control Group		
	Start	End	Start	End	p Value
HbA_1c (%)	7.97 ± 0.36	7.45 ± 0.31 *	8.03 ± 0.34	8.10 ± 0.31	0.0265
FPG (mmol/L)	9.1 ± 0.8	8.0 ± 0.5	8.7 ± 0.7	8.8 ± 0.5	0.29
PPG (mmol/L)	9.2 ± 0.5	8.4 ± 0.6 *	8.7 ± 0.4	9.9 ± 0.6	0.0113
MPG (mmol/L)	9.2 ± 0.6	8.2 ± 0.4 *	8.5 ± 0.6	9.0 ± 0.5	0.02

* Significant difference between the 'functional bread' and the 'control' groups. The reported p values are those resulting from the two-way analysis of variance for repeated measurements, interaction effect.

The HbA_1c values are shown in Figure 1. Between the 'previous' and the 'start' observation time points, no difference between the functional and the control bread groups were observed, both groups showing a slight trend (albeit insignificant) towards worsening of HbA_1c. The observation periods between these two time points were not different between the two groups (treatment group: 6.6 ± 0.6 months; control group: 7.7 ± 1.0 months, $p = 0.34$ between the two).

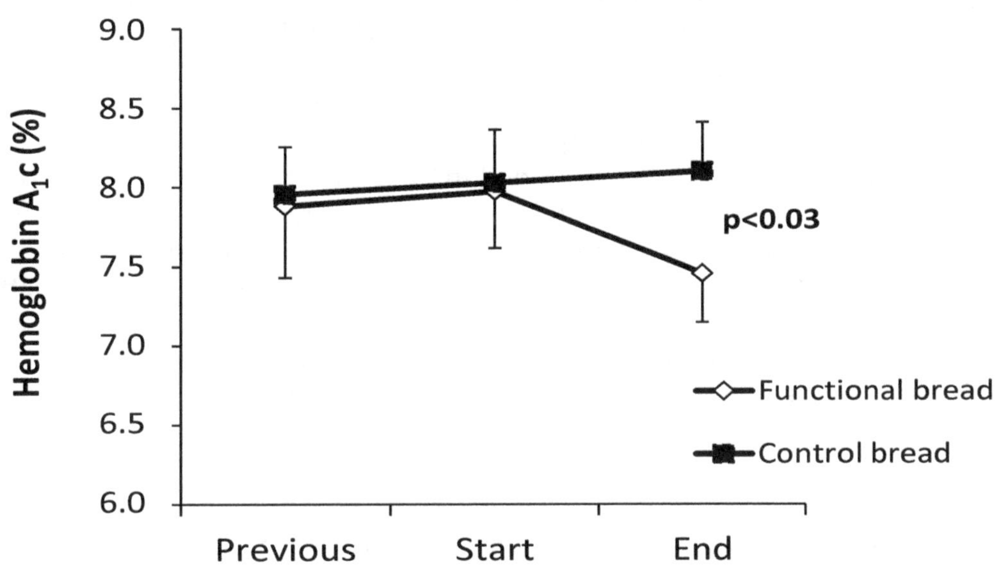

Figure 1. The effect of the functional bread on roughly six-month metabolic control as reflected by HbA_1c. Hemoglobin A_1C values (expressed as percent, mean ± SE) in the seven to eight months before ('previous'), at the beginning ('start') and after six to seven months ('end') of intake of either the functional bread (open symbols) or the control white bread (filled symbols). The data are expressed as mean ± SE. The p value in the figure indicates the significant difference in the changes of HbA_1c % values, before and following the intake of between either the functional bread or the control bread (by ANOVA).

Following the 'start' time point, in the group treated with the functional bread, a −0.52% decrease (as absolute value) of HbA_1c levels ($p < 0.028$ by the pair t test, Figure 1) was observed. In contrast, in the control group HbA_1c did not change (+0.21% ± 0.13%). As a result, there was a significant difference between the two groups in the post-treatment HbA_1c values ($p = 0.027$ by ANOVA, interaction effect). Again, there was no difference in the duration of the observation periods between the 'start' and the 'end' time points, between the treatments and the control group (Table 2). No significant differences between the two groups were however observed in the other clinical and metabolic parameters (Table 4), such a systolic and diastolic blood pressure, total, low-density lipoprotein (LDL) and high-density lipoprotein (HDL) cholesterol.

Table 4. Body weight, systolic and diastolic blood pressure, and fasting lipid concentrations, in the groups treated with either the 'functional' or the 'control' bread, before ('start') and after ('end') the observation periods. Data are expressed as means ± SE.

	Functional Bread		Control Bread	
Parameter	Start	End	Start	End
Weight (kg)	72.9 ± 3.4	73.9 ± 3.5	77.6 ± 3.3	76.9 ± 3.2
Systolic pressure (mm·Hg)	139.7 ± 5.4	138.6 ± 4.2	137.3 ± 4.9	136.4 ± 6.1
Diastolic pressure (mm·Hg)	75.0 ± 3.4	77.3 ± 3.1	78.6 ± 1.7	79.6 ± 1.9
Total cholesterol (mmol/L)	4.60 ± 0.33	4.55 ± 0.48	4.26 ± 0.16	4.32 ± 0.26
HDL cholesterol (mmol/L)	1.50 ± 0.10	1.46 ± 0.12	1.67 ± 0.08	1.57 ± 0.12
LDL cholesterol (mmol/L)	2.23 ± 0.25	2.36 ± 0.48	2.08 ± 0.15	2.26 ± 0.18
Triglycerides (mmol/L)	1.90 ± 0.29 *	1.60 ± 0.16 *	1.11 ± 0.06	1.08 ± 0.12

* $p < 0.05$ between the 'functional' and the 'control' bread groups (by ANOVA, group effect). Abbreviations: HDL: high-density lipoprotein; LDL: low-density lipoprotein.

Although plasma triglyceride concentrations were greater ($p < 0.015$) in the functional than in the control group at the 'start' time point, they did not significantly change in either group between the start and the end periods. Body weight increased by roughly one kilogram in the treatment group ($p = 0.05$ by paired t test vs. baseline), but it did not significantly change in the controls (though without significance differences between the groups by ANOVA).

The data on consumer acceptability are reported in Supplementary material. The overall response was satisfactory, and positive judgments on texture, odor and general acceptance, were delivered, with ranges between 60% and 80%. In contrast, the responses regarding taste were on the whole 'neutral', as they did not elicit any prevalence between sweet and salty taste. As a matter of fact, the functional bread was well accepted by the subjects who completed the study. The relatively large drop-out rate (9 out of originally enrolled 20 subjects) was due to reasons other than bread acceptability (see Methods). Most subjects really appreciated the functional bread and are still continuing to use it regularly.

4. Discussion

Bread is a staple food, and one of the main sources of carbohydrates and energy worldwide. The diet recommended for a person with diabetes should contain 40%–50% energy as carbohydrates, 15% to 20% as proteins and ~30% as fat. A fiber daily intake of 20–40 g is also suggested [3,12]. Foods with a low glycemic index and/or a low glycemic load would be preferred in diabetes, since they blunt post-prandial hyperglycemia [13,14]. Absolute fiber content [15], type (soluble/insoluble), as well as the presence of active compounds interacting with starch, are important modifiers of carbohydrate digestion and absorption particularly in diabetes. Therefore, the design of a flour containing active ingredients, to be employed for bread preparations, is a 'hot' issue today.

In this study, we report the results of roughly six months' administration of a home-prepared 'functional' bread, made up with a flour enriched with fiber (mainly beta glucan), low in starch and salt, as a substitute for common bread, in subjects with type 2 diabetes in everyday life conditions.

We report that this 'functional bread' significantly improved the metabolic control in the T2DM subjects, as shown by significant reductions of glycated hemoglobin, of post-prandial and mean glucose concentrations. In contrast, both HbA_1c and glucose concentrations did not change in the 'control' bread group (Figure 1 and Table 3). Furthermore, in the six to seven months preceding the observation periods, HbA_1c was nearly stable in both groups (Figure 1). Therefore, these data indicate that the intake of the functional bread was effective in the improvement of metabolic control in type 2 diabetes.

This study was conducted on everyday life conditions, and based on data retrieval of a limited number of patients regularly visited at the diabetes Centre. Although larger prospective, controlled studies would be required to confirm these findings, our data nevertheless suggest that daily intake of a functional bread could be useful in subjects with T2DM. Notably, in this group the percent reduction of HbA_1c (−0.52%, as absolute values) was consistent with the concurrent reduction of mean plasma glucose (−17 mg/dL). Indeed, it is well established that a 'one-point' reduction of % HbA_1c is associated with a reduction of 30–40 mg/dL of mean plasma glucose [16]. In addition, the decrease of HbA_1c values here observed is within the range of changes previously observed after high fiber diets in type 2 diabetes [15].

The efficacy of the functional bread here tested could be due to several, concurring factors. First, as reported in Table 1, the starch content was about half that of the reference, regular bread prepared with refined white wheat flour, on a bread-weight basis. However, no patient reported a *decrease* in bread intake (as grams) with the use of the functional bread. Rather, some of them informed the investigators about a (small) increase in the intake of the functional bread, once they realized that the post-prandial glucose values were improved. Thus, a decrease in the intake (as grams) of the functional bread is very unlikely. Second, the functional bread contained beta glucans, that were absent in the reference bread. Third, the beta glucan/starch ratio in the functional bread was 7.6/100. Such a ratio, although lower than that previously reported to be the optimal value to reduce starch digestion/absorption, could have nevertheless produced a favorable effect [9]. On the other hand, greater ratios than those here tested could further improve post-prandial glucose excursions and the metabolic control in T2DM, should bread palatability be preserved. Fourth, the beta-glucans contained in the functional bread, due to their hydrophilic effect, were probably responsible for its greater water content that, on turn, contributed to bread weight despite the lower starch content. Finally, the total fiber content of the functional bread was nearly double that of the reference bread (Table 1). Therefore, several concurrent variables in the composition of the functional bread could have contributed to its beneficial effects. However, the aim of this study was not to analyze separately the impact of each variable on glucose control in type 2 diabetes. We rather tested the effects of the chosen flour product, available in the supermarket, on glucose control and on sensorial aspects in everyday life conditions.

A high (>40 g/day) dietary fiber intake is usually recommended to subjects with type 2 diabetes [3–12]. However, the fiber effect on medium- as well as on long-term metabolic control in T2DM remains controversial [17,18]. A fiber effect had usually been demonstrated when associated to intake of foods with low glycemic index. On the other hand, a high fiber diet may be difficult to be maintained in the long term, because of its poor palatability [19]. In addition, the large gel volume associated to the intake of fibers such as guar gum, despite their efficacy, is often a hurdle in food consumption. In contrast, using beta glucans, the amount of fiber per serving may be increased without either expanding the volume to be ingested or reducing palatability [20]. In this respect, the peculiar composition of the 'functional flour' here reported may represent an optimal balance between fiber intake, starch reduction, bread 'mass' (i.e., weight), and, last but not least, palatability.

Beta glucans have been reported to improve satiety and to decrease caloric intake and appetite [21]. These effects are likely driven by an increased viscosity [22], a delay in CHO absorption [23], and a 'bulking action' [24]. Beta glucans have also been reported to improve glucose and insulin responses [20]. In addition, the consumption of three grams per day of oat or barley beta-glucans daily was sufficient to decrease blood cholesterol levels [25]. Since beta-glucans reduce the rapidly-digestible starch (RDS) fraction, while increasing that of slowly digestibly starch (SDS) [8], these combined effects would result in a relative increase of resistant starch (RS). However, the beta-glucan-associated reduction of starch digestion rate may also be product- and process-dependent [26]. As a matter of fact, the relationships among beta glucan to starch ratio, starch gelatinization and solubility, and RS formation, are quite complex. At beta glucan to starch ratios below 2 [9], starch solubility was lower at the 1.6/10 than at the 1.1/10 ratio, leading to higher RS and lower SDS values. Our beta-glucan to starch ratio of 0.76/10 probably lead to some increase, although not maximal, of the SDS fraction.

Conversely, others reported that a beta glucan to starch ratio of 0.5/10 ratio nevertheless resulted in a significant reduction in starch gelatinization and in its breakdown rate evaluated in vitro [27]. Further research need to be carried out to elucidate these difficult issues.

An association between beta glucan-induced decrease of post-prandial insulin levels, increase satiety and decrease caloric intake, with increase of cholecystokinin, has also been suggested [28]. In our study, neither cholecystokinin nor insulin were measured. Therefore, no conclusions on possible relationships between changes in these two hormones and the observed effects, can be drawn.

Body weight was not significantly different between the two groups (an analyzed by ANOVA). However, a one kilogram positive change in the treatment group was observed ($p = 0.05$ vs. basal value), whereas weight did not change at all in the control groups. As an explanation of such an unexpected finding, as reported above, some subjects of the treatment group admittedly reported that they had increased the bread intake because they realized that their plasma glucose values were improving, as well as because an increased sense of hunger. Nevertheless, the functional bread was capable to improve the metabolic control, thus independently from any major body weight change. It should also be considered that the raw amount and the energy intake of the diet was generally reported to be unchanged in either group.

At variance with the improvement of the glycemic control, other clinical and biochemical parameters, such systolic and diastolic blood pressure, total, LDL, and HDL cholesterol, were unchanged by the functional bread intake, being rather stable in both groups. Lack of any effect of blood pressure might be due to the hypotensive treatment of most of our subjects (Table 2). Conversely, despite the reported hypocholesterolemic effects of beta glucan [25,29], in our study lack of any change in cholesterol could be due to the already near-normal values of our subjects, of total as well as LDL cholesterol, (also in respect to target values) (Table 2). Nevertheless, the hypolipidemic effects of beta glucans t in medium-term studies (four weeks) are controversial [29].

Since high-fiber products may decrease palatability [19], our subjects were accurately tested for sensorial responses. The overall response to the functional bread was however satisfactory, with positive judgments on texture, odor and general acceptance recorded in >50% of the subjects, and a virtually neutral response regarding taste (see Table S1 in the Supplementary material). In this regard, other authors [30,31] reported that beta-glucan inclusion improves both the rheological and the sensory properties of bread.

Although there were some differences in the pharmacological therapy (other than the hypoglycemic agents) between the two groups, with a lower use of statins and ACE-I/ARB, and increased consumption of beta-blockers, in the functional bread group, these differences likely did not affect the results, since no subject modified drug therapy throughout the study. Although statins have been reported to exhibit deleterious effects on plasma glucose [32], plasma glucose was actually unchanged in the control group. Furthermore, the control subjects as well as those of the functional group were on long term therapy with statins. Therefore, statins use per se should not represent a bias in this study.

5. Conclusions

In conclusion, regular intake of a low-starch functional bread, enriched with beta glucan fibers, could improve the medium- to long-term glycemic control in type 2 diabetes mellitus in addition to the drugs used to control of blood glucose.

Acknowledgments: This study was supported by Institutional Grants of the University of Padova (DOR grants) and by a non conditioned grant from the 'Granaio delle Idee'-Maserà di Padova, Italy.

Author Contributions: P.T. designed the study along with A.L., searched for the clinical and biochemical data in the databases, analyzed the results and wrote the paper. A.L. addressed the technological issues of the functional bread, cooperated in the calculation of the results and co-wrote and reviewed the paper.

Abbreviations

The following abbreviations are used in this manuscript:

CHO	carbohydrates
BMI	Body Mass Index
T2DM	Type 2 Diabetes Mellitus
HbA_1c	glycated hemoglobin
CV	cardiovascular
GI	Glycemic Index
ACE-I	angiotensin converting enzyme inhibitors
ARB	angiotensin receptors blockers

References

1. International Diabetes Federation. *IDF Diabetes Atlas*, 7th ed.; International Diabetes Federation: Brussels, Belgium, 2015.
2. Pereira, M.A.; Kartashov, A.I.; Ebbeling, C.B.; van Horn, L.; Slattery, M.L.; Jacobs, D.R., Jr.; Ludwig, D.S.; Jacobs, D.R. Fast-food habits, weight gain, and insulin resistance (the CARDIA study): 15-year prospective analysis. *Lancet* **2005**, *365*, 36–42. [CrossRef]
3. AMD-SID. Standard Italiani per la Cura del Diabete Mellito 2014. Available online: http.//www.standarditaliani.it (accessed on 11 November 2016).
4. Reaven, G.M. Insulin resistance, the insulin resistance syndrome, and cardiovascular disease. *Panminerva Med.* **2005**, *47*, 201–210. [PubMed]
5. Pawar, K.; Thompkinson, D.K. Multiple functional ingredient approach in formulating dietary supplement for management of diabetes: A review. *Crit. Rev. Food Sci. Nutr.* **2014**, *54*, 957–973. [CrossRef] [PubMed]
6. Zarich, S.W. Cardiovascular risk factors in the metabolic syndrome: Impact of insulin resistance on lipids, hypertension, and the development of diabetes and cardiac events. *Rev. Cardiovasc. Med.* **2005**, *6*, 194–205. [PubMed]
7. Grajek, W.; Olejnik, A.; Sip, A. Probiotics, prebiotics and antioxidants as functional foods. *Acta Biochim. Pol.* **2005**, *52*, 665–671. [PubMed]
8. Regand, A.; Tosh, S.M.; Wolever, T.M.; Wood, P.J. Physicochemical properties of beta-glucan in differently processed oat foods influence glycemic response. *J. Agric. Food Chem.* **2009**, *57*, 8831–8838. [CrossRef] [PubMed]
9. Regand, A.; Chowdhury, Z.; Tosh, S.M.; Wolever, T.M.S.; Wood, P. The molecular weight solubility and viscosity of oat beta-glucan affect human glycemic response by modifying starch digestibility. *Food Chem.* **2011**, *129*, 297–304. [CrossRef]
10. Lawless, H.T.; Heymann, H. *Sensory Evaluation of Food: Principles and Practices*; Chapman & Hall: New York, NY, USA, 1998; pp. 341–372.
11. Graziani, M.S.; Ceriotti, F.; Zaninotto, M.; Catapano, A.L.; Medea, G.; Parretti, D.; Gulizia, M.; Averna, M.; Ciaccio, M. La diagnostica di laboratorio delle dislipidemie. Documento di consenso SIBIoC, SISA, SIMG, ANMCO. *Biochim. Clin.* **2014**, *40*, 338–346.
12. Evert, A.B.; Boucher, J.L.; Cypress, M.; Dunbar, S.A.; Franz, M.J.; Mayer-Davis, E.J.; Neumiller, J.J.; Urbanski, P.; Verdi, C.L.; Nwankwo, R. American Diabetes Association. Nutrition therapy recommendations for the management of adults with diabetes. *Diabetes Care* **2013**, *36*, 3821–3842. [CrossRef] [PubMed]
13. Augustin, L.S.; Kendall, C.W.; Jenkins, D.J.; Willett, W.C.; Astrup, A.; Barclay, A.W.; Björck, I.; Brand-Miller, J.C.; Brighenti, F.; Buyken, A.E.; et al. Glycemic index, glycemic load and glycemic response: An International Scientific Consensus Summit from the International Carbohydrate Quality Consortium (ICQC). *Nutr. Metab. Cardiovasc.* **2015**, *25*, 795–815. [CrossRef] [PubMed]
14. Riccardi, G.; Rivellese, A.A.; Giacco, R. Role of glycemic index and glycemic load in the healthy state, in prediabetes, and in diabetes. *Am. J. Clin. Nutr.* **2008**, *87*, 269S–274S. [PubMed]
15. Silva, F.M.; Kramer, C.K.; de Almeida, J.C.; Steemburgo, T.; Gross, J.L.; Azevedo, M.J. Fiber intake and glycemic control in patients with type 2 diabetes mellitus: A systematic review with meta-analysis of randomized controlled trials. *Nutr. Rev.* **2013**, *71*, 790–801. [CrossRef] [PubMed]

16. Rohlfing, C.L.; Wiedmeyer, H.M.; Little, R.R.; England, J.D.; Tennill, A.; Goldstein, D.E. Defining the relationship between plasma glucose and HbA(1c): Analysis of glucose profiles and HbA(1c) in the Diabetes Control and Complications Trial. *Diabetes Care* **2002**, *25*, 275–278. [CrossRef] [PubMed]
17. Beattie, V.A.; Edwards, C.A.; Hosker, J.P.; Cullen, D.R.; Ward, J.D.; Read, N.W. Does adding fiber to a low energy, high carbohydrate, low fat diet confer any benefit to the management of newly diagnosed overweight type II diabetics? *Br. Med. J. (Clin. Res. Ed.)* **1988**, *296*, 1147–1149. [CrossRef]
18. Scott, A.R.; Attenborough, Y.; Peacock, I.; Fletcher, E.; Jeffcoate, W.J.; Tattersall, R.B. Comparison of high fibre diets, basal insulin supplements, and flexible insulin treatment for non-insulin dependent (type II) diabetics poorly controlled with sulphonylureas. *BMJ* **1988**, *297*, 707–710. [CrossRef] [PubMed]
19. Wood, P.J. Cereal beta-glucans in diet and health. *J. Cereal Sci.* **2007**, *46*, 230–238. [CrossRef]
20. Jenkins, A.L.; Jenkins, D.J.; Zdravkovic, U.; Würsch, P.; Vuksan, V. Depression of the glycemic index by high levels of beta-glucan fiber in two functional foods tested in type 2 diabetes. *Eur. J. Clin. Nutr.* **2002**, *56*, 622–628. [CrossRef] [PubMed]
21. Rebello, C.J.; O'Neil, C.E.; Greenway, F.L. Dietary fiber and satiety: The effects of oats on satiety. *Nutr. Rev.* **2016**, *74*, 131–147. [CrossRef] [PubMed]
22. Dikeman, C.L.; Fahey, G.C. Viscosity as related to dietary fiber: A review. *Crit. Rev. Food Sci. Nutr.* **2006**, *46*, 649–663. [CrossRef] [PubMed]
23. Battilana, P.; Ornstein, K.; Minehira, K.; Schwarz, J.M.; Acheson, K.; Schneiter, P.L.; Burri, J.; Jequier, E.; Tappy, L. Mechanism of action of beta-glucan in postprandial glucose metabolism in healthy men. *Eur. J. Clin. Nutr.* **2001**, *55*, 327–333. [CrossRef] [PubMed]
24. Burton-Freeman, B. Dietary fibre and energy regulation. *J. Nutr.* **2000**, *130*, 272S–275S. [PubMed]
25. Tiwari, U.; Cummins, E. Meta-analysis of the effect of beta-glucan intake on blood cholesterol and glucose levels. *Nutrition* **2011**, *27*, 1008–1016. [CrossRef] [PubMed]
26. Brennan, C.S. Dietary fibre, glycaemic response, and diabetes. *Mol. Nutr. Food Res.* **2005**, *49*, 560–570. [CrossRef] [PubMed]
27. Symons, L.J.; Brennan, C.S. The effect of barley beta-glucan fiber fractions on starch gelatinization and pasting characteristics. *J. Food Sci.* **2004**, *69*, FCT257–FCT261.
28. Beck, E.J.; Tosh, S.M.; Batterham, M.J.; Tapsell, L.C.; Huang, X.F. Oat beta-glucan increases postprandial cholecystokinin levels, decreases insulin response and extends subjective satiety in overweight subjects. *Mol. Nutr. Food Res.* **2009**, *53*, 1343–1351. [CrossRef] [PubMed]
29. Zhou, X.; Lin, W.; Tong, L.; Liu, X.; Zhong, K.; Wang, L.; Zhou, S. Hypolipidaemic effects of oat flakes and β-glucans derived from four Chinese naked oat (*Avena nuda*) cultivars in Wistar-Lewis rats. *J. Sci. Food Agric.* **2016**, *96*, 644–649. [CrossRef] [PubMed]
30. Flander, L.; Salmenkallio-Marttila, M.; Suortti, T.; Autio, K. Optimization of ingredients and baking process for improved wholemeal oatbread quality. *LWT* **2007**, *40*, 860–870. [CrossRef]
31. Skendi, A.; Biliaderis, C.G.; Papageorgiou, M.; Izydorczyk, M.S. Effects of two barley beta-glucan isolates on wheat flour dough and bread properties. *Food Chem.* **2010**, *119*, 1159–1167. [CrossRef]
32. Erqou, S.; Lee, C.C.; Adler, A.I. Statins and glycaemic control in individuals with diabetes: A systematic review and meta-analysis. *Diabetologia* **2014**, *57*, 2444–2452. [CrossRef] [PubMed]

Permissions

All chapters in this book were first published by MDPI; hereby published with permission under the Creative Commons Attribution License or equivalent. Every chapter published in this book has been scrutinized by our experts. Their significance has been extensively debated. The topics covered herein carry significant findings which will fuel the growth of the discipline. They may even be implemented as practical applications or may be referred to as a beginning point for another development.

The contributors of this book come from diverse backgrounds, making this book a truly international effort. This book will bring forth new frontiers with its revolutionizing research information and detailed analysis of the nascent developments around the world.

We would like to thank all the contributing authors for lending their expertise to make the book truly unique. They have played a crucial role in the development of this book. Without their invaluable contributions this book wouldn't have been possible. They have made vital efforts to compile up to date information on the varied aspects of this subject to make this book a valuable addition to the collection of many professionals and students.

This book was conceptualized with the vision of imparting up-to-date information and advanced data in this field. To ensure the same, a matchless editorial board was set up. Every individual on the board went through rigorous rounds of assessment to prove their worth. After which they invested a large part of their time researching and compiling the most relevant data for our readers.

The editorial board has been involved in producing this book since its inception. They have spent rigorous hours researching and exploring the diverse topics which have resulted in the successful publishing of this book. They have passed on their knowledge of decades through this book. To expedite this challenging task, the publisher supported the team at every step. A small team of assistant editors was also appointed to further simplify the editing procedure and attain best results for the readers.

Apart from the editorial board, the designing team has also invested a significant amount of their time in understanding the subject and creating the most relevant covers. They scrutinized every image to scout for the most suitable representation of the subject and create an appropriate cover for the book.

The publishing team has been an ardent support to the editorial, designing and production team. Their endless efforts to recruit the best for this project, has resulted in the accomplishment of this book. They are a veteran in the field of academics and their pool of knowledge is as vast as their experience in printing. Their expertise and guidance has proved useful at every step. Their uncompromising quality standards have made this book an exceptional effort. Their encouragement from time to time has been an inspiration for everyone.

The publisher and the editorial board hope that this book will prove to be a valuable piece of knowledge for researchers, students, practitioners and scholars across the globe.

List of Contributors

Mengxiao Ren, Jindan Qi, Anni Hu, Qing Jiang, Yunying Hou, Qianqian Feng and Xiaohua Wang
School of Nursing, Medical College, Soochow University, Suzhou 215006, China

Huaiyu Zhang
School of Medicine, University of California, San Francisco, CA 94110, USA

Omorogieva Ojo
School of Health Sciences, Faculty of Education, Health and Human Sciences, University of Greenwich, London SE9 2UG, UK
Faculty of Education and Health, Department of Adult Nursing and Paramedic Science, University of Greenwich, London SE9 2UG, UK

Renée Wilson, Richard Gearry and Chris Frampton
Department of Medicine, University of Otago, Christchurch 8011, New Zealand

Jinny Willis
Lipid and Diabetes Research Group, Canterbury District Health Board, Christchurch 8011, New Zealand

Paula Skidmore and Elizabeth Fleming
Department of Human Nutrition, University of Otago, Dunedin 9016, New Zealand

Anitra Carr
Department of Pathology, University of Otago, Christchurch 8011, New Zealand

Shuang Tian
Nutrition Department, Longgang Hospital of Traditional Chinese Medicine, Shenzhen 518000, Guangdong, China
National Discipline, Department of Nutrition and Food Hygiene, School of Public Health Harbin Medical University, Harbin 150081, China

Qian Xu, Ruyue Jiang, Tianshu Han, Changhao Sun and Lixin Na
National Discipline, Department of Nutrition and Food Hygiene, School of Public Health Harbin Medical University, Harbin 150081, China

Xin Fang
Unit of Biostatistics, Institute of Environmental Medicine, Karolinska Institutet, Stockholm 17177, Sweden

Hedong Han and Jia He
Department of Health Statistics, Second Military Medical University, Shanghai 200433, China

Mei Li and Chun Liang
Department of Cardiology, Shanghai Changzheng Hospital, Second Military Medical University, Shanghai 200003, China

Zhongjie Fan
Department of Cardiology, Peking Union Medical College Hospital, Peking Union Medical College, Chinese Academy of Medical Sciences, Beijing 100730, China

Jan Aaseth
Faculty of Public Health, Hedmark University of Applied Sciences, Elverum 2411, Norway
Innlandet Hospital Trust, Kongsvinger Hospital Division, Kongsvinger 2226, Norway

Yang Cao
Unit of Biostatistics, Institute of Environmental Medicine, Karolinska Institutet, Stockholm 17177, Sweden
Clinical Epidemiology and Biostatistics, School of Medical Sciences, Örebro University, Örebro 70182, Sweden

Scott Montgomery
Clinical Epidemiology and Biostatistics, School of Medical Sciences, Örebro University, Örebro 70182, Sweden
Clinical Epidemiology Unit, Karolinska University Hospital, Karolinska Institutet, Stockholm 17177, Sweden
Department of Epidemiology and Public Health, University College London, London WC1E 6BT, UK

Paula Nascimento Brandão-Lima
Health Sciences Postgraduate Program, Department of Medicine, Federal University of Sergipe, Rua Cláudio Batista, S/N, Cidade Nova, Aracaju, 49060-108 Sergipe, Brazil

Gabrielli Barbosa de Carvalho and Ramara Kadija Fonseca Santos
Nutrition Sciences Postgraduate Program, Department of Nutrition, Federal University of Sergipe, Avenida Marechal Rondon, S/N, Jardim Rosa Elze, São Cristovão, 49100-000 Sergipe, Brazil

Kiriaque Barra Ferreira Barbosa
Health Sciences Postgraduate Program, Department of Medicine, Federal University of Sergipe, Rua Cláudio Batista, S/N, Cidade Nova, Aracaju, 49060-108 Sergipe, Brazil
Nutrition Sciences Postgraduate Program, Department of Nutrition, Federal University of Sergipe, Avenida Marechal Rondon, S/N, Jardim Rosa Elze, São Cristovão, 49100-000 Sergipe, Brazil
Undergraduate Nutrition Program, Department of Nutrition, Federal University of Sergipe, Avenida Marechal Rondon, S/N, Jardim Rosa Elze, São Cristovão, 49100-000 Sergipe, Brazil

Liliane Viana Pires
Nutrition Sciences Postgraduate Program, Department of Nutrition, Federal University of Sergipe, Avenida Marechal Rondon, S/N, Jardim Rosa Elze, São Cristovão, 49100-000 Sergipe, Brazil
Undergraduate Nutrition Program, Department of Nutrition, Federal University of Sergipe, Avenida Marechal Rondon, S/N, Jardim Rosa Elze, São Cristovão, 49100-000 Sergipe, Brazil

Beatriz da Cruz Santos and Natalia Lohayne Dias-Vasconcelos
Undergraduate Nutrition Program, Department of Nutrition, Federal University of Sergipe, Avenida Marechal Rondon, S/N, Jardim Rosa Elze, São Cristovão, 49100-000 Sergipe, Brazil

Vivianne de Sousa Rocha
Department of Nutrition, Federal University of Sergipe, Avenida Governador Marcelo Déda, 13, Centro, Lagarto, 49400-000 Sergipe, Brazil

Bang-An Luo
Department of Mental Health, Brain Hospital of Hunan Province, Changsha 410007, Hunan, China

Fan Gao
Department of Social Medicine and Health Management, Xiangya School of Public Health, Central South University, Changsha 410078, Hunan, China

Lu-Lu Qin
Department of Social Medicine and Health Management, Xiangya School of Public Health, Central South University, Changsha 410078, Hunan, China
Department of Prevention Medicine, Medical School, Hunan University of Chinese Medicine, Changsha 410208, Hunan, China

Ying-Che Huang
Graduate Institute of Bioresources, National Pingtung University of Science and Technology, Pingtung 91201, Taiwan

Ming-Chang Wu
Graduate Institute of Bioresources, National Pingtung University of Science and Technology, Pingtung 91201, Taiwan
Department of Food Science, National Pingtung University of Science and Technology, Pingtung 91201, Taiwan

Bo-Hua Wu
Department of Food Science, National Pingtung University of Science and Technology, Pingtung 91201, Taiwan

Yung-Lin Chu
International Master's Degree Program in Food Science, International College, National Pingtung University of Science and Technology, Pingtung 91201, Taiwan

Wen-Chang Chang
Department of Food Science, National Chiayi University, Chiayi 60004, Taiwan

Sharon Marie Weldon
Department of Adult Nursing and Paramedic Science, University of Greenwich, London SE9 2UG, UK
Barts Health NHS Trust, The Royal London Hospital, Whitechapel Rd, Whitechapel E1 1BB, UK

Trevor Thompson
Department of Psychology, University of Greenwich, London SE10 9LS, UK

Rachel Crockett
Division of Psychology, Faculty of Natural Sciences, University of Stirling, Scotland FK9 4LA, UK

Xiao-Hua Wang
The School of Nursing, Soochow University, Suzhou 215006, China

Jia Zheng, Xinhua Xiao, Qian Zhang, Tong Wang, Miao Yu and Jianping Xu
Department of Endocrinology, Key Laboratory of Endocrinology, Ministry of Health, Peking Union Medical College Hospital, Diabetes Research Center of Chinese Academy of Medical Sciences & Peking Union Medical College, Beijing 100730, China

Emily Burch, Lauren T. Williams, Harriet Makepeace and Lauren Ball
Menzies Health Institute Queensland, Griffith University, Gold Coast 4215, Australia

Clair Alston-Knox
Office of the Pro-Vice Chancellor, Arts, Education and Law, Griffith University, Mount Gravatt Campus, Brisbane 4222, Australia

Shaminie J Athinarayanan
Virta Health, 535 Mission Street, San Francisco, CA 94105, USA

Sarah J Hallberg
Virta Health, 535 Mission Street, San Francisco, CA 94105, USA
Indiana University Health Arnett, Lafayette, IN 47904, USA
Indiana University School of Medicine, Indianapolis, IN 46202, USA

Tamara L Hazbun
Indiana University Health Arnett, Lafayette, IN 47904, USA
Indiana University School of Medicine, Indianapolis, IN 46202, USA

Victoria M Gershuni
Department of Surgery, Perelman School of Medicine University of Pennsylvania, Philadelphia, PA 19104, USA

Osarhumwese Osaretin Ojo
South London and Maudsley NHS Foundation Trust, University Hospital, Lewisham High Street, London SE13 6LH, UK

Xiao-Hua Wang
The School of Nursing, Soochow University, Suzhou 215006, China

Amanda Rodrigues Amorim Adegboye
Faculty of Education and Health, Department of Psychology, SocialWork & Counselling, University of Greenwich, London SE9 2UG, UK

Carlos Doepking
Department of Nutrition and Dietetics, Faculty of Heath Sciences, University of Atacama, Av. Copayapu 2862, Copiapó, 1530000 Atacama Region, Chile

José C. Fernández-Cao
Department of Nutrition and Dietetics, Faculty of Heath Sciences, University of Atacama, Av. Copayapu 2862, Copiapó, 1530000 Atacama Region, Chile
Nutrition and Public Health, Universitat Rovira i Virgili, C/ Sant Llorenç 21, Reus, 43201 Tarragona, Spain

Marisol Warthon-Medina
Food Databanks National Capability, Quadram Institute Bioscience, Norwich Research Park, Norwich, Norfolk NR4 7UA, UK

International Institute of Nutritional Sciences and Food Safety Studies, University of Central Lancashire, Darwin Building c/o Psychology Scholl Office, Preston, Lancashire PR1 2HE, UK

Nicola M. Lowe
International Institute of Nutritional Sciences and Food Safety Studies, University of Central Lancashire, Darwin Building c/o Psychology Scholl Office, Preston, Lancashire PR1 2HE, UK

Victoria H. Moran
Maternal and Infant Nutrition and Nurture Unit, University of Central Lancashire, Preston, Lancashire PR 1 2HE, UK

Victoria Arija
Research Group in Nutrition and Mental Health (NUTRISAM), Institut d'Investigació Sanitària Pere Virgili (IISPV), Rovira i Virgili University, Reus, 43201 Tarragona, Spain

Lluis Serra-Majem
Research Institute of Biomedical and Health Sciences, University of Las Palmas de Gran Canaria and CHUIMI, Canarian Health Service, 35016 Las Palmas de Gran Canaria, Spain
Consorcio CIBER, M.P. Fisiopatología de la Obesidad y Nutrición (CIBERObn), Instituto de Salud Carlos III (ISCIII), 28029 Madrid, Spain

Paolo Tessari
Department of Medicine (DIMED), University of Padova, 35128 Padova PD, Italy

Anna Lante
Department of Agronomy, Food, Natural Resources, Animals & Environment (DAFNAE), University of Padova, 35123 Padova PD, Italy

Index

www.ingramcontent.com/pod-product-compliance
Lightning Source LLC
LaVergne TN
LVHW060549210926
848485LV00005B/1283